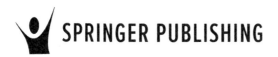 **SPRINGER PUBLISHING**

MW01070515

GET THE MOST FROM YOUR BOOK

Access your included eBook and educator resources today!

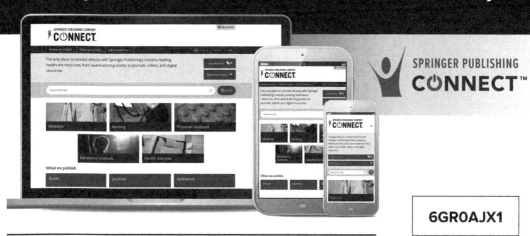

SPRINGER PUBLISHING CONNECT™

6GR0AJX1

eBook Access

Your print purchase of *Epidemiology for the Advanced Practice Nurse: A Population Health Approach,* includes **online access via Springer Publishing Connect™** to increase accessibility, portability, and searchability.

Insert the code at http://connect.springerpub.com/content/book/978-0-8261-8514-3 today!

Educator Resource Access

Let us do some of the heavy lifting to create an engaging classroom experience with a variety of educator resources included in your textbooks SUCH AS:

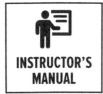
INSTRUCTOR'S MANUAL

POWERPOINTS

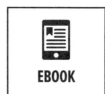
EBOOK

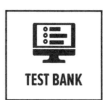
TEST BANK

Visit **https://connect.springerpub.com/** and look for the **"Show Supplementary"** button on your **book homepage** to see what is available to you! First time using Springer Publishing Connect?

Email **textbook@springerpub.com** to create an account and start unlocking valuable resources.

Epidemiology for the Advanced Practice Nurse

Demetrius J. Porche, DNS, PhD, APRN, FNP, PCC, ANEF, FACHE, FAANP, FAAN, is Professor and Dean of Louisiana State University Health—New Orleans School of Nursing. He holds an appointment also in the School of Public Health at Louisiana State University Health—New Orleans. He received his undergraduate Bachelor of Science in Nursing degree from Nicholls State University and his Master of Nursing and Doctor of Nursing Science from Louisiana State University Medical Center. He completed Family Nurse Practitioner postgraduate coursework at Concordia University Wisconsin. Dr. Porche earned a Doctorate of Philosophy from Capella University in Organization and Management with a specialization in Leadership.

Dr. Porche is certified as a Clinical Specialist in Community Health Nursing, Family Nurse Practitioner and Professional Certified Coach. He is board certified in healthcare by the American College of Healthcare Executives. Dr. Porche was inducted as a fellow in the American College of Healthcare Executives, the American Academy of Nurse Practitioners, the American Academy of Nursing, and the National League for Nursing Academy of Nursing Education. He is currently the Chief Editor of *American Journal of Men's Health*. Dr. Porche has authored three editions of *Health Policy: Application for Nurses and Other Healthcare Professionals*.

Dr. Porche currently serves on the American Association of Colleges of Nursing Board, the American Organization of Nursing Leaders Publications Committee, and chairs the Louisiana Health Works Commission and the Louisiana Council of Administrators in Nursing Education (LACANE).

Epidemiology for the Advanced Practice Nurse

A Population Health Approach

Demetrius J. Porche, DNS, PhD, APRN, FNP, PCC, ANEF, FACHE, FAANP, FAAN

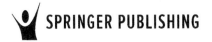 SPRINGER PUBLISHING

Springer Publishing Company, LLC
11 West 42nd Street, New York, NY 10036
www.springerpub.com
connect.springerpub.com/

Acquisitions Editor: Joseph Morita
Senior Content Development Editor: Lucia Gunzel
Compositor: S4Carlisle Publishing Services

ISBN: 978-0-8261-8513-6
ebook ISBN: 978-0-8261-8514-3
DOI: 10.1891/9780826185143

SUPPLEMENTS:
Instructor materials:

A robust set of instructor resources designed to supplement this text is located at http://connect.springerpub.com/content/book/978-0-8261-8514-3. Qualifying instructors may request access by emailing textbook@springerpub.com.

Instructor's Test Bank ISBN: 978-0-8261-8515-0 (Also available on Respondus®.)
Instructor's PowerPoints ISBN: 978-0-8261-8516-7

22 23 24 25 / 5 4 3 2 1

The author and the publisher of this Work have made every effort to use sources believed to be reliable to provide information that is accurate and compatible with the standards generally accepted at the time of publication. Because medical science is continually advancing, our knowledge base continues to expand. Therefore, as new information becomes available, changes in procedures become necessary. We recommend that the reader always consult current research and specific institutional policies before performing any clinical procedure or delivering any medication. The author and publisher shall not be liable for any special, consequential, or exemplary damages resulting, in whole or in part, from the readers' use of, or reliance on, the information contained in this book. The publisher has no responsibility for the persistence or accuracy of URLs for external or third-party Internet websites referred to in this publication and does not guarantee that any content on such websites is, or will remain, accurate or appropriate.

Library of Congress Cataloging-in-Publication Data

Names: Porche, Demetrius J., author.
Title: Epidemiology for the advanced practice nurse : a population health
  approach / Demetrius J. Porche.
Identifiers: LCCN 2021046438 (print) | LCCN 2021046439 (ebook) | ISBN
  9780826185136 (cloth) | ISBN 9780826185143 (ebook)
Subjects: MESH: Epidemiology | Advanced Practice Nursing | Population
  Health | Nurses Instruction
Classification: LCC RA651 (print) | LCC RA651 (ebook) | NLM WA 105 | DDC
  614.4--dc23
LC record available at https://lccn.loc.gov/2021046438
LC ebook record available at https://lccn.loc.gov/2021046439

Contact sales@springerpub.com to receive discount rates on bulk purchases.

Publisher's Note: New and used products purchased from third-party sellers are not guaranteed for quality, authenticity, or access to any included digital components.

Printed in the United States of America.

This book primarily is dedicated in honor of everyone who has died from the COVID-19 pandemic. Let this book serve as a guiding inspiration to learn epidemiology as a strategy to prevent future pandemics and promote the health, welfare, and safety of our international society.

Secondly, this book is dedicated to my best friend and life partner, Dr. James Michael DelPrince; my parents, Hayes James Porche Jr. and Diane Lirette Porche; my two sisters, Anastasia Porche Arceneaux and Chelsealea Porche Lovell; my brothers-in-law, Rory Lovell, Jason Arceneaux Sr., and Anthony DelPrince; and my nephews and nieces, Seth Porche, Sebastian Porche, Jason Arceneaux Jr., Madeline Lovell, and Jasmine Arceneaux.

IN MEMORIAM

This book and my life's work will always be in memory of Reverend Dr. James A. Ertl, my best friend and partner, for a life of adventure, travel, smiles, laughter, and love that ended all too soon. In my thoughts every day. In memory, with love until we meet again.

CONTENTS

CONTRIBUTORS

Donald E. Mercante, PhD
Professor of Biostatistics
School of Public Health
Louisiana State University Health Sciences Center
New Orleans, Louisiana

Clair P. Millet, DNP, APRN, PHCNS-BC
Assistant Professor of Clinical Nursing
Director of Nursing Professional Development
Robert Wood Johnson Public Health Nurse Leader
Louisiana State University Health Sciences Center
New Orleans, Louisiana

**Demetrius J. Porche, DNS, PhD, APRN, FNP,
PCC, ANEF, FACHE, FAANP, FAAN**
Professor and Dean
Louisiana State University Health Sciences Center
New Orleans School of Nursing
New Orleans, Louisiana

Oghenemaro C. Ugbeme, BSc, BSN, RN
Registered Nurse
Neuro Progressive Unit
Ochsner Medical Center, Jefferson
New Orleans, Louisiana

PREFACE

The COVID-19 pandemic emphasized the critical need for epidemiology and public health measures to control and prevent the transmission of known and novel diseases. This pandemic has exposed our vulnerabilities as an academic, scientific healthcare community and global society. Epidemiology has served as the basic foundational knowledge to understand the distribution of COVID-19 on an international scale and the evolving nature of this pandemic within disparate communities. Epidemiologic science evolved to strengthen our understanding of the determinants of COVID-19 to discern high-risk populations, along with knowledge of the long-term COVID-19 sequelae. We have witnessed the impact of pharmacologic and nonpharmacologic measures to control a pandemic. We have built on our past knowledge from previous pandemics and developed new knowledge for potential future epidemics or future pandemics. Through this pandemic we have witnessed the intersection of health, healthcare systems, science, policy, and politics. Living during this pandemic has challenged the resilience of our public health system and scientific community, individuals on a personal level, and the fabric of our society. This pandemic has demonstrated that epidemiology is a core public health science critical to all aspects of human interaction and healthcare practice. Epidemiology helps us "know the unknown to reduce fear" and makes sense out of chaos through the systematic analysis of disease occurrence patterns and distribution while also informing us of the associated determinants of health and illness.

Epidemiology for the Advanced Practice Nurse: A Population Health Approach explores the principles of epidemiology within a population health framework. The book is written in a concise, to the point, easy-to-read format. Each chapter identifies competencies and essential epidemiologic terminology relevant to the chapter topics. At the conclusion of each chapter, summary points and critical reasoning questions are proposed. As epidemiology is a core science of public health practice, this book serves as essential core information to the practice of advanced practice nursing regarding educational level or role preparation. Each chapter has a judicious use of tables and figures to emphasize and summarize relevant information.

Epidemiologic content is covered in four book sections. Section I, Advanced Practice Nursing Population Health, sets the population-based framework from which to conceptualize the practice of epidemiology. Chapter 1, Population Health, defines populations and population health, introduces principles of population level prevention, and summarizes the core public health functions. This chapter explores the relationship between epidemiology and population health. Chapter 2, Determinants of Health, describes several categories of health determinants inclusive of the social determinants of health. The beginning characterization of risk factors is described including both modifiable and nonmodifiable risk factors. The national Healthy People initiatives are presented and elucidate the interaction between the individual and population health. Health disparities and inequities are defined along with their measures. Chapter 3, Advanced Practice Nursing Roles and Competencies in Epidemiology and Population Health, articulates the meaning and roles within advanced practice nursing. Competency or practice standard relevant to population health and epidemiology for each advanced practice role—certified nurse midwife, nurse practitioner, clinical nurse specialist, and nurse anesthetist—is presented.

Section II, Epidemiology, presents the core epidemiology content. Chapter 4, Epidemiology Primer, defines epidemiology as a discipline and practice. Descriptive and analytical epidemiology is defined and compared. The epidemiologic process is outlined as a clinical reasoning process. Epidemiology as a science is presented along with the six scientific method steps. The epidemiologic approach and investigation process is also presented as a critical reasoning strategy for the advanced practice nurse. The epidemiologic triad of agent, host, and environment framework is linked to the chain of infection. Basic epidemiologic tools of case counts, frequencies, and proportions and rates are introduced. Chapter 5, Historical Epidemiologic Perspectives, presents relevant historical figures who laid the foundation for epidemiologic practice. A historical epidemiologic timeline outlines the evolution of epidemiology, public health, and infectious diseases. Historical epidemiologic studies that provided foundational epidemiologic principles are reviewed. The chapter concludes with a review of historical pandemics. Chapter 6, Etiology and Natural History of Disease and Illness, provides the foundation and basic level of information needed about a health condition in order to practice epidemiology. Some relevant topics in this chapter are natural history of disease, stages of disease, immunity types, chain of infection, transmission modes, iceberg theory, prevention levels, and contact tracing. The chapter concludes with linking some of the content presented to date in sections of the web of causation or association. Chapter 7, Disease Occurrence: Morbidity and Mortality, provides the basics of epidemiologic measurement for morbidity and mortality information. This chapter also presents information on epidemiologic surveillance systems. Chapter 8, Diagnostic and Screening Tests: Validity and Reliability, differentiates screening and diagnostic testing. The determination of appropriate screening and diagnostic tests for populations is characterized through the presentation of methods to measure test sensitivity, specificity, positive predictive value, and negative predictive value. Chapter 9, Risk Assessment and Estimation, focuses on the assessment of health risk. The calculation of risk estimation formulas (relative risk, odds, and attributable risk) are described. The communication of risk and process of risk management to prevent disease is a function of the advanced practice nurse.

Section III, Tools and Epidemiologic Study Designs, provides the research and biostatistical processes that generates epidemiologic evidence. This section presents the original research study designs to generate epidemiologic data used in the epidemiologic reasoning process. Chapter 10, Observational Epidemiologic Research: Introduction to Observational Research—Descriptive, Case Studies, Case Series, Ecological, and Cross-Sectional, serves as an introduction to observational research. This chapter presents common aspects to research such as sampling, type I and type II error, and the components of a research proposal and report. Chapter 11, Cohort Studies, presents the research study designs for both prospective and retrospective cohort studies, along with some additional content on risk ratio. Chapter 12, Case Control, Other Study Designs, and Research Appraisal, presents content research designs such as case control, nested case control, methodical research, historical research, and triangulation. Strategies to critically appraise research studies are introduced in this chapter with additional tools listed in the Appendix. The gold standard for experimental research is presented in Chapter 13, Experimental Studies: Quasi-Experimental, Experimental, and Randomized Clinical Trials. This chapter presents the traditional experimental designs inclusive of randomization. There is no perfect research study design as each research study has potential for the introduction of bias and has inherent design or method limitations. Chapter 14, Epidemiologic Design Bias, Confounders, and Interaction, identifies various types of bias that could impact research findings. Additionally, research variables can confound and interact with each other to impact study findings. Chapter 15, Biostatistics Primer, presents foundational statistical information to the calculation of population level data. This chapter presents a scale of measurement, descriptive statistics, probability, and risk estimation. Chapter 16, Field, Forensic, and Legal Epidemiology, presents the practical application of epidemiologic knowledge, skills, and methods to resolve population-based public health problems. Two evolving specialty areas of epidemiology—forensic and legal—are presented as a role for advanced practice nurses.

Section IV, Fields of Epidemiology in Practice, further extends the practice of epidemiology as an opportunity for advanced practice nurses. This section contains several chapters on epidemiologic practice specialties: Pandemic Epidemiology (Chapter 17), Social Epidemiology (Chapter 18), Infectious Disease Epidemiology

(Chapter 19), Genetic and Environmental Epidemiology (Chapter 20), Occupational Epidemiology (Chapter 21), and Reproductive and Maternal Health Epidemiology (Chapter 22). The final chapter of this section, Chapter 23, Clinical and Healthcare Epidemiology and Evidence-Based Healthcare, presents epidemiology as a basic science for clinical practice. This chapter addresses content on antibiograms, describes the role of the hospital epidemiologist, healthcare epidemiologist, and methods nosocomial infection measurement.

Section V, Policy and Ethics, contains two chapters. Chapter 24, Epidemiology in Health Policy and Program Evaluation, introduces the basics of policy formulation and epidemiologic data as a measure of program evaluation. Chapter 25, Epidemiologic Ethical and Professional Issues, provides the ethical principles and guidelines along with professional standards that guide the advanced practice nurses' practice of epidemiology.

The book concludes with supporting appendices with content such as an integrated epidemiologic and community assessment, morbidity and mortality formula summaries, environmental health hazards, critical appraisal of epidemiologic studies, reportable diseases, epidemiological data presentation, and epidemiologic resources.

 A robust set of instructor resources designed to supplement this text is located at http://connect.springerpub.com/content/book/978-0-8261-8514-3. Qualifying instructors may request access by emailing textbook@springerpub.com.

ACKNOWLEDGMENTS

The ability to write a book on epidemiology originates from my doctoral studies in epidemiology under the mentorship and guidance of Myrtis J. Snowden, DrPH, RN, FAAN, and Margaret Oalmann, DrPH, at Louisiana State University Medical Center (now Health Sciences Center). This book is a natural evolution from my life experiences, nursing practice, and knowledge developed by multiple colleagues, nursing faculty, and my students throughout my career. This book is a result of essential feedback from graduate students regarding public health and epidemiology. To all my colleagues and students, thanks for challenging and transforming my thinking about nursing, advanced practice nursing, administration, public health, and epidemiology.

A special thanks to my administrative assistant, Karen Smith, for her support and assistance with various aspects of composing this book.

INSTRUCTOR RESOURCES

 SPRINGER PUBLISHING CONNECT™ | A robust set of instructor resources designed to supplement this text is located at http://connect.springerpub.com/content/book/978-0-8261-8514-3. Qualifying instructors may request access by emailing **textbook@springerpub.com.**

Available resources include:

- **Test Bank:**
  - Multiple-Choice Questions With Answers/Rationales
- **Chapter-Based PowerPoint Presentations**

Section I:
Advanced Practice Nursing Population Health

Chapter 1

POPULATION HEALTH

Clair P. Millet

The day may soon dawn when we Americans can enjoy a measure of life and health that is consistent with our extraordinary resources and the intelligence of our people. The pioneers have begun their work; it is far from finished. New fields, new enterprises, are visible. The times call for the high spirit of the courageous pioneers among physicians, scientists, and nurses.

—Lillian Wald

CHAPTER COMPETENCIES

At the conclusion of this chapter, the reader will be able to:

1. Articulate the defining characteristics of a population and population health
2. Describe the determinants of health categories
3. Differentiate population health strategies and population management strategies
4. Describe the relationship of population health and epidemiology

ESSENTIAL TERMINOLOGY

Essential population health terms are:

- Population
- Cohort
- Population health
- Public health
- Health

POPULATION HEALTH

The United States' healthcare system is rapidly evolving and tremendously complex. Most would agree there needs to be a solution to address gaps and fragmented services in healthcare delivery. Population health is one of those solutions and is a broad concept that encompasses the elimination of disease and factors that influence health. The term *population health* is not new

and was originally defined as the "health outcomes of a group of individuals, including the distribution of such outcomes within the group" (Kindig & Stoddardt, 2003, p. 381). Kindig and Stoddardt also posit that the field of population health includes health outcomes, patterns of health determinants, and policies and interventions that link these two together. Population health can be a strategy for understanding the health of populations or an approach that focuses on interconnected conditions and factors that influence the health of populations over the life course, identifies systematic disparities in their patterns of occurrence, and applies resulting knowledge to develop and implement policies and interventions to improve the health and well-being of populations (Magnusson et al., 2019). Population health is both a concept as already defined, as well as a field of study. Multiple determinants or factors affecting health outcomes must be explored in this field of study, such as behaviors, medical care, interventions, and environment.

Epidemiology is often referred to as population medicine due to its focus on the health of groups of people. A crucial role of epidemiology provides evidence of deviations that take place over time in the health issues within a community. While the original definition of population health focused on outcomes, the area of population health has evolved more broadly to include collaborative activities or interventions that result in an improvement of a population's health status. In epidemiology, the patient is synonymous to the group or cohort. A cohort is a group of individuals that is observed to study causes and the degree to which health problems impact population health. Epidemiology collects, analyzes, and interprets data regarding the distribution and determinants of disease among populations (Nash et al., 2021).

There are several terms that need to be introduced to fully grasp the concept of population health. A population can be the number of individuals living in a geographically defined area (Young, 1998). A population can also be identified by common characteristics or common risk factors. A geographically defined population may be within a city, parish/county, or state. Common characteristics can be features such as religion or ethnicity. Common risk factors can be those such as smoking or obesity. It is important to understand the manner in which the term *population* is used and in what context. The World Health Organization (WHO) defines health as "a state of complete physical, mental, and social well-being and not merely the absence of disease or infirmity" (1994). The limits of the definition of health continue to evolve and sometimes can be unclear. Population health requires systems thinking and necessitates consideration of the implications of health problems affecting our entire society as well as the health issues of marginalized, vulnerable, or high-risk groups.

It is important to note that population health is not identical with public health. Public health is a core component of population health. Public health is concerned with protecting the health of populations and focuses on assessment, assurance, and policy development—core functions that ultimately impact the health of individuals, families, and communities. Population health efforts generate information to inform public health strategies that can be deployed where needed.

Drivers (Determinants) of Population Health and Population Health Status

The drivers of health are complex and interconnected. Health is influenced by many factors that can be classified into six broad categories: (a) genetics, (b) behavior, (c) physical environment, (d) medical care, (e) social factors, and (f) policymaking.

Genetics: Some genetic factors that can adversely affect population health may be more prevalent in certain populations. Some examples of genetic factors include age, gender, and inherited conditions.

Behavior: Behavior affects individual and population health outcomes. Some examples of behaviors are smoking, physical activity, and diet.

Physical Environment: The physical environment is inclusive of the physical and built environment. Some examples of physical environment are an individual's school, work, or home environment.

Medical Care: Access to healthcare and the quality of that care impact health. Barriers to access healthcare include lack of availability, lack of insurance coverage, high costs, and/or limited language access.

Social Factors: Social factors and physical conditions and social determinants of health affect individual, family, community, and population health. Some examples of social determinants of health are education, income, safe neighborhoods, transportation, and housing.

Policymaking: Local, state, and federal policies affect individual and population health. Over extended periods of time, policies can positively impact population health. An example is the 1966 National Traffic and Motor Vehicle Safety Act which reduced the rates of injuries and death from motor vehicle accidents.

It is important to note that health inequities are differences in health status or in the distribution of health resources among different population groups (WHO, 2018). Health inequities contribute to poorer health outcomes for certain populations, are unfair, and could be mitigated by utilization of population health strategies and policies that address health for all. Structural racism is a fundamental cause of persistent health disparities in the United States and restricts the ability of disenfranchised groups to live long and healthy lives. Determinants of health are discussed in more detail in Chapter 2.

Population Health Strategies

Improvement in specific populations requires interventions on multiple determinants, such as personal health behavior, access to healthcare, and changes in environments. No single entity can be held accountable for achieving desired outcomes. Collaboration across healthcare sectors and businesses must occur to be successful in improving health. Collaborators need to assess their approach to health and how resources are allocated to demonstrate shared accountability for better outcomes.

Health in All Policies (HiAP) is a collaborative approach that integrates and articulates health considerations into policymaking across sectors to improve the health of all communities and people (Centers for Disease Control and Prevention [CDC], 2016b). The HiAP population health strategy recognizes that health is created by several determinants and beyond the scope of traditional public health activities. Population health strategy can be utilized in population management strategy. An example of this would be using the HiAP approach to achieve The National Prevention Strategy (NPS) and Healthy People 2030 to improve health outcomes and population health and health equity.

The passing of the Affordable Care Act (ACA) in 2010 was the impetus for creating the National Prevention Council and the development of the NPS to appreciate the benefits of prevention for a healthier country and to improve population health. The NPS was created by the Office of the Surgeon General with input from an advisory group, stakeholders, and the public. The NPS provides evidence-based recommendations for improving health and wellness and addressing leading causes of disability and death (National Prevention Council, 2011). The NPS recommends policy, program, and systems approaches for four strategic directions: (a) healthy and safe community environments, (b) clinical and community preventive services, (c) empowered people, and (d) elimination of health disparities, and seven priorities: (a) tobacco free living, (b) preventing drug abuse and excessive alcohol use, (c) healthy eating, (d) active living, (e) injury- and violence-free living, (f) reproductive and sexual health, and (g) mental and emotional well-being.

In 2014, the Robert Wood Johnson Foundation (RWJF) implemented its vision to engage all Americans in a national population health movement toward building a Culture of Health that gives all members of our society the opportunity to lead healthier lives (Plough, 2014). A Culture of Health means that everyone has an opportunity to be healthier. This initiative required addressing the social determinants of health and removing obstacles that affect the health and well-being of individuals. The obstacles to good health include poverty, discrimination, and their consequences including powerlessness and lack of access to good jobs with fair pay, quality education, housing, safe environments, and healthcare (WHO, 2017).

The RWJF's Culture of Health is essentially an action framework that focuses on well-being and equity with the goal of empowering and supporting people to lead healthier lives now and in generations to come (RWJF, 2015). The overall goal of the Culture of Health initiative is to improve the nation's population health, well-being, and equity through activities in four different action areas including (a) making health a shared value; (b) fostering cross-sector collaboration to improve well-being; (c) creating healthier, more equitable communities; and (d) strengthening integration of health services and systems (2015).

Each of these four action areas includes a number of "drivers" that would be the factors to advance a Culture of Health. The RWJF describes these drivers as a set of investment priorities that are deemed important areas for activity in the action area, which are required for sustained health improvement and well-being (Chandra et al., 2016). For example, within the action area of "making health a shared value," the drivers include mindset and expectations, sense of community, and civic engagement. Each of the action areas also includes a set of measures against which Culture of Health–related outcomes can be followed.

Healthy People 2030 is the fifth iteration of the Healthy People initiative. Healthy People 2030 is targeted at novel challenges and builds on lessons learned from the previous four iterations. It provides a strategic framework for a national agenda that communicates a vision for improving health and achieving health equity. Healthy People sets national health objectives for a 10-year period based on scientific evidence. Healthy People 2030 contains 12 topic areas and 355 objectives with the following overarching goals:

- Attain healthy, thriving lives and well-being, free of preventable disease, disability, injury, and premature death.
- Eliminate health disparities, achieve health equity, and attain health literacy to improve the health and well-being of all.
- Create social, physical, and economic environments that promote attaining full potential for health and well-being for all.

- Promote healthy development, healthy behaviors, and well-being across all life stages.
- Engage leadership, key constituents, and the public across multiple sectors to take action and design policies that improve the health and well-being of all (U.S. Department of Health and Human Services Office of Disease Prevention and Health Promotion, 2020).

The Healthy People initiative serves as a guide for population health efforts and introduces methods to transform culture and elevate the health status of populations.

Population Management Strategies

Population health science is the analysis of conditions that shape distributions of health within and across populations and how they manifest as the health of individuals (Keyes, 2016). Population management strategies can be applied to drive improvement of population health, health equity, and healthcare costs. Reimbursement strategies historically have guided how healthcare services are delivered. Fee-for-service is the most common method for reimbursement and not focused on outcomes. This method reimburses providers for each service rendered via claims successfully submitted to the insurer. It does not matter if the patient had the correct outcome or the most optimal care. The fee-for-service model supports volume to produce revenue, not value.

The Institute for Healthcare Improvement (IHI) developed the Triple Aim as a framework which is particularly useful for population management. The IHI defines population management as positioning payment and the delivery of healthcare services toward the achievement of specific healthcare related metrics and outcomes for a particular population (Loehrer et al., 2016). The Triple Aim addresses three major problems facing the U.S. healthcare system today: high cost, low quality, and poor health outcome. Population management drives outcomes for which a system is held financially accountable and are largely within its control. Essentially, a healthcare entity is paid to improve health outcomes.

Population health is one of the three pillars of the IHI Triple Aim for optimizing health system performance. The other two pillars are patient experience of care and per capita cost (IHI, 2016). The goal of the Triple Aim is to improve the patient care experience, improve population

health, and reduce per capita healthcare costs. This model has been effective in guiding improvements to the healthcare system over the years; however, an additional aspect that has been adopted by many providers is that of the improved clinical experience leading to the creation of the Quadruple Aim in 2007. The assumption is that without an improved clinical experience, the other three pillars from the Triple Aim will not be fully realized. The Triple Aim was instrumental for change in the United States by motivating healthcare delivery systems to focus on cost reduction and improving patient care experiences and moving from a volume-based to a value-based strategy.

There is consensus that nurse care coordination is the most effective strategy for reducing costs and improving outcomes. Care coordination is foundational to improving the qualit care for individuals and populations via the efficient and effective use of resources (American Nurses Association, 2016). Care coordination also contributes to better management of chronic disease and reduced medical errors. Intensity and type of care coordination/management varies according to the complexity of the patient. Care coordination is one of the six priorities identified by the National Quality Strategy to reduce care fragmentation and improve the quality of life for patients with chronic illness and disability (Agency for Healthcare Research and Quality, 2016).

Navigating the multiple silos of healthcare providers and services is very complex for individuals and their families. Fragmentation of healthcare and social services is a major factor in patient noncompliance, polypharmacy, and medical errors resulting in suboptimal outcomes. Interprofessional team case management is frequently the primary focus of integrated care, a necessary strategy to improve population health outcomes.

Community health needs assessments (CHNAs) are a key intervention to addressing the needs of a population. The Public Health Accreditation Board defines community health assessment as a "systematic examination of the health status indicators for a given population that is used to identify key problems and assets in a community" (Public Health Accreditation Board, 2013, p. 10). The ultimate goal of a community health assessment is to develop strategies to focus on the community's health needs and identified problems. There is diversity in the instruments and methods that can be used to conduct a community health assessment. The key elements in CHNAs are community engagement and collaborative participation. Public health agencies are essential partners in population health initiatives. Partnerships can be key to leveraging epidemiologic and public health data with shared resources to improve population health.

Another population health management strategy is the CDC's 6/18 Initiative: Accelerating Evidence into Action. In this initiative, the CDC and partners targeted six common and costly health conditions with 18 proven interventions. Collaborating partners are healthcare providers, public health professionals, insurers, and employers who purchase insurance to improve health and control costs of healthcare by:

- giving partners rigorous evidence about high-burden health conditions and related interventions,
- highlighting disease prevention interventions to increase their coverage and quality, and
- aligning proven preventive practices with value-based ways of paying for healthcare (CDC, 2016a).

To improve health and control costs, the CDC has prioritized six high disease burden health conditions and effective interventions: (a) prevent unintended pregnancy, (b) control high blood pressure, (c) reduce tobacco use, (d) control asthma, (e) improve antibiotic use, and (f) prevent type 2 diabetes (CDC, 2016a). The 6/18 Initiative's six ways to spend smarter for healthier people is an evidence-based approach to population health management.

Prevention and Population Health

Epidemiologic data are used to identify subgroups in the population who are at high risk for disease (Celentano & Szklo, 2019). Identification of those that are high-risk assists in targeting preventive interventions such as screening for early detection of disease. Once these groups are identified, the specific causative factors or determinants that put them at high risk can be mitigated. Examples are smoking or diet which can be modified once identified as a targeted intervention for high-risk groups.

There are three consistent types of prevention: primary, secondary, and tertiary prevention.

Primary prevention occurs before disease takes place. It is the goal we hope to achieve where everyone is healthy and free of disease. A classic example of primary prevention is immunizations. Immunizations are given to prevent disease. This is how diseases that were once prevalent such as polio eradicated and those such as tetanus and influenza diminished. Other examples of primary prevention are altering risky behaviors, such as poor nutrition, smoking, and banning substances or exposures associated with illness or disease. Three lifestyle modifications: (a) reducing or eliminating tobacco use, (b) portion control of healthy foods, and (c) increasing regular physical activity are consistently identified in population-based epidemiologic research as most likely to reduce the prevalence of chronic conditions (Nash et al., 2021). A focus on primary prevention strategies intends to improve population health and decrease healthcare costs.

Secondary prevention occurs after disease develops but before signs and symptoms develop. This level of prevention is aimed at early disease detection or reduction of risk factors while the individual is asymptomatic. Examples of secondary prevention are regular blood pressure screenings, screenings for cholesterol measurements for cardiovascular disease, pap smears for cervical cancer in women, or prostate specific antigen (PSA) levels for prostate cancer in men. Early identification of disease and initiation of early intervention are more effective and tend to prolong life.

Tertiary prevention occurs once the individual is symptomatic and assists in disease management to slow or stop the disease progression. Tertiary prevention aims to minimize complications from disease and utilizes evidence-based interventions, for example, speech therapy and occupational therapy for victims of cerebrovascular accident (stroke). Other examples of tertiary prevention are measures such as chemotherapy or rehabilitation. Tertiary prevention is critical to reducing healthcare costs in addition to coordinating and providing continuity of care. Levels of prevention are discussed again in Chapter 6.

Epidemiology and Population Health

Improvement efforts for population health are informed by data from a variety of sources. Sources can include birth and death records, claims data, electronic medical records, population-based surveys, focus groups, and many others. Epidemiologic data are used to identify health issues that need to be addressed, to identify those groups and subgroups affected, to monitor and evaluate intervention efforts, and to identify factors contributing to disease and death (Nash et al., 2021). The knowledge produced by epidemiology needs to be translated into interventions to ultimately improve the health of the population.

The ACA of 2010 has made the utilization of epidemiology in healthcare system planning, allocation of resources, and provision of services a necessity. Healthcare systems are now responsible for ensuring the health of the populations they serve and have been forced to depend on epidemiologic data to focus on population health outcomes.

Measurements of the health of a population are called *population health status measures*. Two measurements became the standard for summarizing the health status of populations in the 20th century: infant mortality rate and life expectancy (Riegelman, 2020). Data are retrieved utilizing birth certificates, death certificates, and census surveys. The infant mortality rate estimates the rate of death in the first year of life per 1,000 live births. It was used as a primary measurement of child health for several years. Many preventive measures and interventions to impact infant mortality over the years has decreased infant mortality rates worldwide. Mortality rate reduction in children 2 to 5 years old have not been as successful. This is an excellent example of why additional measures of population health status evolve over time. Consequently, this new measure of under 5 years old mortality is now the standard measure by the WHO of child health (2020).

Life expectancy measures the overall death experience of the population. The probability of dying was also incorporated into each year of life. Quite simply, life expectancy is the average period that a person may expect to live and tells us how well a jurisdiction (city, region, state, country) is doing in terms of death in a particular year. It is important to note that life expectancy cannot be used to predict a population's life span as prediction requires that no change will occur. We have seen life expectancy rise with improvements in living standards, lifestyle, education, and greater access to quality healthcare services. The life expectancy in the United States in 2019 was 78.8 years, an increase of 0.1% from 2018. The 2021 life expectancy for the world population is 72.8 years (CDC National Center for Health Statistics, 2021).

CONCLUSION

Population health has great potential to mitigate health disparities. It is evident that the need for epidemiology to guide population health continues to grow. It is imperative that epidemiology is utilized to not only identify risk factors but to target the right care to the right individuals at the correct time—now called precision medicine (Khoury, 2015). Effective population health improvement requires attention to prevention, determinants of health, and the utilization of population health and population health strategies. The population health lens can be used at the individual, practice, institutional, systems, and community levels to drive improvements to health outcomes.

END-OF-CHAPTER RESOURCES

SUMMARY POINTS

- The term *population health* is not new and was originally defined as the "health outcomes of a group of individuals, including the distribution of such outcomes within the group."
- A cohort is a group of individuals that is observed to study causes and the degree of health problems to impact population health.
- A population can be the number of individuals living in a geographically defined area.
- Health is "a state of complete physical, mental, and social well-being and not merely the absence of disease or infirmity" WHO (1994).
- Public health is concerned with protecting the health of populations and focuses on assessment, assurance, and policy development core functions that ultimately impact the health of individuals, families, and communities.
- The drivers of health are complex and interconnected.
- Health is influenced by many factors that can be classified into six broad categories: (a) genetics, (b) behavior, (c) physical environment, (d) medical care, (e) social factors, and (f) policymaking.
- Population health strategy can be utilized in population management strategy.
- A Culture of Health means that everyone has an opportunity to be healthier.
- The Triple Aim addresses three major problems facing the U.S. healthcare system today: high cost, low quality, and poor health status.
- The goal of the Triple Aim is to improve the patient care experience, improve population health, and reduce per capita healthcare costs.
- Care coordination is foundational to improving the quality of care for individuals and populations via the efficient and effective use of resources.
- Community health needs assessments (CHNAs) are a key intervention to addressing the needs of a population.
- To improve health and control costs, the CDC has prioritized six high disease-burden health conditions and effective interventions: (a) prevent unintended pregnancy, (b) control high blood pressure, (c) reduce tobacco use, (d) control asthma, (e) improve antibiotic use, and (f) prevent type 2 diabetes.

EPIDEMIOLOGY CRITICAL REASONING QUESTIONS

1. Identify a population of interest. What epidemiologic health conditions are associated with this population? Consider the impact of the drivers (determinants) of population health as related to this population and the health condition.
2. Determine the common population health improvement strategies among Health in All Policies (HiAP), Culture of Health, the ACA, and Healthy People 2030.
3. Explain the following statements:
   a. Epidemiology is the foundation of population health.
   b. Population health is epidemiology.

ADDITIONAL RESOURCES

 A robust set of instructor resources designed to supplement this text is located at http://connect. springerpub.com/content/book/978-0-8261-8514-3. Qualifying instructors may request access by emailing textbook@springerpub.com.

REFERENCES

Agency for Healthcare Research & Quality. (2016). *National healthcare quality and disparities report chart book on care coordination.* AHRQ Pub. No. 16-0015-6-EF.

American Nurses Association. (2016). *The value of nursing care coordination: A white paper of the American Nurses Association.* https://www.nursingworld.org/~4afc0d/globalassets/practiceandpolicy/health-policy/care-coordination-white-paper-3.pdf

Celentano, D., & Szklo, M. (2019). *Gordis epidemiology* (6th ed.). Elsevier.

Centers for Disease Control. (2016a). *CDC's 6/18 initiative: Accelerating evidence into action.* www.CDC.gov/sixeighteen/index.html

Centers for Disease Control. (2016b). *Health in all policies.* https://www.cdc.gov/policy/hiap/index.html

Centers for Disease Control National Center for Health Statistics. (2021). *NCHS fact sheet*. https://www.cdc.gov/nchs/data/factsheets/factsheet_NVSS.pdf

Chandra, A., Miller, C., Acosta, J., Weilant, S., Trujillo, M., & Plough, A. (2016). Drivers of health as a shared value: Mindset, expectations, sense of community, and civic engagement. *Health Affairs, 35*(11), 1959–1963. https://doi.org/10.1377/hlthaff.2016.0603

Institute for Healthcare Improvement. (2016). *Triple aim for populations 2016*. http://www.ihi.org/Topics/TripleAim/Pages/default.aspx

Keyes, K. (2016). Setting the agenda for a new discipline: Population health science. *American Journal of Public Health, 106*(4), 633–634. https://doi.org/10.2105/AJPH.2016.303101

Khoury, M. J., & Evans, J. P. (2015). A public health perspective on a national precision medicine cohort: Balancing long-term knowledge generation with every health benefit. *JAMA, 313*(21): 2117–2118. https://doi.org/10.1001/jama.2015.3382

Kindig, D., & Stoddart, G. (2003). What is population health? *American Journal of Public Health, 93*(3), 380–383. https://doi.org/10.1016/j.pop.2019.07.001

Loehrer, S., Lewis, N., & Bogan, M. (2016). Improving the health of populations: A common language is key. *Healthcare Executive, 31*(2), 82–83.

Magnusson, D., Eisenhart, M., Gorman, L., Kennedy, V., & Davenport, T. (2019). Adopting population health frameworks in physical therapist practice, research, and education: The urgency of now. *Physical Therapy, 99*, 1039–1047. https://doi.org/10.1093/ptj/pzz048

Nash, D., Skoufalos, A., Fabius, R., & Oglesby, W. (2021). *Population health: Creating a culture of wellness* (3rd ed.). Jones & Bartlett Publishing.

National Prevention Council. (2011). *National prevention strategy*. U.S. Department of Health & Human Services, Office of the Surgeon General. https://www.hhs.gov/sites/default/files/disease-prevention-wellness-report.pdf

Plough, A. (2014). Building a culture of health: Challenges for the public health workforce. *American Journal of Preventive Medicine, 47*(5S3), S388–S390. https://doi.org/10.1016/j.amepre.2014.07.037

Public Health Accreditation Board. (2013). *Public health accreditation board: Acronyms & glossary of terms, version 1.5* (p. 10). https://www.phaboard.org/wp-content/uploads/2018/11/FINAL_PHAB-Acronyms-and-Glossary-of-Terms-Version-1.5.pdf

Riegelman, R. (2020). *Population health: A primer*. Jones & Bartlett Publishing.

Robert Wood Johnson Foundation. (2015). *From vision to action: Measures to mobilize a culture of health*. Author.

U.S. Department of Health and Human Services Office of Disease Prevention and Health Promotion. (2020). *Healthy People 2030 framework*. https://www.healthypeople.gov/2020/About-Healthy-People/Development-Healthy-People-2030/Framework

World Health Organization. (1994). *Constitution of the World Health Organization* (40th ed.). Author.

World Health Organization. (2017). *Social determinants of health*. www.who.int/social_determinants/en/

World Health Organization. (2018). *Health inequities and their causes*. https://www.who.int/news-room/facts-in-pictures/detail/health-inequities-and-their-causes

Young, T. (1998). *Population health concepts and methods*. Oxford University Press.

Chapter 2

DETERMINANTS OF HEALTH

Clair P. Millet

The most important practical lesson that can be given to nurses is to teach them what to observe.
–Florence Nightingale

CHAPTER COMPETENCIES

At the conclusion of this chapter, the reader will be able to:

1. Describe the determinants of health
2. Articulate how risk factors affect health
3. Describe the social determinants of health and their relationship to health inequities
4. Differentiate between health and healthcare disparities

ESSENTIAL TERMINOLOGY

Essential determinants of health terms are:

- Determinants of health
- Risk factor
- Health equity
- Health literacy
- Social determinants of health
- Health and healthcare disparities

What makes some people healthy and others unhealthy? Addressing critical health issues requires utilization of tools, such as epidemiology, to assist in determining why people get sick, disabled, or die. Answering "why" this happens requires one to understand the determinants of health. The World Health Organization (WHO) identifies the determinants of health as (a) the social and economic environment, (b) the physical environment, and (c) the person's individual characteristics and behaviors (2017). This premise is based on the idea that the context of an individual's life determines their health. An individual's socioeconomic status can be defined by numerous factors such as education, job or occupation, and income which impacts the health of the individual as well as the community with which they interact. The physical environment affects individual and population health. Determinants such as safe water, clean air, healthy workplaces, safe communities, and safe roads all contribute to positive health outcomes.

WHO defines a risk factor as any attribute, characteristic, or exposure of an individual that increases the likelihood of developing disease or injury. Risk factors can be modifiable or nonmodifiable. Modifiable risk factors can be changed by taking measures to address them. Examples include smoking, high blood pressure, poor diet, and obesity. Nonmodifiable risk factors include those we cannot control such as age, gender, race, and family history. Many of these risk factors and determinants of health are interconnected; however, it is important to note that some may not be under an individual's control. The way in which we conceptualize the determinants of health has evolved over time. The field of epidemiology investigates how disease is distributed in populations and the factors that determine the distribution. An essential purpose of epidemiology is to identify the etiology of disease and the risk factors that increase a person's risk for disease. Several factors, whether considered alone or combined, affect the health of individuals and communities. Multiple determinants or factors affecting health outcomes must be explored such as risks, behaviors, medical care, interventions, and environment.

THE HEALTHY PEOPLE INITIATIVE AND DETERMINANTS OF HEALTH

The Healthy People initiative is designed to guide national health promotion and disease prevention efforts to improve the nation's health. The Healthy People initiative sets national health goals and objectives for a 10-year period based on scientific evidence. Goals and objectives are tracked over a decade. End-of-decade assessments and applied epidemiology are conducted to track progress toward achieving the national objectives. Resultant of these efforts, numerous changes are made based on feedback from an extremely broad and diverse group of individuals and organizations. Health priorities change over time and are reflected across the initiative. Each Healthy People release encompasses determinants of health and considers health risk factors. The first was Healthy People 1990, released in the 1980s, focusing on decreasing deaths throughout the life span and on increasing independence of older adults. Healthy People 2000 was guided by three overly broad goals: (a) increase the span of healthy life, (b) reduce health disparities, and (c) achieve access to preventive services for all. Healthy People 2010 had an increased focus on improving quality of life and targeted elimination of health disparities, rather than reducing them.

It was not until Healthy People 2020 that the initiative began to explore the relationships between health status and biology, individual behavior, health services, social factors, and policies. The emphasis was on an ecological approach to disease prevention and health promotion. Healthy People 2020 defined the determinants of health as the range of personal, social, economic, and environmental factors that influence health status (Office of Disease Prevention and Health Promotion [ODPHP], n.d.-a).

Healthy People 2020 identified the determinants of health under five broad categories: (a) policymaking, (b) social factors, (c) health services, (d) individual behavior, and (e) biology and genetics. The premise is that the interaction among these factors is what determines individual and population health. Policymaking at all levels (i.e., local, state, federal) affect individual and population health. Social determinants of health are the social factors and physical conditions of the environment in which people are born, live, learn, play, work, and age. These conditions can be defined by the amount of money, power, or resources that people have, all of which are influenced by policy choices. Health services are dependent upon access to care and the quality of healthcare services received which impact health. Individual behavior also affects health. There are many public health interventions focused on changing individual behaviors such as physical activity, diet, and substance use such as alcohol, cigarettes, and illicit drugs. Hand washing is another example of an individual behavior to reduce transmission of potentially infectious material which may cause another to become ill or even die. Biology and genetics play a significant role in one's health. Biological and genetic factors affect certain populations more than others. Older adults are biologically predisposed to be in worse health than adolescents due to the diminished physical and cognitive effects of the aging process. While there are many causes of disease, family history is often a strong predictor of risk for common diseases such as cancer, diabetes, autoimmune disorders, cardiovascular disease, and mental illnesses.

Healthy People 2030 launched in August 2020 and was formulated to build upon the knowledge gained from the previous work. The focus of the fifth iteration is on health equity, social determinants of health, and health literacy with a focus on well-being. Health equity is defined as an ideal state marked by fairness and the achievement of optimal health and well-being for all populations, where disparities in health are eliminated (Association of Public Health Nurses, 2014). The premise of health equity is that all people can attain their full health potential, and no one is disadvantaged from achieving this potential because of their position in society or some other socially determined circumstance. Health literacy is based on whether a person can acquire, process, and comprehend basic health information and services that are necessary to make appropriate health decisions.

The social determinants of health (SDOH) are the conditions in which people are born, grow, live, learn, work, worship, and age that affect an individual's health and quality of life. Examples include education, employment, health services, housing, income, public safety, and environment, both physical and social. SDOH affect everyone via the conditions in which they are in. At their best, SDOH can have a protective effect on health, where conversely, at their worst, they can contribute to illness and death. The SDOH are a major factor in health inequities and are multilayered. It is important to identify risk factors present in the context of the SDOH to effectively target interventions to improve health and reduce health disparities.

One of the five overarching goals of Healthy People 2030 is related to SDOH. The goal is to "create social, physical, and economic environments that promote attaining the full potential for health and well-being for all" (ODPHP, n.d.-b). The SDOH are grouped into five domains: (a) economic stability, (b) education access and quality, (c) healthcare access and quality, (d) neighborhood and built environment, and (e) social and community context. Social, economic, and environmental conditions in addition to health behaviors, are related to an estimated 80% of health outcomes in the United States (Bradley et al., 2016). Aligning the right resources to address the SDOH effectively remains a challenge for healthcare.

HEALTH DISPARITIES

The National Institutes of Health (NIH) defines health status disparities as "differences in the incidence, prevalence, mortality and burden of diseases and other adverse conditions that exist among specific populations" (2000). The NIH further defines healthcare disparities as the differences in access to or availability of facilities and services. Healthy People 2020 also defined health disparity as, "a particular type of health difference that is closely linked with social, economic, and/or environmental disadvantage" and notes that disparities adversely affect groups of individuals who have "systematically experienced greater obstacles to health based on their racial or ethnic group; religion; socioeconomic status; gender; age mental health; cognitive, sensory, or physical disability; sexual orientation or gender identity; geographic location; or other characteristics historically linked to discrimination or exclusion" (U.S. Department of Health and Human Services [DHHS], 2010). The Centers for Disease Control and Prevention (CDC) further defines health disparities as "preventable differences in the burden of disease, injury, violence, or opportunities to achieve optimal health that are experienced by socially disadvantaged populations" (2017).

Vulnerable populations and underserved groups have faced longstanding disparities in health over the years. Recognition of health disparities began in the early 2000s and introduced the concepts of disparities in tobacco use and mental health care in two Surgeon General's reports (Ndugga & Artiga, 2021). While some improvements in population health have occurred, many disparities have persisted and, in some cases, grown. The COVID-19 pandemic is an example that has shown that people of color had worse health outcomes when compared to Whites. There are also longstanding disparities in healthcare. The Affordable Care Act (ACA) of 2010 created expansions in healthcare coverage, creating increased access to care across groups; however, it has not solved the issues related to health disparities.

Almgren (2018) posits that the measures of disparities involve three broad categories of health and healthcare delivery: burden of disease, access to care, and quality of care. These measures of disparity often overlap across categories. An example of this would be the incidence rate of disease that is sensitive to preventive measures, such as cardiovascular disease. These can serve as measures of a population's burden of disease and those disparities can be explicated in healthcare access and quality. Measuring the burden of disease occurrence is the prevalence and distribution of diseases, disabilities, and mortality in a population.

Racial and Ethnic Disparities

Racial and ethnic minorities tend to receive poorer quality care compared to those that are not in the minority. The sources of racial and ethnic health disparities include differences in geography, lack of access to adequate health coverage, communication difficulties between patient and provider, cultural barriers, provider stereotyping, and lack of access to providers (American College of Physicians, 2010). The populations that have been primarily underserved in the U.S. healthcare system include African Americans, Latinos, Native Americans, and Asian Americans (DHHS, Agency for Health Care Research and Quality, 2019). The *National Healthcare Quality and Disparities Report of 2019* indicates that some disparities were getting reduced from 2000 to 2018, yet disparities persist and some even worsened for poor and uninsured population in priority areas. SDOH are significant for health disparities among racial and ethnic minorities.

CONCLUSION

Epidemiology is a discipline that deals with the determinants of health. There is increased realization that focusing on the determinants of health and health disparities is an important aspect of improving the health of populations and improving healthcare outcomes. Inequities in education, housing, job security, and environmental health must be eradicated if health disparities are to be addressed effectively. More research and data collection related to determinants of health and health disparities are needed for stakeholders and healthcare providers to implement preventive measures to protect all individuals from illness, disability, and death.

END-OF-CHAPTER RESOURCES

SUMMARY POINTS

- The World Health Organization (WHO) identifies the determinants of health as (a) the social and economic environment, (b) the physical environment, and (c) the person's individual characteristics and behaviors.
- WHO defines a risk factor as any attribute, characteristic, or exposure of an individual that increases the likelihood of developing disease or injury.
- The Healthy People initiative is designed to guide national health promotion and disease prevention efforts to improve the nation's health.
- The Healthy People initiative sets national health goals and objectives for a 10-year period based on scientific evidence.
- Health equity is defined as an ideal state marked by fairness and the achievement of optimal health and well-being for all populations, where disparities in health are eliminated.
- Social determinants of health (SDOH) are the conditions in which people are born, grow, live, learn, work, worship, and age that affect an individual's health and quality of life.
- The National Institutes of Health (NIH) defines health status disparities as "differences in the incidence, prevalence, mortality and burden of diseases and other adverse conditions that exist among specific populations."
- The Centers for Disease Control and Prevention (CDC) further defines health disparities as "preventable differences in the burden of disease, injury, violence, or opportunities to achieve optimal health that are experienced by socially disadvantaged populations."

EPIDEMIOLOGY CRITICAL REASONING QUESTIONS

1. Identify a population of interest. What determinants of health are associated with this population? Consider the impact of associated risk factors and the determinants of health as related to this population and the health condition(s).
2. Determine strategies required to address health inequities focusing on determinants of health for population health improvement among disparate populations.

3. Explain the following statement:
   a. Utilizing an epidemiologic approach to disease occurrence targeting risk factors and addressing determinants of health can improve population health.

ADDITIONAL RESOURCES

 A robust set of instructor resources designed to supplement this text is located at http://connect.springerpub.com/content/book/978-0-8261-8514-3. Qualifying instructors may request access by emailing textbook@springerpub.com.

REFERENCES

Almgren, G. (2018). *Health care politics, policy and services* (3rd ed.). Springer Publishing Company.

American College of Physicians. (2010). *Racial and ethic disparities in health care updated 2010: Policy Paper*. https://www.acponline.org/system/files/documents/advocacy/current_policy_papers/assets/racial_disparities.pdf

Association of Public Health Nurses. (2014). *The public health nurse's role in achieving health equity: eliminating inequalities in health (Position Paper)*. https://www.phnurse.org/assets/docs/2015%20PHN%20Role%20in%20Achieving%20Health%20Equity.pdf

Bradley, K., Esposito, D., Romm, I., Loughnane, J., & Ajayi, T. (2016). *The business case for community paramedicine: Lessons from Commonwealth Care Alliances Pilot Program*. Center for Health Care Strategies (Issue Brief). https://www.chcs.org/resource/business-case-community-paramedicine-lessons-commonwealth-care-alliances-pilot-program/

Center for Disease Control and Prevention. (2017). *Health disparities*. https://www.cdc.gov/aging/disparities/index.htm

National Institutes of Health. (2000). *Addressing health disparities*. https://www.google.com/url?sa=t&rct=j&q=&esrc=s&source=web&cd=&ved=2ahUKEwiBw8Ge14HxAhUQSK0KHVyjAFEQFjACegQICRAD&url=https%3A%2F%2Fhsric.nlm.nih.gov%2Fhsric_public%2Ftopic%2Fdisparities%2F&usg=AOvVaw1ymVZnuCdJ_JJDJzrdtnUk

Ndugga, N., & Artiga, S. (2021). *Disparities in health and healthcare* [Issue Brief]. https://www.kff.org/racial-equity-and-health-policy/issue-brief/disparities-in-health-and-health-care-5-key-question-and-answers/

Office of Disease Prevention and Health Promotion. (n.d.-a). *Determinants of health. Healthy People 2020.* U.S. Department of Health & Human Services. https://www.healthypeople.gov/2020/about/foundation-health-measures/Determinants-of-Health

Office of Disease Prevention and Health Promotion. (n.d.-b). *Social determinants of health. Healthy People 2030.* https://health.gov/healthypeople/objectives-and-data/social-determinants-health

U.S. Department of Health and Human Services. (2010). *The Secretary's Advisory Committee on National Health Promotion and Disease Prevention Objectives for 2020.* Phase I report: Recommendations for the framework and format of Healthy People 2020. https://www.healthypeople.gov/2020/about/foundation-health-measures/Disparities

U.S. Department of Health and Human Services, Agency for Health Care Research and Quality. (2019). *National health care disparities report 2019.* https://www.ahrq.gov/sites/default/files/wysiwyg/research/findings/nhqrdr/2019qdr-final-es.pdf

World Health Organization. (2017). *The determinants of health.* https://www.who.int/news-room/q-a-detail/determinants-of-health

ADVANCED PRACTICE NURSING ROLES AND COMPETENCIES IN EPIDEMIOLOGY AND POPULATION HEALTH

Clair P. Millet

You must never so much think as whether you like it or not, whether it is bearable or not; you must never think of anything except the need, and how to meet it.

–Clara Barton

CHAPTER COMPETENCIES

At the conclusion of this chapter, the reader will be able to:

1. Articulate the meaning of advanced practice nurse and advanced practice nursing
2. Describe the role of the advanced practice nurse in epidemiology and population health
3. Understand the advanced practice nurse's competencies required for population health

ESSENTIAL TERMINOLOGY

Essential advanced practice nursing/nurse terms in epidemiology and population health are:

- Advanced practice nursing
- Advanced practice nurse
- Evidence-based practice
- Competency
- Advanced practice nursing functional role competencies

Nurses play a key role in the field of epidemiology and in population health. Population-focused nursing demands application of nursing theory and practice while integrating the tenets of public health to contribute to the improvement of community and population health.

While advanced practice nurses (APNs) not all specialize in public health, it is essential that APNs have a foundational knowledge of concepts on the health and illness continuum from a population perspective.

ADVANCED PRACTICE NURSING

APNs play an integral role in healthcare. Advanced practice nursing is the application of an expanded range of competencies to improve health outcomes for patients and populations in a specialized clinical area of the larger discipline of nursing (Hamric, 2019). An APN is a licensed nurse who has completed an advanced graduate-level education program and/or certification by a nationally recognized certifying body in one or more roles and population foci. An APN practices in one of the following four functional roles: nurse midwife (NM), nurse practitioner (NP), clinical nurse specialist (CNS), and certified registered nurse anesthetist (CRNA). APNs by virtue of their education, qualifications, competencies, knowledge, skills, and abilities are uniquely poised to directly contribute to population health. These nurses are prepared by education and certification to assess, diagnose, and manage care of individuals, groups, and populations.

Advanced Practice Nursing Roles in Epidemiology and Population Health

An essential and significant role of the APN is that of the direct clinical care provider. APNs use clinical reasoning to bring together their clinical knowledge with specific observations, perceptions, and facts from a particular situation to impact the health of individuals, groups, and populations. Improving the health of populations cannot be accomplished by nurses alone as coordination and collaboration across disciplines are critical to success. Evidence-based care coordination or transition management models can be applied to a variety of settings to improve population health (Fraher et al., 2015). APNs can lead in linking individuals with diverse parts of the healthcare system and coordinate transitions of care for effective management of disease and risk reduction.

APNs are expert *coaches* and provide expert guidance and teaching to other healthcare providers and to individual patients to mitigate risks, perform assessments and interventions, as well as manage illness and evaluate systems of care. Nursing assessment utilizing an epidemiologic approach is critical for APNs to be able to identify gaps in services and the causes of poor health for certain groups and populations.

Evidenced-based practice (EBP) is the judicious integration of the best evidence with clinical expertise. APNs use reliable EBP information for their clinical decision-making, current referral, and management guidelines. For example, EBPs such as protocols and clinical practice guidelines are utilized to support nursing practice and to provide the most optimal outcomes. APNs are skilled in performing literature review(s) relevant to epidemiology, disease, and health to ascertain the best and current evidence. EBP assists APNs to evaluate and improve nursing practice through research, thereby contributing to knowledge. APNs engage in scholarly inquiry and participate in formal and collaborative research to validate and/ or create new knowledge that contributes to population health.

APNs are *leaders* who exemplify professional, clinical, and systems leadership through coordination of care delivery and provision of community leadership. Facilitation of individual practice and healthcare system change through participation in quality improvement initiatives are key to the role of the APN. Advanced communication and leadership skills can be utilized to evaluate practice and effect change in population health.

APNs provide reliable information to others and act as both internal and external consultants. Consultation can occur as either formal or informal consultation. All nurses, including APNs, must be advocates for the patients and the populations they serve.

APNs are skilled collaborators, evidenced through collaboration with other healthcare professionals, patients, and families. Baggs and Schmitt (1988) identified six critical elements of physician–nurse collaboration: cooperation, assistiveness, shared decision-making, communication, planning, and coordination. Collaboration between health care professionals increases awareness of the others' knowledge and skills, leading to continued improvement in decision-making and care to improve population health.

Complex decisions are made on a regular basis in both the practice of population health and clinical medicine; however, the process for decision-making, including the framework, and reasoning that support ethical choices, may not always be clear. The central ethical requirement of routine clinical practice is competence. APNs should be competent to perform the functions of their professional scope of practice and make continuing efforts to maintain their level of competence.

Advanced Practice Nursing Competencies in Epidemiology and Population Health

All APNs share the same core knowledge criteria and competencies, although the actual clinical skill set varies and is dependent on the needs of the APN's specialty patient population (Hamric, 2019). A core concept in APN practice is that direct clinical practice is the central competency of any APN role and informs all other competencies. In a seminal work on competency assessment, Wright (1998) defined core competencies as the "knowledge, skills, abilities and behaviors needed to carry out a job" (p. 56). Subsequently, possession of appropriate competencies fulfills the organizational, departmental, and work setting requirements under the varied circumstances that may occur. Core competencies are based on key essential job functions and are typically articulated in competency statements that are measurable in some way.

APNs must understand epidemiology and epidemiological concepts, including the use of epidemiologic data to effectively assess for and treat illness, and manage disease processes holistically. A comprehensive approach is integral to consider for an individual's or group's environment and the determinants of health that affect them. Competencies in assessment and early detection of health problems give cause to early intervention resulting in treatment and resolution with reductions in healthcare costs.

APN Roles National Competencies Analysis for Population Health

Each of the advanced practice nursing role competencies were analyzed for population health applicability utilizing the national competencies for the NP, National Organization of Nurse Practitioner Faculties (NONPF) 2017 Core Competencies for Nurse Practitioners; CNS, National Association of Clinical Nurse Specialist (NACNS) 2019 Clinical Nurse Specialist Core Competencies; NM, American College of Nurse Midwives (ACNM) 2020 Core Competencies for Basic Midwifery Practice; and CRNA, American Association of Nurse Anesthetists (AANA) 2020 Scope of Nurse Anesthesia Practice. The utilization of the AANA 2020 Scope of Nurse Anesthesia Practice was decided on as the AANA did not have an identified core competency document. The American Nurses Association (ANA, 2010) defined the scope of nursing practice as "The description of the *who, what, where, when, why,* and *how* of nursing practice" (p. 67). This refers to the legal authority granted to the APN to provide healthcare services. Scope of practice is closely tied to state statutes or the Nurse Practice Act for the state and varies for each APN role. The national competencies for each APN concentration and role are identified in the following for application to population health.

Nurse Practitioner—NONPF (2017)

NPs have clinical expertise in diagnosing and treating health conditions with an emphasis on disease prevention and population health management. The NP competencies are population-focused competencies divided into nine competency areas: (a) scientific foundation competencies, (b) leadership competencies, (c) quality competencies, (d) practice inquiry competencies, (e) technology and information literacy competencies, (f) policy competencies, (g) health delivery system competencies, (h) ethics competencies, and (i) independent practice competencies. Each of these competency areas include applicability to population health and are identified as follows. The core competency is listed with the correlating number as listed in the NONPF document.

Scientific Foundation Competencies

1. Critically analyzes data and evidence for improving advanced nursing practice. For example, comparing patient data with evidence-based standards to improve care; 2. Integrates knowledge from the humanities and sciences within the context of nursing science; 3. Translates research and other forms of knowledge to improve practice processes and outcomes; and 4. Develops new practice approaches based on the integration of research, theory, and practice knowledge. Population health theories, conceptual frameworks and principles for practice, evidence-based care, evidence appraisal, research and quality improvement methods, and monitoring of health outcomes are some suggested crucial population health content for the NP curriculum.

Leadership Competencies

Core competencies that can influence and affect population health are: 1. Assumes complex and advanced leadership roles to initiate and guide change; 2. Provides leadership to foster collaboration with multiple stakeholders (e.g., patients, community, integrated healthcare teams, and policy makers) to improve healthcare; 3. Demonstrates leadership that uses critical and reflective thinking; 4. Advocates for improved access, quality, and cost-effective healthcare; and 7. Participates in professional organization and activities that influence APN and/or health outcomes of a population focus.

Quality Competencies

1. Uses best available evidence to continuously improve quality of clinical practice; 2. Evaluates

the relationships among access, cost, quality, and safety and their influence on healthcare; and 3. Evaluates how care processes, financing and policy decisions impact the quality of care. These identified quality competencies can all contribute to improved population health.

Practice Inquiry Competencies

1. Provides leadership in the translation of new knowledge into practice; 2. Generates knowledge from clinical practice to improve practice and patient outcomes; 3. Applies clinical investigative skills to improve health outcomes; 4. Leads practice inquiry, individually or in partnership with others; 5. Disseminates evidence from inquiry to diverse audiences using multiple modalities; and 6. Analyzes clinical guidelines for individualized application into practice. These competencies can be addressed in patient management and evaluation of outcomes affecting population health.

Technology and Information Literacy Competencies

1. Integrates appropriate technologies for knowledge management to improve healthcare; 2. Translates technical and scientific health information appropriate for various users' needs; and 5. Uses technology systems that capture data on variables for the evaluation of nursing care. Utilization of technology and information literacy competencies has application in available technology in clinical practice. Tools such as population-appropriate clinical indicators incorporated into electronic health records, telehealth and electronic data sets are examples in which epidemiologic approaches to improve population health could be utilized effectively. Use of technologies to monitor and evaluate clinical problems such as blood pressure, vital signs, glucose, or weight, for example, can also be beneficial in population health strategies.

Policy Competencies

All the listed NP core competencies in the policy area have implications for population health: 1. Demonstrates an understanding of the interdependence of policy and practice; 2. Advocates for ethical policies that promote access, equity, quality, and cost savings; 3. Analyzes ethical, legal and social factors influencing policy development; 4. Contributes to the development of health policy; 5. Analyzes the implications of health policy across disciplines; 6. Evaluates the impact of globalization on healthcare policy development; and 7. Advocates for policies for safe and healthy practice environments. NPs can conduct policy analysis to evaluate outcomes at local, state, national, and international levels while advocating for patients. Areas for health policy and healthcare reform such as national health priorities and vulnerable populations and needs are examples of population health management. Global issues such as infectious disease, immigration, disasters, and terrorism all have potential population health implications.

Health Delivery System Competencies

1. Applies knowledge of organizational practices and complex systems to improve healthcare delivery; 3. Minimizes risk to patients and providers at the individual and systems level; 5. Evaluates the impact of healthcare delivery on patients, providers, other stakeholders, and the environment; and 7. Collaborates in planning for transitions across the continuum of care. Interprofessional collaborative partnerships and use of data to improve practice can improve outcomes. Needs assessments of populations served, planning, delivering, and/or evaluating models of care address competencies to improve population health. Competency in legislative and regulatory issues that affect health, such as determinants of health, policy, and advocacy are all factors NPs need to possess for effective population health management.

Ethics Competencies

1. Integrates ethical principles in decision-making; 2. Evaluates the ethical consequences of decisions; and 3. Applies ethically sound solutions to complex issues related to individuals, populations, and systems of care. Ethical decision-making and considerations in decision-making in clinical practice can have an impact on population health. Sources of information that facilitate ethical decision-making require population health contemplation, such as clinical research, cultural sensitivity, legal statutes, and scope of practice. Population-, spiritual-, or system-specific resources may also be complex and affect population health strategies or management.

Independent Practice Competencies

All independent practice competencies have a direct impact on individual and population health: 1. Functions as a licensed independent practitioner; 2. Demonstrates the highest level of accountability for professional practice; 3. Practices independently managing previously diagnosed and undiagnosed patients to include providing the full spectrum of healthcare services across the life span, utilization of advanced health assessment skills, employing screening and diagnostic strategies in the diagnosing and treatment of patients and families over time within scope of practice; 4. Provides patient-centered care recognizing cultural diversity including the establishment of patient relationship and mutually acceptable plan of care; 5. Educates professional and lay caregivers to provide culturally and spiritually sensitive, appropriate care; 6. Collaborates with both professional and other caregivers to achieve optimal health outcomes; 7. Coordinates transitional care services across care settings; and 8. Participates in the development, use and evaluation of professional standards and evidence-based care.

Clinical Nurse Specialist—NACNS (2019)

CNSs have advanced clinical expertise in diagnosis and intervention to prevent, remediate, or alleviate illness and promote health with a defined specialty population (NACNS, 2019). The totality of CNS expert clinical practice is evidenced in the advanced care of patients and impacts populations. The core CNS competencies are the foundation of CNS practice. The three spheres of impact are patient direct care, nurses and nursing practice, and organizations/systems. The CNS core competencies with application to population health are identified in the following by the sphere of impact as noted in Chapter 3 of the *NACNS Statement on CNS Practice and Education, Third Edition.*

Patient/Direct Care (P)

The patient for the CNS represents a patient, family, healthcare surrogate, community, and population. All sixteen competencies (P.1–16) listed in the patient/direct care sphere have population health implications. The CNS builds relationships for health and wellness promotion. They synthesize assessment data and evidence using their advanced knowledge, clinical expertise, critical thinking and clinical judgment to diagnose, design, and implement evidence-based, cost-effective interventions to meet multifaceted needs of complex patients. The CNS considers the social determinants of health in designing and implementing strategies for effective patient care. The CNS also analyzes the ethical impact of scientific advances, including cost and clinical effectiveness and advocates for patients' preferences and rights. These core competencies are characterized by a holistic perspective in the advanced nursing

management of health, illness, and disease states and directly contribute to population health (NACNS, 2019).

Nurse and Nursing Practice Sphere (N)

The CNS advances nursing practice to achieve the optimal outcomes by ensuring evidence-based practices are utilized and meet the needs of patients and/or populations. N.1 Offering expert specialty consultation to nurses related to complex patient care needs; N.8 Using evidence-based knowledge as a foundation for nursing practice to enable optimal nurse-sensitive outcomes; N.9 Mentoring nurses and nursing staff in using evidence-based principles; N.11 Assessing the outcomes of nursing practice using methods that provide valid data; and N.14 Mentoring nurses to analyze legislative, regulatory, and fiscal policies that affect nursing practice and patient outcomes.

Organizations/Systems Sphere (O)

The CNS articulates the value of nursing care, influences system changes that facilitate improvement of quality, cost-effective patient outcomes and advocates for professional nursing. The following core competencies contribute to population health: O.2 Using leadership, collaboration, and conflict resolution to build partnerships within and across systems and/or communities; O.4 Leading systematic quality improvement and safety initiatives based on identification of a precise problem, gap analysis, and process evaluation; O.5 Leading the interprofessional team in finding, creating, implementing, and assessing evidence-based practices and research opportunities; O.6 Working with research-focused colleagues to translate, conduct, and disseminate research that improves clinical knowledge and practice; O.7 Leading and participating in selecting, integrating, managing, and evaluating technology and products to promote optimal health outcomes; O.8 Facilitating change in response to community needs in a dynamic healthcare environment; O.12 Promoting nursing's unique contributions to advancing health to stakeholders, such as the community, public, and policymakers; and O.13 Promoting equitable health care by participating in professional organizations and public policy activities.

Nurse Midwife—ACNM (2020)

Nurse midwives provide integrated, accessible healthcare services and are accountable for addressing most healthcare needs, developing a sustained partnership with clients, and practicing within a context of family and community (ACNM, 2020). The core competencies are arranged into five sections: (a) hallmarks of midwifery; (b) components of midwifery care: professional responsibilities; (c) components of midwifery care: midwifery management process; (d) components of midwifery care: fundamentals; and (e) components of midwifery care: primary, preconception, gynecologic/reproductive/sexual health, antepartum, intrapartum, and postpregnancy care. The identified competencies attributed to population health as noted in the ACNM Core Competencies for Basic Midwifery Practice document are identified in the following.

Hallmarks of Midwifery

C. Incorporation of evidence-based care into clinical practice; G. Promotion of continuity of care; H. Utilization of health promotion, disease prevention, and health education; I. Application of a public health perspective; J. Utilizing an understanding of social determinants of health to provide high-quality care to all persons including those from underserved communities; L. Integration of cultural safety into all care encounters; M. Incorporation of evidence-based integrative therapies; N. Skillful communication, guidance, and counseling; P. Ability to collaborate with and refer to other members of the interprofessional health care team; and Q. Ability to provide safe and effective care across settings.

Components of Midwifery Care: Professional Responsibilities

The professional responsibilities related to population health include: D. Knowledge of national and international issues and trends in women's and transgender and nonconforming individuals' perinatal and neonatal care; E. Support for legislation and policy initiatives that promote quality healthcare; F. Knowledge of health disparities; G. Knowledge of issues and trends in healthcare policy and systems; H. Advocacy for health equity, social justice, and ethical policies in healthcare; I. Appropriate use of technology and informatics to improve the quality and safety of healthcare; L. Ability to evaluate, apply, interpret, and collaborate in research; N. Development of critical thinking and leadership skills; and T. Ability to consult, collaborate, and refer with other healthcare professionals as part of the healthcare team.

Components of Midwifery Care: Midwifery Management Process

The midwifery management process guides all areas of clinical care. All competencies noted in this section by the ACNM have direct impact on population health. A. Obtains all necessary data for complete evaluation of the client; B. Identifies problems or diagnoses and healthcare needs based on correct interpretation of data; C. Anticipates potential problems or diagnoses that may be expected based on identified risk factors; D. Evaluates the need for immediate intervention and/or consultation, collaborative management, or referral as dictated by the client's condition; E. Develops a comprehensive evidence-based plan of care; F. Assumes responsibility for safe and efficient implementation of a evidenced-based plan of care including the provision of treatments and interventions as indicated; and G. Evaluates the effectiveness of treatments and/or interventions.

Components of Midwifery Care: Fundamentals

Knowledge of the following subject areas is fundamental to the practice of midwifery and contributes to population health outcomes. C. Reproductive and perinatal epidemiology and basic epidemiologic methods relevant to midwifery practice; D. Research and evidence-based practice; I. Clinical genetics and genomics; and J. Diversity, equity and inclusion.

Components of Midwifery Care: Primary, Preconception, Gynecologic/Reproductive/Sexual Health, Antepartum, Intrapartum, and Postpregnancy Care

Midwifery care includes the independent management of primary health screening, health promotion and the provision of care from adolescence through the life span, as well as the neonatal period using the midwifery management process (ACNM, 2020). Competencies relative to population health in which a midwife demonstrates knowledge, skills and abilities include *Primary Care*: A1. Applies nationally defined goals and objectives for health promotion and disease prevention; A2. Provides age-appropriate physical, mental, genetic, environmental, sexual, and social health assessment; A3. Utilized nationally defined screening and immunization recommendations to promote health and detect and prevent diseases; A4. Applies management strategies and therapeutics to facilitate health and promote healthy behaviors; A5. Utilizes advanced health assessment skills to identify normal and abnormal findings; and A6. Applies management strategies and therapeutics for treatment of common health problems and deviations from normal, such as infections utilizing consultation, collaboration, and referral as indicated.

Components of Midwifery Care: Preconception Care

B1. Performs thorough evaluation including complete health history, family history, relevant genetic history, and physical exam; and B4. Performs health and laboratory screenings.

Components of Midwifery Care: Gynecologic/Reproductive/Sexual Health Care

C2. Utilizes common screening tools and diagnostic tests; C3. Manages common gynecologic and urogynecologic problems; C5. Screens for and treats sexually transmitted infections including partner evaluation, treatment, and referral as indicated; and C8. Identifies deviation from normal and appropriate interventions utilizing consultation, collaboration, and/or referral as indicated.

Components of Midwifery Care: Antepartum Care

D4. Uses management strategies and therapeutics to promote normal pregnancy; D5. Utilizes nationally defined screening tools and diagnostics as indicated; D7. Examines the influence of the environmental, cultural, and occupational factors, health habits and maternal behaviors on pregnancy outcomes; D8. Screens for health risks; and D11. Identifies deviations from normal and institutes appropriate interventions.

Components of Midwifery Care: Intrapartum Care

E3. Identifies deviations from normal and implements appropriate interventions.

Components of Midwifery Care: Postpregnancy Care

F2. Utilizes management strategies and therapeutics to facilitate a healthy puerperium and F9. Identifies deviations from normal and appropriate interventions.

Components of Midwifery Care: Care of the Well Neonate

G4. Evaluates the neonate including initial physical and behavioral assessment; gestational age assessment; ongoing assessment, and management of term, well neonate during the first 28 days; and identification of deviations from normal and consultation and/or referral as indicated. G5d. Provision of preventive care such as therapeutics according to local and national

guidelines; testing and screening according to local and national guidelines; and the need for ongoing preventive care. G5f. Provision of appropriate interventions and referrals for abnormal condition, such as infection and health education specific to the needs of the neonate and family.

Certified Registered Nurse Anesthetists—AANA (2020)

CRNAs are independent practitioners who plan and deliver anesthesia, pain management, and related care to patients of all health complexities across the life span (AANA, 2020). CRNAs provide the preoperative services related to population health by performing a comprehensive history and physical examination, assessment, and evaluation, and developming a comprehensive patient-specific plan of care to avoid complications which is imperative to health outcomes. Selecting, ordering, prescribing, administering, and monitoring the patient are critical competencies in anesthesia care. Providing comprehensive patient-centered pain management to optimize recovery is integral to improved health outcomes.

CRNAs should be patient advocates when indicated to positively impact population health. Being aware of the community served better positions CRNAs to understand what resources may be needed to target the healthcare needs of the patient. Health outcomes data and evidence-based protocols are utilized by CRNAs to provide patients with effective anesthesia and pain management care (AANA, 2021).

Advanced Practice Nursing Management of Disease Occurrence

APNs must understand the population of interest and identify core factors involved in the disease process. Comprehension of the basics of disease modes of transmission, pathogenicity, and patterns of occurrence are essential for APNs. The identification of the mode of transmission of a disease can significantly impact the plan of action to treat and contain the spread of disease. The study of the disease agent, host, and the environment, later discussed as the epidemiologic triad components of a disease, helps the APN plan for an effective intervention and reduction of communicable disease. The APN must also understand and have familiarity with epidemiologic data and measures of disease occurrence such as morbidity and mortality, life expectancy, and fatality rates to comprehend disease distribution and health outcomes. Assessment of changing patterns of disease incidence is analyzed by the APN to reduce the spread of disease and death in and across populations.

CONCLUSION

APNs contribute to achieving better care for individuals, improved population health outcomes, and lower healthcare costs. Advance practice nursing competencies required to positively impact population health outcomes have been presented in this chapter to include each of the national APN functional roles. Consistent themes emerge across all functional roles of advanced practice nursing. Advanced assessment and analytical skills to include use of epidemiologic data and concepts to better understand disease occurrence and distribution are crucial to optimal health outcomes. Other key population health advanced nursing competencies include leadership, systems thinking, public health science, and policy analysis/development.

END-OF-CHAPTER RESOURCES

SUMMARY POINTS

- Population-focused nursing demands application of nursing theory and practice while integrating the tenets of public health to contribute to the improvement of community and population health.
- APNs play an integral role in healthcare.
- Advanced practice nursing is the application of an expanded range of competencies to improve health outcomes for patients and populations in a specialized clinical area of the larger discipline of nursing.
- An APN is a licensed nurse who has completed an advanced graduate-level education program and/or certification by a nationally recognized certifying body in one or more roles and with a population focus.
- An APN practices in one of the following four functional roles: nurse midwife, nurse practitioner, clinical nurse specialist and certified registered nurse anesthetist.
- Evidence-based practice is the judicious integration of the best evidence with clinical expertise.
- All APNs share the same core criteria and competencies, although the actual clinical skill set varies and is dependent on the needs of the APN's specialty patient population.
- APNs must understand epidemiology and epidemiologic concepts, including the use of epidemiologic data to effectively assess for and treat illness and manage disease processes holistically.
- Advanced assessment and analytic skills to include use of epidemiological data and concepts to better understand disease occurrence and distribution are crucial to optimal health outcomes.

CRITICAL REASONING QUESTIONS

1. Choose an infectious disease outbreak. Discuss the epidemiology of the infection and describe the role of APN to manage it.
2. How can prevention activities lessen the burden of disease in communities or populations and reduce healthcare costs? How can APNs play a significant role in this endeavor?
3. Explain the following statement: APNs are critical catalysts for change in building population health.

ADDITIONAL RESOURCES

 A robust set of instructor resources designed to supplement this text is located at http://connect. springerpub.com/content/book/978-0-8261-8514-3. Qualifying instructors may request access by emailing textbook@springerpub.com.

REFERENCES

American Association of Nurse Anesthetists. (2020). *Scope of nurse anesthesia practice.* https://www.aana.com/docs/default-source/practice-aana-com-web-documents-(all)/professional-practice-manual/scope-of-nurse-anesthesia-practice.pdf?sfvrsn=250049b1_6

American Association of Nurse Anesthetists. (2021). *The CRNA's role in addressing racial and ethnic disparities in anesthesia care* [Position Statement]. https://www.aana.com/docs/default-source/practice-aana-com-web-documents-(all)/professional-practice-manual/2021-disparities-position-statement-final-_bod.pdf?sfvrsn=f45c2514_7

American College of Nurse Midwives. (2020). *ACNM core competencies for basic midwifery practice.* https://www.midwife.org/acnm/files/acnmlibrarydata/uploadfilename/000000000050/ACNMCoreCompetenciesMar2020_final.pdf

American Nurses Association. (2010). Nursing's *social policy statement* (3rd ed.). Author.

Baggs, J., & Schmitt, M. (1988). Collaboration between nurses and physicians. *Journal of Nursing Scholarship, 20*(3), 145–149. https://doi.org/10.1111/j.1547-5069.1988.tb00055.x

Fraher, E., Spetz, J., & Naylor, M. (2015). *Nursing in a transformed health care system: New roles, new rules.* Interdisciplinary Nursing Quality Research Initiative [Research Brief]. http://ldi.upenn.edu/sites/default/files/pdf/inqri-ldi-brief-nursing.pdf

Hamric, A. (2019). A definition of advanced practice nursing. In A. Hamric, C. Hanson, M. Tracy, & E. O'Grady (Eds.), *Advanced practice nursing: An integrative approach* (6th ed.). Saunders Elsevier.

National Association of Clinical Nurse Specialists. (2019). *Statement on clinical nurse specialist practice and education* (3rd ed.). NACNS.

National Organization of Nurse Practitioner Faculties. (2017). *Nurse practitioner core competencies.* https://cdn.ymaws.com/www .nonpf.org/resource/resmgr/competencies /2017_NPCoreComps_with_Curric.pdf

Wright, D. (1998). *The ultimate guide to competency assessment in health care* (2nd ed.). Creative Health Care Management.

Section II:
Epidemiology

Chapter 4

EPIDEMIOLOGY PRIMER

Demetrius J. Porche

The science on which public health decisions are based is epidemiology, or the study of the distribution of diseases, health problems, or risk factors in the population and action taken to alleviate those problems. The science of demography augments epidemiology and studying population problems.

–William Foege

CHAPTER COMPETENCIES

At the conclusion of this chapter, the reader will be able to:

1. Demonstrate an understanding of the definition and scope of epidemiology
2. Describe a comparison of descriptive and analytic epidemiology
3. Demonstrate an understanding of the epidemiologic process
4. Compare the similarities and differences in the epidemiologic approach and scientific methods
5. Analyze a health- or disease-related condition using the epidemiologic triad
6. Describe the differences in the epidemiologic tools

ESSENTIAL TERMINOLOGY

The essential epidemiology primer terminology consists of:

- Agent
- Analytic epidemiology
- Count
- Descriptive epidemiologic study
- Descriptive epidemiology
- Environment
- Epidemiologic reasoning
- Epidemiologic triad
- Epidemiology
- Experimental analytic study
- Frequency
- High-risk approach
- Host
- Observational analytic study
- Population-based approach
- Proportion
- Rate
- Ratio
- Science
- Scientific method
- Substantive epidemiology

EPIDEMIOLOGY DEFINED

The term *epidemiology* is derived from the Greek words *epi* which means upon, *demos* which means people, and *logos* which means science. Epidemiology is considered a basic public health science. Advances in population health science and population health management are grounded in the utilization of epidemiologic information. Therefore, epidemiology is also considered foundational to population health. Epidemiology is also considered a core science of public health and public health nursing practice.

Throughout time, multiple definitions of epidemiology have been proposed. The definitions have evolved from describing the focus of epidemiology to including defining aspects for the utilization of epidemiologic information to prevent health conditions. Table 4.1 presents a summary of some of the definitions. The study of the distribution and determinants of health and

Table 4.1 Epidemiology Definitions

Definition	Author
The study of health and populations in relation to their environment and ways of living	Morris (2007)
The study of the prevalence and dynamics of stages of health in populations	Frerichs and Neutra (1978)
The science of the dynamics of health in populations	Rich (1979)
It is concerned with the patterns of disease occurrence in human populations and the factors that influence these patterns	Lilienfeld and Lilenthal (1980)
The discipline of epidemiology is the aggregate principles of studying illness occurrence and related states and events	Miettinen (1985)
The study of the distribution and determinants of disease frequency in human populations	Hennekens and Buring (1987)
The quantitative analysis of the circumstances under which disease processes occur in population groups, factors that affect the incidence, distribution, and host responses, and utilization of this knowledge to prevent and control disease	Evans (1979)
The study of the distribution and determinants of health-related states or events in specified populations and the application of this study to the control of health problems	Last (2000)
The study of health status of populations	Schwabe et al. (1977)

Source: From Frerot, M., Lefebvre, A., Aho, S., Callier, P., Astruc, K., & Aho Glélé, L. S. (2018). What is epidemiology? Changing definitions of epidemiology 1978–2017. *PLoS One, 13*(12), e0208442. https://doi.org/10.1371/journal .pone.0208442

health-related conditions or events in populations to promote and preserve population health while preventing and controlling health-related conditions or events in specific populations is the definition of epidemiology embraced in this book.

COMPONENTS OF EPIDEMIOLOGY

The term *epidemiology* has been defined to describe the types of data or information collected and the purpose for collecting the specific population-related data or information. In addition, the term *epidemiology* has been used to describe specific methods and strategies to develop the epidemiologic body of knowledge. Epidemiology can be categorized into three component types: substantive, descriptive and analytic.

Substantive epidemiology is considered the cumulative collection of epidemiologic knowledge generated through epidemiologic methods. Some authors also refer to this as descriptive epidemiology. Others consider substantive and descriptive epidemiology different, with descriptive epidemiology considered the body of information or knowledge that describes the health conditions and the associated factors that

lead to or contribute to the health condition (risk factors). Descriptive epidemiology describes the manner in which epidemiologic data are organized and analyzed to understand health conditions or disease frequency within a population over time and the extent to which the health condition or disease varies in a population. Descriptive epidemiology is characterizes health conditions according to person, place, and time. Box 4.1 presents the characteristics examined with descriptive epidemiology. Descriptive

---

BOX 4.1. Descriptive Epidemiology Characteristics: Person, Place, Time

- **Person:** Characteristics (such as age, sex, occupation, income) of the individual affected by the health condition
- **Place:** Geographical location of the affected individual (such as residence, work location, leisure activity location)
- **Time:** When the health event occurred (beginning of symptoms/signs, testing time, diagnostic time, reporting of health condition time)

epidemiology has also been characterized as the "who, what, when, and where" of epidemiology. Box 4.2 presents the descriptive epidemiologic process. Analytical epidemiology uses descriptive epidemiologic information to analyze the determinants of health conditions, such as the association between an exposure and health condition or disease, or the causes and effects of health conditions or diseases. Analytic epidemiology has been characterized as the "why and how" of epidemiology. Table 4.2 compares descriptive and analytic epidemiology.

EPIDEMIOLOGIC SCIENCE AND EPIDEMIC SCIENCE

Science has several applicable definitions. Science is defined as the pursuit and application of knowledge. It is also described as the rigorous methods used to understand the natural and social worlds. Science is also known as a methodology to develop knowledge through the scientific method. The scientific method is characterized into six steps. To generate knowledge that is considered "science" many disciplines require that these six scientific steps should be utilized in some manner. Box 4.3 presents a review of the scientific method.

Epidemiologic science is described and characterized as the body of knowledge accumulated through epidemiology, the methods used to collect epidemiologic data, and the underpinning philosophical and theoretical information that guides epidemiologic thinking and data collection. Similarly, epidemiology frequently investigates disease outbreaks within a defined population, known as epidemics. Epidemic science is evolving as a branch of epidemiology science. Epidemic science includes the rigorous epidemiologic methods used to study epidemics and the knowledge base gained from the study of an epidemic within a specific population (Rojek & Horby, 2016).

BOX 4.2. Descriptive Epidemiology Process

- Define the population
- Define the health condition or disease under investigation
- Describe the health condition or disease in terms of person, place, and time
- Measure the health condition or disease
- Compare health condition or disease measurement to known epidemiologic data
- Generate an etiological hypothesis about health condition or disease in the population

---

BOX 4.3. Scientific Method

- Define the purpose of the investigation
- Construct an hypothesis
- Collect data to test the hypothesis
- Analyze data
- Propose conclusions from the data and integrate the information into the existing state of knowledge
- Communicate findings through peer-reviewed dissemination

Table 4.2 Descriptive and Analytic Epidemiology Comparison

Descriptive Epidemiology	Analytic Epidemiology
Describes distribution of disease by person, place, time	Measures the association between an exposure and the health condition or disease
Generates hypotheses about risk factors and disease causes	Tests hypotheses about determinants of health condition/disease such as risk factors and causes, and analyzes the distribution of exposure and health conditions/disease
Focus on who, what, when, and where	Focuses on how and why
Analyzed by population level data	Analyzed by comparative population groups
Methods include incidence, prevalence, case reports, case series, descriptive studies	Methods include observational and experimental studies

GOAL AND OBJECTIVES OF EPIDEMIOLOGY

The primary goals of epidemiology are to prevent and control health conditions that impact the health of individuals and the population and to develop the science of epidemiology to continually improve epidemiologic methods and the epidemiologic knowledge base. Epidemiological goals are accomplished through multiple interrelated objectives. Box 4.4 presents an outline of the multiple objectives of epidemiology.

EPIDEMIOLOGIC APPROACH

The epidemiologic approach to conducting an investigation consists of two approaches. These two approaches are a population-based and a high-risk approach. In a population-based approach, a specific population is characterized and defined. Once the population is characterized and defined, epidemiologic methods are used to analyze the epidemiologic data within the specific population. In contrast, a high-risk approach targets the epidemiologic investigation at those persons within a defined aggregate group or community who are known to possess the identified high-risk characteristic. Nurses should have a clear perspective as to what constitutes the population of interest prior to initiating the epidemiologic approach and reasoning.

EPIDEMIOLOGIC REASONING

Epidemiologic reasoning is the thought process utilized by epidemiologists to approach or resolve a health condition. The epidemiologic reasoning process uses the scientific method as a foundation to guide the reasoning process. Box 4.5 summarizes the epidemiologic reasoning process. Risk factor determination and disease association and causation use the epidemiologic reasoning process to understand the dynamics of the health condition. The first step in epidemiologic reasoning is to characterize the population structure. The population structure consists of the make up or composition of a population, which is generally representative of demographic characteristics. Next, epidemiologic reasoning must characterize the exposure to a risk factor within a population and the presence of a health condition or disease within a population. The third step characterizes the person characteristics of the population and the health condition within the population, determining whether there is an association that exists between the risk factor or exposure and the population. Once the risk factor or exposure is linked to the persons within the population, further analysis attempts to characterize the strongest associations between the risk factor or exposure by the population structure. The determination of an association does not indicate causation.

After this association is characterized, the epidemiologist develops appropriate inferences about the associative or causal relationships based on the distribution patterns of the disease within the population. During this analysis, the epidemiologist further develops inferential

---

BOX 4.4. Epidemiology Objectives

- Study the natural history and prognosis of health conditions/diseases
- Identify syndromes and classification of health conditions/diseases
- Examine effective screening and diagnostic testing strategies
- Determine the extent of health conditions/diseases in a population
- Survey health conditions/diseases in a population
- Identify and prevent or decrease the impact of the risk factors of health conditions/diseases
- Identify and prevent the cause or etiology of a health condition/disease
- Evaluate the efficacy and effectiveness of preventive and therapeutic measures
- Evaluate the efficacy, outcome, and impact of various modes of healthcare delivery
- Provide epidemiologic information that informs the development of health-related and public policy

---

BOX 4.5. Epidemiologic Reasoning Process

- Determine the population structure
- Characterize the exposure or risk factor in the population or characterize the health condition within the population
- Determine if there is an association between the exposure or risk factor, the population characteristics, and health condition
- Infer an hypothesis about the causal or associative relationships between the population characteristics, exposure or risk factor, and the health condition
- Examine the impact of preventive or therapeutic strategies on the exposure or risk factor within the population and on the health condition

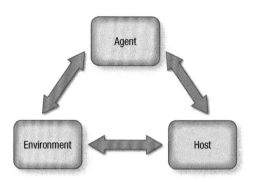

Figure 4.1 Epidemiologic triad.

BOX 4.6. Agent, Host, Environment Factors Influencing Disease Development

Agent
■ Infectivity
■ Pathogenicity
■ Antigenic stability

Host
■ Age
■ Gender/sex
■ Genotype
■ Behavior
■ Health status
■ Lifestyle factors
■ Nutritional status

Environment
■ Weather
■ Temperature
■ Housing
■ Geography
■ Air quality
■ Occupational setting

---

hypothesis about the associate and causal relationship between the disease patterns according to the population structure. Lastly, the epidemiologist develops preventive or therapeutic strategies targeting the exposure or risk factors to alter the presence of the health condition within the population.

EPIDEMIOLOGIC TRIAD (TRIANGLE)

Human disease occurs through the interaction of three dynamic systems, known as the epidemiologic triad or triangle. The epidemiologic triad is represented by the interaction among an agent, a host, and the environment (Figure 4.1). The agent is an offending microorganism such as a bacterium or virus. The host is the human who is susceptible to disease transmission. The environment consists of the air, water, soil, chemicals, diet, and other factors that facilitate disease transmission.

The epidemiologic triad model can explain the principles of communicable disease transmission by which the interaction of the three factors results in the development of a disease process. The interaction of the agent, host, and environment is sometimes facilitated through a vector. A vector is an agent or organism that can promote the interaction of the agent, host, and environment to cause the establishment of a disease, such as a mosquito with malaria or deer tick with Lyme disease. In addition to the vector, there are characteristics of the agent, host, and environment that impact whether a disease occurs (Box 4.6). These three epidemiologic triad factors are critical to disease transmission and are key to the development of prevention strategies. Breaking the linkages of the epidemiologic triad can break the chain of infection (Chapter 5).

It is also important to note that human disease also results from the interaction of genetic, behavioral, and environmental factors.

THINKING EPIDEMIOLOGICALLY

Thinking epidemiologically integrates the scientific method, epidemiologic reasoning, and the epidemiologic triad into a coherent thought pattern. Epidemiologic thinking uses an integrative investigative approach to understanding the distribution of health conditions and determinants of health conditions within a population to develop preventive and therapeutic population-based strategies. Figure 4.2 is offered as an integrative epidemiologic thinking process.

EPIDEMIOLOGICAL TOOLS

Epidemiological analysis requires the use of several tools that will be presented throughout this book. The tools of epidemiology facilitate an understanding of the data to understand the complex distribution and determinants of health within a population. Measures of health and disease provide evidence to develop or confirm hypotheses generated during the epidemiologic reasoning process. The overall purpose of

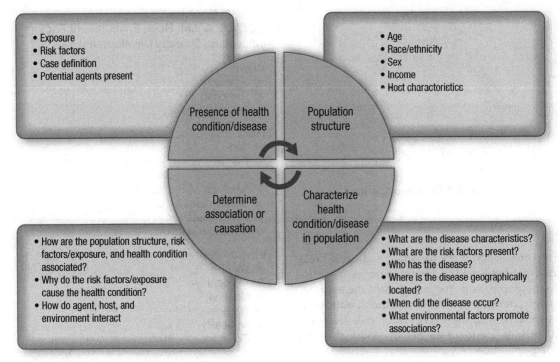

Figure 4.2 Integrative epidemiologic thinking process.

epidemiology is measurement of health and disease occurrence. The primary tools of epidemiology consist of measurement and epidemiologic studies. Epidemiologic tools permit the healthcare provider to count, divide, and compare population data. The measurement tools are:

- **Counts:** The raw number of events; these counts represent the most basic descriptive epidemiologic measure;
- **Frequency:** Compares one part of the distribution to another part of the distribution or the entire population. Common frequency measures are proportions, ratios, and rates. Frequency measures have a basic formula:

$$\frac{\text{Numerator}}{\text{Denominator}} \times 10^n$$

- **Ratio:** A measure in which the numerator is not part of the denominator. Odds ratio is a type of ratio that determines the ratio of the odds of a disease in one group to the odds in another group of the population. In ratio, the numerator and denominator can be different categories of the same variable such as males and female or persons aged 30 to 39 and 40 to 49 years of age. In some ratios, the numerator and denominator can be completely different

variables such as the number of pharmacies in a county and the size of the population residing in the county. Ratio measures have the basic formula:

$$\frac{\text{Number or rate of events in one group}}{\text{Number or rate of events in another group}}$$

- **Proportion:** A measure that compares a part to the whole; in a proportion, the numerator is included in the denominator. The basic proportion measure formula is:

$$\frac{\begin{array}{c}\text{Number of persons or events with}\\\text{a characteristic or attribute}\end{array}}{\begin{array}{c}\text{Total number of persons or events}\\\text{of which the numerator is a}\\\text{component or subset}\end{array}} \times 10^n$$

- **Rates:** A proportion with a specified period of time; a rate measures the frequency of an event in a specific defined population over a specified period of time. Rates provide critical epidemiologic data that are useful for comparing disease frequency in different locations, among different groups of the population, and at different time periods with the element of time considered. Rate is considered a measure of risk. Two common rates used in epidemiology are incidence and prevalence (Mortimer & Borenstein, 2006).

Epidemiologic studies provide another set of tools to assist the epidemiologist to understand the distribution and determinants of health in a population. Epidemiologic studies can be divided into three categories: descriptive, observational analytic, and experimental analytic; or two categories, observational and experimental analytic. Research studies as an epidemiologic tool are used in the following manner:

- **Descriptive epidemiologic studies** describe the distribution of disease by person, place, and time facilitating the generation of hypotheses. Descriptive and exploratory research designs are within this category;
- **Observational analytic studies** describe the distribution of disease in a comparative manner to provide a basis to generate new hypotheses or test existing hypotheses. Observational analytic studies consist of case-control and cohort;
- **Experimental analytic studies** test existing hypotheses with the desire to determine causal associations. Experimental analytic studies consist of experimental and randomized controlled clinical trials (Mortimer & Borenstein, 2006).

END-OF-CHAPTER RESOURCES

SUMMARY POINTS

- Epidemiology is considered a basic public health science.
- Epidemiology is also considered foundational to population health.
- Epidemiology is the study of the distribution and determinants of health and health-related conditions or events in populations to promote and preserve population health while preventing and controlling health-related conditions or events in specific populations.
- Epidemiology can be categorized into three component types: substantive, descriptive, and analytic.
- Substantive epidemiology is considered the cumulative collection of epidemiologic knowledge generated epidemiologicamethods.
- Descriptive epidemiology is considered the body of information or knowledge that describes the health conditions and the associated factors that lead to or contribute to the health condition (risk factors).
- Analytical epidemiology uses descriptive epidemiologic information to analyze the determinants of health conditions such as the association between an exposure and health condition or disease, or the causes and effects of health conditions or diseases.
- Science is defined as the pursuit and application of knowledge.
- Epidemiology science is described and characterized as the body of knowledge accumulated through epidemiology, the methods used to collect epidemiologic data, and the underpinning philosophical and theoretical information that guides epidemiologic thinking and data collection.
- Epidemic science is the rigorous epidemiologic methods used to study epidemics and the knowledge base gained from the study of an epidemic within a specific population.
- The primary goals of epidemiology are to prevent and control health conditions that impact the health of individuals and the population and to develop the science of epidemiology to continually improve epidemiologic methods and the epidemiologic knowledge base.

- In a population-based approach, a specific population is characterized and defined.
- A high-risk approach targets the epidemiologic investigation at those persons within a defined aggregate group or community who are known to possess the identified high-risk characteristic.
- Epidemiologic reasoning is the thought process utilized by epidemiologists to approach or resolve a health condition.
- The epidemiologic triad is represented by the interaction among an agent, a host, and the environment.
- The tools of epidemiology facilitate a comprehension of the data to understand the complex distribution and determinants of health within a population.
- The overall tool of epidemiology is measurement of health and disease occurrence.
- Counts represent the most basic descriptive epidemiologic measure.
- A frequency compares one part of the distribution to another part of the distribution or the entire population.
- Ratio is a measure in which the numerator is not part of the denominator.
- Proportion is a measure that compares a part to the whole.
- Rates are expressed as a proportion with a specified period of time.

EPIDEMIOLOGY CRITICAL REASONING QUESTIONS

1. Review the definition of epidemiology proposed for this book and the definitions provided in Table 4.1. Compose a definition of epidemiology relevant to your healthcare practice.
2. Differentiate substantive, descriptive, and analytic epidemiology relative to your practice.
3. Identify a recent health-related event. Analyze the health-related event in terms of person, place, and environment, using the principles of the epidemiologic triad.
4. Describe the epidemiologic triad for both an infectious and noninfectious health condition.

5. Compose a three-column table that aligns the scientific process in column 1 with the epidemiologic approach in column 2. In column 3, provide an exemplar from your practice on the meaning of each of these processes.
6. Use the epidemiologic integrative thinking process to analyze a health-related condition or event of interest.
7. Provide examples from the literature of the utilization of the following epidemiologic tools:
   a. Counts
   b. Ratio
   c. Rate

ADDITIONAL RESOURCES

 SPRINGER PUBLISHING CONNECT™ A robust set of instructor resources designed to supplement this text is located at http://connect. springerpub.com/content/book/978-0-8261-8514-3. Qualifying instructors may request access by emailing textbook@springerpub.com.

REFERENCES

Evans, A. (1979). Definitions of epidemiology. *American Journal of Epidemiology, 109*(3), 379–382. https://doi.org/10.1093/oxford journals.aje.a112692

Frerichs, R., & Neutra, R. (1978). Definitions of epidemiology. *American Journal of Epidemiology, 108*(1), 74–75. https://doi.org/10.1097/MCC .0b013e32832e47af

Frerot, M., Lefebvre, A., Aho, S., Callier, P., Astruc, K., & Aho Glélé, L. S. (2018). What is epidemiology? Changing definitions of epidemiology 1978–2017. *PLoS One, 13*(12), e0208442. https://doi.org/10.1371/journal .pone.0208442

Hennekens, C., & Buring, J. (1987). *Epidemiology in medicine.* Lippincott Williams and Wilkins.

Last, J. (2000). *A dictionary of epidemiology* (4th ed.). Oxford University Press.

Lilienfeld, A., & Lilenthal, D. (1980). *Foundations of epidemiology.* Oxford University Press.

Miettinen, O. (1985). *Theoretical epidemiology: Principles of occurrence research in medicine.* Wiley.

Morris, J. (2007). Uses of epidemiology. *International Journal of Epidemiology, 36*(6), 1165–1172. https://doi.org/10.1093/ije/dym227

Mortimer, J., & Borenstein, A. (2006). Tools of the epidemiologist. *Alzheimer Disease & Associated Disorders, 20*(Suppl. 2), S35–S41. https://doi.org/10.1097/00002093-200607001-00004

Rich, H. (1979). More definitions of epidemiology. *American Journal of Epidemiology, 109*(1), 102–103. https://doi.org/10.1093/oxford journals.aje.a112653

Rojek, A., & Horby, P. (2016). Modernising epidemic science: Enabling patient-centered research during epidemics. *BioMed Central Medicine, 14,* 212–219. https://doi .org/10.1186/s12916-016-0760-x

Schwabe, C., Riemann, H., & Franti, C. (1977). *Epidemiology in veterinary practice.* Lea & Febiger.

Chapter 5

HISTORICAL EPIDEMIOLOGIC PERSPECTIVES

Demetrius J. Porche

A small body of determined spirits fired by an unquenchable faith in their mission can alter the course of history.

–Mahatma Gandhi

CHAPTER COMPETENCIES

At the conclusion of this chapter, the reader will be able to:

1. Describe important historic events in epidemiology
2. Demonstrate an understanding of historical epidemiologic discoveries and events that have impacted modern-day epidemiology
3. Discuss historical leaders who have contributed to the development of epidemiology and epidemiology science
4. Recognize the historic development of epidemiologic study designs

ESSENTIAL TERMINOLOGY

Essential historical epidemiological terms are:

- Cowpox
- Dairy maids
- Demography
- Inoculation
- Miasm
- Pellagra
- Public health nursing
- Puerperal fever
- Shoe-leather epidemiology

History is the foundation of the future. If we are not to repeat the errors of the past, one must be knowledgeable about the historical developments that have led to the current modern-day

state of affairs. The history of epidemiology has been influenced by many historical leaders from a diverse background of professions and disciplines. These historical leaders shared the purposeful mission to prevent and control health-related events with the desire to promote health among populations. This chapter focuses on historical leaders and events that have shaped modern-day epidemiology.

HISTORICAL PERSONS

Lillian Wald

Lillian Wald (Figure 5.1) was born in 1867 in Cincinnati, Ohio, of Jewish descent and died in 1940 in Westport, Connecticut. Lillian Wald is considered an influential social reformer of the 20th century. She attended the New York Hospital School of Nursing. After experiencing firsthand the poverty and hardship experienced by immigrants on the Lower East Side of New York, she established the Henry Street Settlement. She lived and began working in the Henry Street Settlement to help the industrial working poor. She and her colleagues provided healthcare services to the residents on a "sliding fee scale" based on their ability to pay for the healthcare services. Later she added the provision of social services and healthcare education.

Lillian Wald is credited with coining the term "public health nursing" to describe the practice of team nursing outside of the hospital in the

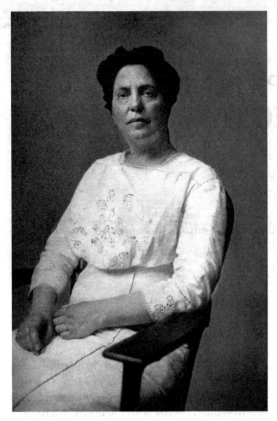

Figure 5.1 Lillian Wald.

Source: From Public domain, via Wikimedia Commons.

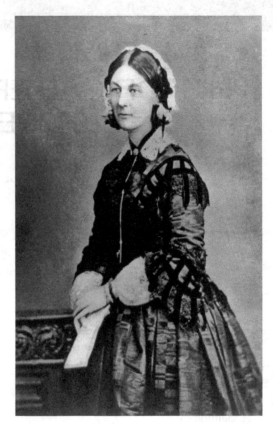

Figure 5.2 Florence Nightingale.

Source: From Library of Congress, Public domain, via Wikimedia Commons.

community setting. Some historical references identify Lillian Wald as the founder of community health nursing. These terms were used to describe nursing care that was integrated into the public community to a group of patients. Lillian Wald also established school health nursing, placing nurses within the public schools. Lillian Wald's work would be considered a form of population health today.

Lillian Wald had a vision for a national health insurance plan. She partnered with the Metropolitan Life Insurance Company to develop an insurance partnership that served as a model for health insurance. She started the Visiting Nurse Service of New York at the Henry Street Settlement. She is known as an advocate for children, labor, immigrants, civil and women's rights. She participated in the development of the National Association for the Advancement of Colored People, United States Children's Bureau, the National Child Labor Committee, and the National Women's Trade Union League.

Florence Nightingale

Florence Nightingale (Figure 5.2) was born in Florence, Italy, in 1820 of English descent. She died in 1910 in Mayfair, London, England. Florence Nightingale is known as the "mother of modern nursing." She is also known favorably as "The Lady With the Lamp" and "The Angel of the Crimea." She is considered to be a British nurse, social reformer, and statistician. Some historians describe Florence Nightingale's collection of data as that of an epidemiologist rather than of a statistician. She has also been considered a sanitarian.

In 1844, Nightingale enrolled as a nursing student at the Lutheran Hospital of Pastor Fliedner in Kaiserwerth, Germany. In the 1850s, she returned to London to work as a nurse in the Middlesex Hospital for ailing governesses. Nightingale had to provide care during the cholera outbreak in London. During this time, she began to recognize that unsanitary conditions

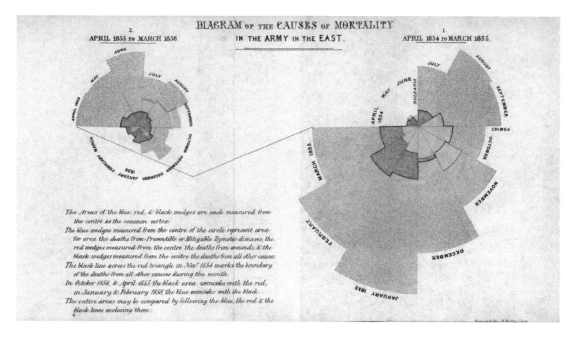

Figure 5.3 Example of a "Nightingale Rose Diagram" or a polar area diagram by Florence Nightingale (1820–1910).

Source: From Florence Nightingale, Public domain, via Wikimedia Commons.

were conducive to the rapid spread of cholera. She desired to reduce the mortality rate from cholera by improving hygienic practices.

In 1853, the Crimean War broke out with the British Empire at war against the Russian Empire for control of the Ottoman Empire. In the latter part of 1854, the Secretary of War, Sidney Herbert, requested that Nightingale organize a corps of nurses to provide nursing care to the sick and fallen soldiers in the Crimea. Nightingale assembled a team of 34 nurses from a variety of religious orders. Nursing during the Crimean War has been considered the greatest challenge of Nightingale's nursing career.

In the Crimea, she experienced the unsanitary conditions. Known for her organizational skills, during her tenure in the Crimea, she developed numerous patient care services and structured the provision of health care services in the hospital to promote qualities such as exposure to fresh air and sunlight. Nightingale collected meticulous records of each soldier patient entrusted to her care during this time, what some would later refer to as early epidemiologic or statistical data. Nightingale helped create the Royal Commission with the support of Queen Victoria. The Royal Commission employed leading statisticians such as William Farr

and John Sutherland to analyze military mortality data. She is accredited for translating data into a visual diagram (Figure 5.3) known as the "Nightingale Rose Diagram." This diagram was accredited with demonstrating how the Commission's work decreased the mortality rate and lead to new sanitary standards for the military. Nightingale was the first female member of the Royal Statistical Society (History.com, 2020).

Edward Jenner

Edward Jenner (Figure 5.4) was born in 1749 and died in 1823 in Berkeley, Gloucestershire, United Kingdom. He was orphaned during his childhood and developed a strong interest in nature and science during his early school years. At the early age of 13 years old, Jenner apprenticed with a country surgeon and apothecary in Sodbury. Historical records indicate that Jenner overhead dairymaids discussing "I shall never have smallpox for I have had cowpox. I shall never have an ugly pockmarked face." During that time, it was a commonly held belief that dairymaids were in some manner protected from smallpox (Riedel, 2005).

At the age of 21, he completed his apprenticeships with a sound knowledge of surgical and

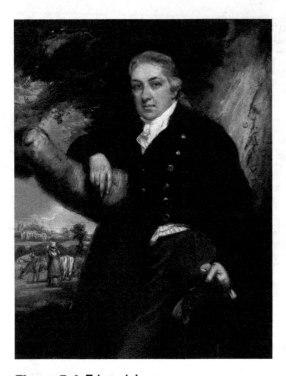

Figure 5.4 Edward Jenner.

Source: From John Raphael Smith, Public domain, via Wikimedia Commons.

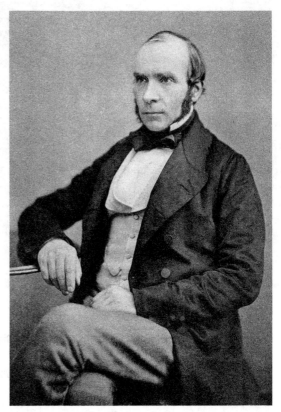

Figure 5.5 John Snow.

Source: From Public domain, via Wikimedia Commons.

medical practice. As an English physician and scientist, he became a student of John Hunter on staff at St. George's Hospital in London. Under the further apprenticeship of George Harwicke, he began the process of studying smallpox protection that occurred naturally from cowpox in 1796. He began to conclude that cowpox not only protected against smallpox but could also be transmitted from one person to another person deliberately to develop some immunologic protection. In May 1796, Jenner identified a young dairymaid, Sarah Nelms, who had fresh cowpox lesions on her hand and arms. On May 14, 1796, using some matter from Nelm's lesions, he inoculated an 8-year-old boy, James Phipps. At this time, this process was known as variolation. The boy developed some symptoms such as mild fever, axillae discomfort, and loss of appetite, then began to feel better. In July 1796, Jenner inoculated the boy again with matter from smallpox lesions. The young boy did not develop any disease; therefore, Jenner concluded that protection from cowpox did provide protection from smallpox. Jenner is best known for his contributions to immunizations and the ultimate eradication of smallpox. His scientific contributions to immunizations laid the foundation for immunology (Riedel, 2005).

John Snow

John Snow (Figure 5.5) was born in 1813 in York, United Kingdom, into a laborer family of farmers. He died in 1858 in Sackville Street, London, United Kingdom. He apprenticed as a surgeon at 14 years old. In 1836, he moved to London to begin his formal education in medicine. In 1838, he became a member of the Royal College of Surgeons and graduated from the University of London in 1844. He was admitted into the Royal College of Physicians in 1850. Snow is known as a leader in anesthesia, medical hygiene, and toxicology. Epidemiologically, he is most known for the identification of the mode of cholera transmission. He is also famously known for administering chloroform to Queen Victoria during childbirth (Vinten-Johansen et al., 2003).

During the middle of the 19th century, cholera was a major problem in England. In

September 1854, it was estimated that about 600 people living within close proximity of the Broad Street water pump in London had died of cholera. The Registrar at this time was William Farr. Farr and Snow disagreed about the cause of cholera. Farr was a proponent of the theory that cholera was spread by "bad air," known as the miasmatic theory, which proposed that cholera was spread via a cloud of bad air or miasm. Snow did not support this theory based on the fact of the geographic proximity of cholera cases to the Broad Street water pump. Snow believed if this theory were true, the cases of cholera spread through the air would be more geographically dispersed (Vinten-Johansen et al., 2003).

Snow proposed that cholera was transmitted through water. At this time in London, the water intakes for the water pumps were located in a polluted area of the Thames River. Some of the water companies during this time were trying to move the water intake area up the Thames River to a less polluted area. Snow began what now is called the development of "shoe-leather epidemiology," that is going from house to house to collect epidemiologic data on cholera case counts, mortality, and determining each household's water supply. Snow pioneered disease mapping, developing maps of the London water pumps, plotting the cholera cases and deaths by household (Vinten-Johansen et al., 2003).

There were two major water companies supplying water to the pumps, the Southwark and Vauxhall Company and the Lambeth Company. The number of deaths for the Southwark and Vauxhall Company were 315 per 10,000 houses compared to Lambeth Company which was 38 deaths per 10,000 houses. Through his mapping of cholera cases and the water pumps, Snow deducted that access to the water pumps was associated with the number of cholera cases. Specifically, homes supplied with water by the Southwark and Vauxhall Waterworks Company had the largest number of cholera cases. Snow removed the handle of the water pump near Broad Street. With the removal of this water handle, the number of cholera cases in the area decreased over time. It was later determined that the Broad Street water pump had been placed 3 feet from an old cesspit that leaked fecal bacteria in the water (Figure 5.6). Through his diligent work with geographic mapping of cholera cases, conducting house-to-house investigations of cholera cases, and preventive strategy of removing the water pump handle, John Snow is known as the father of epidemiology (Vinten-Johansen et al., 2003).

Sir Richard Doll

Sir William Richard Shaboe Doll was born in 1912 in Hampton, United Kingdom, and died in 2005 in Oxford, United Kingdom. He is considered by some as the world's most distinguished medical epidemiologist. Sir Richard Doll is credited with demonstrating that cigarette smoking was a causative factor in the development of lung cancer. He developed a short questionnaire that was administered by social workers to 650 male patients in London hospitals. These patients were admitted with suspected lung, liver, or bowel cancer. After the diagnosis was confirmed, Sir Richard Doll demonstrated that lung cancer was confirmed in the men who were smokers and those without the cancer diagnosis were nonsmokers. During his career, he also demonstrated the associative relationship between smoking and bladder and other cancers and cardiovascular disease (Richmond, 2005).

Joseph Goldberger

Joseph Goldberger (Figure 5.7) was born in 1874 in the Kingdom of Hungary. He died in 1929 in Washington, DC. Goldberger was an American physician and epidemiologist in the United States Public Health Service. Pellagra was identified in 1735 as a loathsome skin disease, frequently misdiagnosed as leprosy. Pellagra is known as the four Ds disease—dermatitis, diarrhea, dementia, and death. In 1914, Goldberger designed two experiments to evaluate if improvements in the diet of institutionalized children and adults would prevent pellagra. The first group of institutions were two orphanages in Jackson, Mississippi, that had a high incidence of pellagra. Goldberger determined that pellagra affected children mostly between the age of 6 and 12 years of age. He also determined that their diet was poor in lean meat and other forms of animal protein. He conducted another experiment in two women's wards (one ward of Black women and one ward of White women) in the Georgia State Sanitarium. His experiment at the orphanage and sanitarium included a diet enriched with an increased proportion of fresh meat and leguminous protein foods such as milk, buttermilk, eggs, beans, and peas. After the

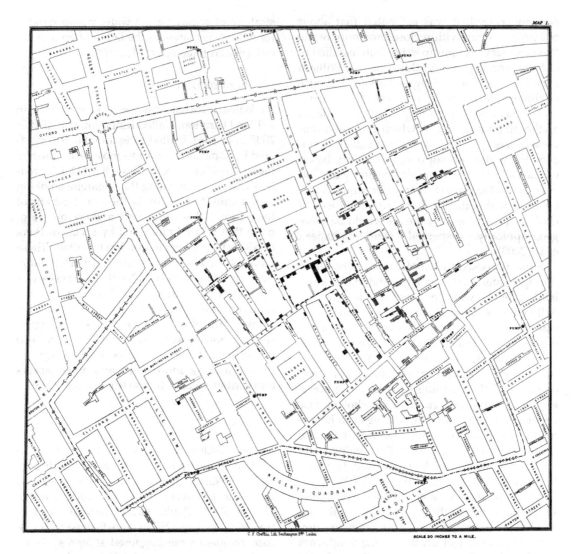

Figure 5.6 Original map made by John Snow in 1854. Cholera cases are highlighted in black.

Source: From John Snow, Public domain, via Wikimedia Commons.

introduction of this diet, the recurrence of pellagra cases drastically decreased or ceased. This experiment further determined the linkage of vitamin B niacin (nicotinic acid) deficiency and the development of pellagra. The body's synthesis of vitamin B is dependent upon an essential amino acid, tryptophan, which is found in milk, cheese, fish, meat, and eggs (Morabia, 2006).

John Graunt

John Graunt was born in 1620 and died in 1674 in London, United Kingdom. Gaunt is known as an English statistician and demographer.

He is considered the founder of the science of demography. A prosperous haberdasher and businessman, he studied the death records of the London parishes since 1532. Through his analysis of death records, he was able to identify certain phenomenon of death statistics. He began classifying the death rates according to different categorical causes of death. Gaunt noted that death rates were higher in urban than rural areas and also noted that male death rates were higher than female death rates. His interest in death rates and survivorship of illnesses led him to develop tables based on age and life expectancy known as life tables. Gaunt is credited

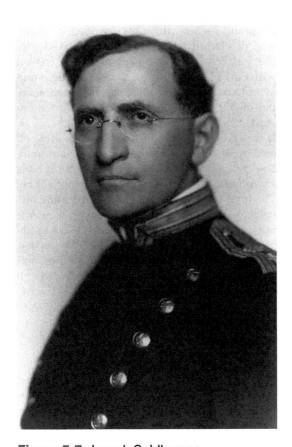

Figure 5.7 Joseph Goldberger.

Source: From Public domain, via Wikimedia Commons.

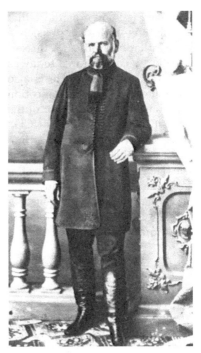

Figure 5.8 Ignaz Semmelweis.

Source: From Unknown author, Public domain, via Wikimedia Commons.

with developing the innovation of life tables that present mortality in terms of years of survivorship. His work on the data extracted from the Bills of Mortality, the analysis of 50 years of data, were summarized into a book in 1662 entitled, *Natural and Political Observations Made Upon the Bills of Mortality* (Morabia, 2013).

Ignaz Semmelweis

Ignaz Philipp Semmelweis (Figure 5.8) was born in 1818 in Budapest, Hungary, and died in 1865 in Oberdobling, Vienna, Austria. Semmelweis was a physician with a specialty in obstetrics. He was interested in the major public health problem of that time, childhood fever, which was also known as puerperal fever. Puerperal fever is fever associated with childbirth or the immediate period after childbirth. In the early 19th century, puerperal fever was a major cause of death among women after childbirth with a mortality rate of about 25% to 30% (Zoltan, 2020).

He observed that the morality rate of women in the first division of the clinic was two to three times higher than the mortality rate of women in the second division of clinic. The two clinic divisions were identical with the exception that students were taught in the first division of the clinic and midwives in the second division of the clinic. From this observation, he proposed that students carried something to their patients during labor. The students were known to go directly from the dissection room to the maternity ward. From these observations, he ordered students to wash their hands in a chlorinated lime solution before each examination of a maternity patient. After the implementation of this hand washing practice, the mortality rate in the first division decreased from about 18.2% to 1.2%. Semmelweis is credited with discovering the cause of puerperal fever and introducing asepsis into medical practice (Zoltan, 2020).

William Farr

William Farr was born in 1807 in Kenley, United Kingdom, in a poverty-stricken family. He died in 1883 in Maida Vale London,

United Kingdom. Farr is known as the father of medical statistics. As a British physician, Farr pioneered quantitative studies of disease incidence and deaths, what is known today as morbidity and mortality statistics. He is also known for developing a disease classification system that some consider the precursor of the International Classification of Diseases (ICD). Farr did not agree with John Snow regarding the cause of cholera and believed cholera was caused by miasm. He is considered a major figure of the social medicine movement in Victorian England and a major author of the history of health statistics. He also constructed the first English life table (Morabia, 2013).

Smith and Spalding

H. Smith and J. Spalding served as temporary advisors to the World Health Organization investigating an outbreak of paralysis in Morocco in the 1950s. Similar outbreaks were also reported in Switzerland, Germany, and the United States. The Moroccan local health authorities collected incidence data along with characteristics of each case to include clinical presentation, laboratory data, geographic distribution of cases, socioeconomic factors, and case follow-up reports. The clinical symptoms consisted of muscle weakness and loss of superficial sensations in the hands and legs, with some experiencing fever and diarrhea. The clinical presentation began with aching pain in the calf, followed by sensory disturbance in the lower limbs, persisting for a day or two, with some symptoms disappearing. Then motor weakness would set into the lower limbs. No signs of infection were detected in the cases. All blood and cerebrospinal fluid analyses were negative. From these data, an infectious cause was ruled out with a diagnosis of acute peripheral neuritis. The condition occurred in both sexes and all age groups with the chief incidence being in adult women, adult men, and older children. There were no cases among the Europeans, Jews, or the "better-to-do" Muslims (Smith & Spalding, 1959).

Smith and Spalding suspected there was some type of poisoning that caused the neuritis. It was found that cooking oil labeled as "olive oil" was being sold in the old Arab town. The epidemiologic data collected indicated the neuritis primarily affected persons living in conditions of poverty. A family proposed that dark olive oil sold in lower socioeconomic communities was the causative factor. Therefore, this family fed their dog food cooked with the dark olive oil. After eating the food cooked with dark olive oil, the dog developed signs and symptoms consistent with paralysis and acute peripheral neuritis. This "olive oil" demonstrated the presence of phosphates and cresols. It was later determined that the dark olive oil sold in the lower socioeconomic community was contaminated with ortho-cresyl phosphate, a synthetic oil used for jet engine lubrication. The toxic oil was a "man-made lubricating oil" being sold as cooking oil to lower socioeconomic individuals that contained 33% vegetable oil and 3% of mixed cresyl and phosphates. This epidemiologic investigation by Smith and Spalding demonstrated the teamwork and collaboration that occurs among clinical scientists during an epidemiological investigation (Smith & Spalding, 1959).

Clark and Anderson

E. Aileen Clarke and Terence W. Anderson compared 212 cases of invasive cervical cancer to 1,060 age-matched controls. Five years before the year of invasive cervical cancer diagnosis, 32% of the cases had been screened by the Papanicolaou (Pap) smear, compared with 56% of the controls. Clark and Anderson determined there was a statistical significance at $p < .0001$ with a relative risk of invasive cancer of 2.7 with 95% confidence limits of 2.0 to 3.7 in women who had not been screened with the Pap smear. The differences between the cases and controls persisted with stratification of the data by age, income, education, marital history, smoking habit, employment status, and access to medical care. Clarke and Anderson are credited with establishing that the Pap smear is an effective screening procedure for invasive cervical cancer (Clarke & Anderson, 1979).

Jonas Salk

Jonas Salk (Figure 5.9) was born in 1914 in New York, New York, and died in 1995 in La Jolla, California. Salk was an American virologist and medical researcher. Salk is known for the successful development of the polio vaccine. In 1947, Salk was appointed the Director of the Virus Research Laboratory at the University of Pittsburgh School of Medicine. With funding from the National Foundation of

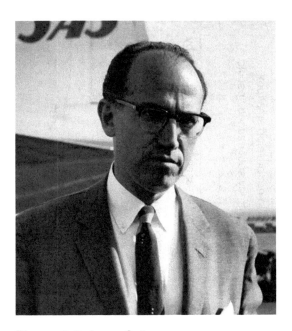

Figure 5.9 Jonas Salk.

Source: From SAS Scandinavian Airlines, Public domain, via Wikimedia Commons.

Infantile Paralysis, now known as the March of Dimes Birth Defects Foundation, he studied techniques that would lead to the development of a vaccine for paralytic poliomyelitis. Salk is known for administering "killed polio virus" to himself and other volunteers who had not had polio, his laboratory colleagues, and his wife and children. Salk determined that all inoculated with the "killed polio vaccine" developed antibodies to polio with no reported negative reactions to the vaccine. Salk is also known for founding the Salk Institute of Biological Studies in La Jolla in 1963 with the grant aid of the National Science Foundation and March of Dimes. Prior to his death in 1995, he worked tirelessly to search for a vaccine for the human immunodeficiency virus (HIV; Salk, 2020).

HISTORICAL EPIDEMIOLOGIC STUDIES

Historical epidemiologic studies serve as the origin of the development the discipline of epidemiology. Table 5.1 outlines historical events that have defined the development and evolution of the practice of epidemiology over time. Several formidable historical epidemiologic studies are recounted in the following.

Classification of Fevers

Thomas Sydenham lived from 1624 to 1689, a graduate of Oxford Medical School. Sydenham conducted detailed analyses of observations regarding diseases occurring throughout London. From these detailed observations, he was able to identify and recognize different diseases and symptoms associated with the respective diseases. A major contribution of his work at that time was the classification of fevers into three classes: continued fevers, intermittent fevers, and smallpox. This early classification of fevers, although criticized by many, lead to the differentiation of treatments based on fever symptomatology (Garrison, 1926).

Scurvy

James Lind was a Scottish naval surgeon who lived from 1716 to 1794. During this time, there was a concern that men in the navy were dying more from disease than of the "sword." Lind's 1754 book, *A Treatise on Scurvy*, detailed the symptoms of scurvy along with the association of the disease occurring after months at sea. He noted that scurvy presented as spongy bleeding gums, bleeding under the skin, and extreme fatigue. Additionally, he noted that presence of scurvy mostly in the months of April, May, and June along with the presence occurring more commonly in weather conditions such as cold, rain, fog, and thick weather. After this first observed association with the presence of scurvy symptoms with the environment, Lind observed that the sea diet for mariners was extremely gross and hard on their digestive systems.

In 1747, Lind conducted an experiment on 12 ill men with symptoms of scurvy. He divided the sailors into six groups of two. He added a dietary intervention to each of the six group's diet. Two men received a quart of cider, two men took two spoonfuls of vinegar three times a day, two men had a half-pint of seawater every day, two men were given lemons and oranges, and two men received an elixir of garlic, mustard seed, and horseradish. Lind identified that the most sudden and visible effects were among the two men who received lemons and oranges with both men being fit for duty after 6 days of treatment. This led to the inclusion of lemons, oranges, and other citrus fruits as a requirement for the mariner diet (Schneider & Lilienfeld, 2015).

Table 5.1 Historical Epidemiological Timeline

Time Period	Historic Development
460–377 BC	Hippocrates was considered the first epidemiologist; he proposed a rational perspective of disease rather than a supernatural basis, observed differences in geographical presentation of diseases, is considered the Father of Medicine
910	Rhazes, Persian physician, identifies smallpox
1489	Leonardo da Vinci dissects corpses
1546	Girolamo Fracastroro, Italian physician, proposed that contagions were rapidly spread by seedlike entities that were spread through direct contact, air, or contaminated clothing
1590	Zacharius Jannssen invents the microscope
1662	John Gaunt, English statistician, published books that analyze mortality rolls in London, reported temporal trends for diseases, and calculated life tables and life expectancy
1670	Anton van Leeuwenhoek discovers blood cells
1683	Anton van Leeuwenhoek observes bacteria
1701	Giacomo Pylarini gives first smallpox inoculation
1747	James Lind publishes treatise stating that citrus fruit prevents scurvy
1754	James Lind, Scottish naval surgeon, identified symptoms of scurvy and determines its common presence in sailors
1774	Benjamin Jesty, English farmer and dairyman, noticed milkmaids develop cowpox from cows but do not develop smallpox
1775	Percivall Pott, English surgeon, was the first person who identified environmental carcinogens; chimney soot caused specific cancers
1847	Ignaz Semmelweis discovered the prevention of puerperal fever
1850	Lemuel Shattuck published report on sanitation and public health issues in the Commonwealth of Massachusetts, considered by some as the beginning of epidemiology in the United States
1854	John Snow, English physician, identified contaminated water as the cause of cholera in London, one of the most influential contributors to epidemiology
1857	First United States quarantine convention regarding the prevention of typhus, cholera, and yellow fever; Louis Pasteur identified germs as the cause of disease
1867	Joseph Lister developed use of aseptic surgical methods
1870	Robert Koch and Louis Pasteur established the germ theory of disease
1870–1879 1882–1883	Robert Koch, German physician, demonstrated that anthrax bacillus causes anthrax infection; proposed Koch's postulates of causation

(continued)

Table 5.1 Historic Epidemiological Timeline *(Continued)*

Time Period	Historic Development
1879	First vaccine for cholera developed
1881	Louis Pasteur developed first vaccine for anthrax
1882	Louis Pasteur developed first vaccine for rabies
1887	T. K. Takaki, Japanese naval surgeon, eradicated beriberi by adding vegetables, meat, and fish to sailors' diet
1890	Emil von Behring discovered antitoxins, developed tetanus and diphtheria vaccines
1896	First vaccine for typhoid fever developed
1897	First vaccine for bubonic plague developed
1906	United States developed standards methods of water analysis
1913	Pasteurization of milk implemented to prevent disease; Harvard School of Public Health established as first public health school in the United States
1918	H1N1 pandemic
1921	Edward Mellanby discovered that vitamin D deficiency causes rickets
1923	First vaccine for diphtheria developed
1926	First vaccine for whooping cough developed
1927	First vaccine for tuberculosis and tetanus developed
1928	Sir Alexander Fleming developed penicillin
1930	Influenza virus isolated from persons proving that influenza is caused by a virus, not a bacterium
1933	Andrewes Smith and Laidlaw isolated influenza A in ferrets
1935	First vaccine for yellow fever developed
1936	Francis isolated influenza B virus; Burnet discovered that influenza virus can be grown in hen's eggs
1937	First vaccine for typhus developed
1938	Term "clinical epidemiology" introduced
1945	First vaccine for influenza developed
1955	Jonas Salk developed first polio vaccine
1957–1958	H2N2 pandemic
1964	First vaccine for measles developed

(continued)

Table 5.1 Historic Epidemiological Timeline *(Continued)*

Time Period	Historic Development
1966	FDA licensed amantadine, antiviral medication for prophylactic treatment of influenza A
1967	Term "neuroepidemiology" introduced; first vaccine for mumps developed
1968	H3N2 pandemic
1970	First vaccine for rubella
1974	First vaccine for chicken pox developed
1977	First vaccine for pneumonia developed
1980	Smallpox eradicated
1981	First vaccine for hepatitis B developed
1982	Term "molecular cancer epidemiology" introduced
1983	Human immunodeficiency virus (HIV) identified
1992	First vaccine for hepatitis A developed
1994	Rimantadine approved by the FDA for treatment of influenza A
1999	Neuramindase inhibitors oseltamivir and zanamivir licensed to treat influenza infection
2003	First nasal spray influenza vaccine licensed
2007	Term "e-epidemiology" introduced; FDA approved first vaccine for avian influenza A (H5N1) virus
2009	H1N1 pdm09 virus pandemic; first doses of H1N1 vaccine administered
2010	Term "molecular pathological epidemiology" used
2014	FDA approves first intravenous influenza medication peramivir
2019	Novel coronavirus (COVID-19) pandemic

Source: From Centers for Disease Control and Prevention. (2019). *Influenza historic timeline.* https://www.cdc.gov/flu/pandemic-resources/pandemic-timeline-1930-and-beyond.htm; Hajar, R. (2015). History of medicine timeline. *Heart Views, 16*(1), 43–45. https://doi.org/10.4103/1995-705X.153008; Morabia, A. (2013). Epidemiology's 350th anniversary: 1662–2012. *Epidemiology, 24*(2), 179–183. https://doi.org/10.1097/EDE.0b013e31827b5359

Anthrax

Louis Pasteur was a French chemist who lived from 1822 to 1895. Pasteur was convinced that bacteria identified as anthrax was associated with disease. He noted that anthrax bacteria was present on necropsy (autopsy) of sheep who had died of anthrax. He postulated the association between earthworms and anthrax. He noted that anthrax spores or bacteria were brought up to the surface of the Earth where sheep who had died of anthrax were buried.

Pasteur continued his studies to include the prevention of anthrax infections and anthrax-related deaths in sheep by inoculating live sheep with a his new anthrax vaccine. The inoculated sheep lived and the unvaccinated sheep died. Therefore, Pasteur was noted to provide evidence that vaccination was an effective measure to control diseases such as anthrax and provided evidence to support anthrax bacteria as the cause of the disease (Garrison, 1926).

Occupational Health and Epidemiology

Bernardino Ramazzini (1633–1714) was an Italian physician who lived and studied in Germany and Italy. Ramazzini observed the association with men who worked in the cesspits having bloodshot and dim eyes. After this observation, he studied the effects of working in cesspools and privies. Through this epidemiologic observation, he was interested in the relationship between work and health conditions. Ramazzini wrote the book, *The Diseases of Workers* in 1690, published in 1703. This was the first book to characterize work-related health conditions. He made a significant contribution to occupational epidemiology by describing his observations about work-related health conditions and the need to develop prevention efforts to eliminate the work-related health conditions (Garrison, 1926; Rosen, 1958).

Typhoid Mary

Typhoid fever is an infectious disease characterized by continued fever, physical and mental depression, rose colored spots on the chest and abdomen, diarrhea, and other intestinal-related conditions. Mary Mallon, an Irish cook known as "Typhoid Mary," was believed to be associated with over 53 cases of typhoid fever in a 15-year period. Mary Mallon was a cook in many of the New York homes that experienced typhoid fever. The presence of typhoid was associated with her assuming employment in a family's home but never preceded her employment as a cook. Examination of Mary Mallon's stool sample identified she was a chronic carrier of typhoid (*Health News*, 1968).

From 1907 to 1910, she was confined by public health officials, based on a New York Supreme Court decision that upheld the community's right to confine her to custody and required her isolation. In 1910, she was released from confinement. Within 2 years of her release, there was a typhoid outbreak in New Jersey and New York hospitals. It was determined that Mary Mallon under the assumption of another name had secured employment in the New Jersey and New York hospitals as a cook. Eventually, she accepted voluntary isolation and refrained from working as a cook.

The incident of Typhoid Mary taught public health officials about the importance of record-keeping and keeping track of disease carriers. This is considered by some historians as the original case of investigating, tracking, and controlling of certain diseases by what is now known as contact tracing. This case also emphasized the importance of protecting the public food supplies and importance of the investigative aspects of epidemiology (*Health News*, 1968).

The Shattuck Report

Lemuel Shattuck, who lived from 1793 to 1859, was a Boston historian, sociologist, statistician, and politician. He published the first report on sanitation and public health problems in the Commonwealth of Massachusetts. The Shattuck Report is historical since it set forth and identified the need for many public health programs. This report clarified the importance of and called for the establishment of state and local boards of health. His report also recommended the organization and collection of vital statistics, the exchange of health information, the need for sanitary inspections, research on tuberculosis, and the integration of sanitation and prevention in medical school curricula. As a result of the Shattuck Report, boards of health were established with state and local health departments soon to follow (Shi & Johnson, 2013).

Morbidity Statistics Study

Edgar Sydenstricker was an American statistician who lived from 1881 to 1936. He was concerned that morbidity statistics in the United States were developing methods of analysis slower than mortality statistics. He recognized that morbidity statistics were not regularly collected and identified as there were several barriers to the collection of homogeneous morbidity data. Sydenstricker conducted a morbidity study under the direction of the U.S. Public Health Service from 1921 to 1924. This was considered the first morbidity study that identified the variations of incidence of disease or illness according to age categories. He is also known for identifying five categories or groups of morbidity statistics: reports of communicable diseases; hospital and clinical records; insurance, industrial, and school illness records; illness surveys; and illness records in frequently observed populations (Sydenstricker, 1926).

Framingham Heart Study

A cardiovascular disease study was launched in Framingham, Massachusetts, in 1948. The purpose of the study was to identify risk factors that contributed to the development of cardiovascular disease. This study spanned a period of 30 years collecting medical exams, survey information, and related medical tests and activities. The Framingham heart study used a prospective cohort study design. This study led to the refinement of research study design methods such as cohort tracking, population selection, sampling, and developing population and community support for epidemiologic research (Dawber et al., 1963).

Lung Cancer and Cigarette Smoking

Lung cancer increased after World War II. In the early 1950s, the first epidemiologic studies began to link lung cancer and cigarette smoking. By 1964, there were several case-control and prospective cohort studies published that indicated a significant relationship between cigarette smoking and lung cancer. These case-control and prospective cohort studies were the first to identify the association between cigarette smoking and lung cancer while establishing the significant contribution that case-control and prospective cohort epidemiologic study designs can make to science (Doll & Hill, 1950).

Nurses' Health Study

The Nurses' Health Study (NHS) is among the largest prospective epidemiologic studies conducted to identify risk factors of major chronic illnesses in women. There have been three different Nurses' Health Studies to date. Nurses were selected as optimal candidates for a prospective study based on their knowledge about health and their ability to provide complete and accurate information regarding various disease processes.

The original NHS was established in 1976 by Dr. Frank Speizer. This original NHS prospective epidemiologic study was conducted to investigate the long-term consequences of oral contraceptives in women. Other factors explored were smoking, cancer, and heart disease. Eventually the follow-up questionnaires contained more information on lifestyle, diet, and nutrition. A quality-of-life supplemental questionnaire was also added. The nurses included in this study were between 30 and 55 years old, married, and lived in one of the following states: California, Connecticut, Florida, Maryland, Massachusetts, Michigan, New Jersey, New York, Ohio, Pennsylvania, and Texas. Nurses were recruited from a roster obtained from the American Nurses Association with state board of nursing review and approval. The nurse cohorts are surveyed at least every 2 years. This original NHS study also collected toenail and blood samples from the nurses.

The NHS II was established in 1989 by Dr. Walter Willett. This second cohort study included a younger sample of nurses, single and married, 25 to 42 years old, with the intent to explore the impact of oral contraceptives initiated during adolescence, diet and physical activity in adolescence, and lifestyle factors such as smoking, along with a food questionnaire administered. Other information collected includes pregnancy history and menopause status along with the collection of blood and urine samples.

The Nurses' Health Study 3 (NHS3) was established in 2010 by Drs. Jorge Chavarro, Walter Willett, Janet Rich-Edwards, and Stacye Missmer. This third study includes licensed practical nurses or licensed vocational nurses (LPN/LVN) and registered nurses 19 to 46 years old. A goal of this third study is to increase the number of nurses from diverse ethnic backgrounds. This study continues the focus of the previous two studies along with exploring women's health issues related to new hormone preparations for birth control and fertility and pregnancy issues with an increased focus on adolescent diet and breast cancer risk.

Significant contributions have been made from the Nurses' Health Studies. These three cohorts of nurses have assisted in the generation of epidemiologic science regarding the association of diet, smoking, physical activity levels, obesity, oral contraceptive use, hormone therapy, endogenous hormones, dietary factors, sleep, genetics and other lifestyle and behaviors associated with the development of chronic disease. For further information regarding the findings of the NHS, the reader is directed to the *American Journal of Public Health's* September 2016 issue. Some of the significant findings are:

- One of the first prospective cohort studies to demonstrate an association between circulating sex hormones and postmenopausal breast cancer risk;
- One of the first prospective cohort studies to observe an association between higher vitamin D levels and lower risks of both colon polyps and colon cancer; and

- Assisted in the identification of genetic variations involved in cancers and cancer-related factors including mammographic density, body mass index, height, skin pigmentation, and circulating biomarkers.

HISTORIC PANDEMICS

Pandemics have occurred throughout the ages significantly causing illness and deaths. Pandemics significantly impact a country and population on multiple levels simultaneously. Table 5.2 presents an account of historic pandemics. Our challenge is to learn from and expand our capability to respond to and prevent future pandemics.

Table 5.2 Historic Pandemics

Unit of Time	Pandemic
430 BC	Plague of Athens
165–180	Antonine plague, possible smallpox Romain Empire
250–271	Cyprian plague
541–588	Plague of Justinian, Yersinia pestis Byzantine Empire
1346–1353	Black Death, Yersinia pestis
1519–1520	Smallpox outbreak Mexico
1545–1548	Cocoliztli 1 (Great Pestilence) Mexico
1576–1578	Cocoliztli 2 (Great Pestilence) Mexico
1793	Yellow fever Philadelphia, United States
1889–1890	Russian flu, Influenza A
1894–1922	Yersinia pestis, Third plague
1899–1923	Cholera
1915	Encephalitis lethargica
1916	American polio epidemic
1918–1920	Spanish flu, Influenza H1N1
1929	Psittacosis
1957–1958	Asian flu, Influenza H2N2
1968	Hong Kong flu, Influenza H3N2
1981–Present	HIV infection
2002–2004	Severe acute respiratory syndrome
2009–2010	Swine flu, H1N1
2009	Mumps
2012–Present	Middle East respiratory syndrome, Coronavirus
2015–Present	Zika virus
2019–Present	COVID-19, Coronavirus

END-OF-CHAPTER RESOURCES

SUMMARY POINTS

- History is the foundation of the future.
- Historical leaders shared the purposeful mission to prevent and control health-related events with the desire to promote health among populations.
- Lillian Wald coined the term *public health nursing* and described the practice of team nursing.
- Nightingale is known for her contributions to collecting detailed statistical/morbidity data and sanitary practices.
- Jenner contributed to the development in immunization immunology through inoculation with cowpox.
- Snow assisted with identifying the cause of cholera in London and removed a water pump handle as a preventive strategy.
- Doll is considered the world's most distinguished medical epidemiologist.
- Goldberger made significant contributions to pellagra.
- Graunt categorized causes of death.
- Semmelweis introduces asepsis into medical practice.
- Farr pioneered quantitative studies of disease incidence and deaths, what is known today as morbidity and mortality statistics.
- Smith and Spalding demonstrated the teamwork needed and collaboration that occurs among clinical scientists during an epidemiologic investigation.
- Clarke and Anderson are credited with establishing that the Pap smear as an effective screening procedure for invasive cervical cancer.
- Salk is known for administering "killed polio virus" to himself and other volunteers who had not had polio, his laboratory colleagues, and his wife and children.
- Scurvy was first associated with an intervention of lemons and oranges.
- Anthrax vaccination in sheep contributed knowledge regarding disease prevention.
- Occupational health was developed based on inquiry about symptoms present in specific types of workers.
- Typhoid Mary contributed to the development of contact tracing as a public health measure.
- The Shattuck Report called for the establishment of boards and departments of health.
- The Framingham heart study was a prospective cohort study.
- Early lung cancer and cigarette smoking confirmed the importance of case-control and prospective cohort studies.

EPIDEMIOLOGY CRITICAL REASONING QUESTIONS

1. Identify the historical events that are relevant to your health practice.
2. Describe the epidemiologic triad that is evident in the epidemiologic historic events.
3. List the aspects of the epidemiologic approach and thinking that were integral to these historic events.

ADDITIONAL RESOURCES

 A robust set of instructor resources designed to supplement this text is located at http://connect. springerpub.com/content/book/978-0-8261-8514-3. Qualifying instructors may request access by emailing textbook@springerpub.com.

REFERENCES

Clarke, E., & Anderson, T. (1979). Does screening by "Pap" smears help prevent cervical cancer? A case-control study. *The Lancet, 314*(8132), 1–4. https://doi.org/10.1016/s0140-6736(79)90172-7

Dawber, T., Kannel, W., & Lyell, L. (1963): An approach to longitudinal studies in a community: The Framingham study. *Annuals of the New York Academy of Sciences, 107*, 539–556. https://doi.org/10.1111/j.1749-6632.1963.tb13299.x

Doll, R., & Hill, A. (1950). Smoking and carcinoma of the lung: Preliminary report. *British Medical Journal, 2*, 739. https://doi.org/10.1136/bmj.2.4682.739

Garrison, F. (1926). *History of medicine*. Saunders.

Health News. (1968). *Medical milestones: Mary Mallon, Typhoid Mary, November 1968*. New York Department of Health.

History.com. (2020). *Florence Nightingale.* https://www.history.com/topics/womens-history/florence-nightingale-1

Morabia, A. (2006). *Joseph Goldberger's research on the prevention of pellagra.* JLL Bulletin: Commentaries on the History of Treatment Evaluation. https://www.jameslindlibrary.org/articles/joseph-goldbergers-research-on-the-prevention-of-pellagra/

Morabia, A. (2013). Epidemiology's 350th anniversary: 1662–2012. *Epidemiology, 24*(2), 179–183. https://doi.org/10.1097/EDE.0b013e31827b5359

Richmond, C. (2005). Sir Richard Doll. *British Medical Journal, 331*(7511), 295. https://doi.org/10.1136/bmj.331.7511.295

Riedel, S. (2005). Edward Jenner and the history of smallpox and vaccination. *Baylor University Medical Center Proceedings, 18*(1), 21–25. https://doi.org/10.1080/08998280.2005.11928028

Rosen, G. (1958). *History of public health.* MD Publications.

Salk, J. (2020). *History of Salk: About Jonas Salk.* https://www.salk.edu/about/history-of-salk/jonas-salk/

Schneider, D., & Lilienfeld, D. (2015). *Lilienfeld's foundations of epidemiology* (4th ed.). Oxford.

Shi, L., & Johnson, J. (2013). *Novick & Morrow's Public health administration: Principles for population-based management.* Jones & Bartlett.

Smith, H., & Spalding, J. (1959). Outbreak of paralysis in Morocco due to ortho-cresyl phosphate poisoning. *Lancet, 2*(7110), 1019–1021. https://doi.org/10.1016/S0140-6736(59)91486-2

Sydenstricker, E. (1926). A study of illness in a general population. *Public Health Reports, 61*, 12. https://doi.org/10.2307/4578020

Vinten-Johansen, P., Brody, H., Paneth, N., Rachman, S., & Rip, M. (2003). *Cholera, chloroform, and the science of medicine: A life of John Snow.* Oxford University Press.

Zoltan, I. (2020). *Ignaz Semmelweis—German-Hungarian physician.* Encyclopedia Britannica. https://www.britannica.com/biography/Ignaz-Semmelweis

Chapter 6

ETIOLOGY AND NATURAL HISTORY OF DISEASE AND ILLNESS

Demetrius J. Porche

...I will prevent disease whenever I can, for prevention is preferable to cure....
—*The Hippocratic Oath, Modern Version, Hippocrates (460–377 B.C.)*

CHAPTER COMPETENCIES

At the conclusion of this chapter, the reader will be able to:

1. Diagram an interrelated natural disease history model to include the natural stages of the disease with integrated incubation time periods, subclinical and clinical, prepathogenic and pathogenic, and targeted disease specific interventions
2. Develop population-based prevention strategies that integrate several types of immunity and prevention levels
3. Implement prevention strategies to break the chain of infection for specific diseases
4. Instruct cases and potential contacts regarding isolation and quarantine measures
5. Construct a web of association

ESSENTIAL TERMINOLOGY

Essential etiology and natural history of disease and illness terminology are:

- Active carrier
- Active immunity
- Acute phase
- Association
- Causation
- Clinical presentation
- Cocooning
- Community immunity
- Contact tracing
- Convalescence
- Herd immunity
- Iceberg theory
- Immunity
- Immunogenicity
- Incubation period
- Infectivity
- Isolation
- Latent stage
- Modes of transmission
- Natural history of disease
- Passive carrier
- Passive immunity
- Pathogenicity
- Persistent stage
- Preclinical stage
- Primary prevention
- Primordial prevention
- Prodromal
- Quarantine
- Quaternary prevention
- Secondary prevention
- Subclinical stage
- Susceptibility
- Tertiary prevention
- Virulence

NATURAL HISTORY OF DISEASE

A disease has a typical course of progression in a human. This natural course of disease progression that occurs over a period of time is known as the natural history of disease. The natural history of disease consists of five stages:

susceptibility, incubation, prodromal, acute, and convalescence. Figure 6.1 presents the exposure, minimum incubation period, and prodromal period for hantavirus in a Chilean population. This figure demonstrates the time period in days from hantavirus exposure to the development of symptoms and prodromal period.

Susceptibility is considered a predisease state. At the susceptibility stage, the individual has not developed the disease. At some point, an individual has an exposure. The individual may or may not develop a disease depending on their level of susceptibility. Susceptibility is considered the period of time that the individual is at risk for developing a disease dependent upon potential etiologic exposure. From the period of exposure to an agent to the time the individual develops the onset of signs and symptoms, is known as the incubation period. Each disease

has a specific incubation period. The incubation period is critical to determining the length of time preventive strategies are necessary such as isolation and quarantine. Infectious disease incubation periods are dependent upon the rate or organism growth in the host, exposure dosage to the infectious agent, portal of entry, and host immune response. The term *latency period* is sometimes used interchangeably with incubation period. Latency period is also sometimes differentiated as the time period from infection to infectiousness. Table 6.1 presents biologic characteristics of organisms that impact the development of an infectious disease.

Stages of Disease

The prodromal period is characterized by increased replication of the pathogen and initial

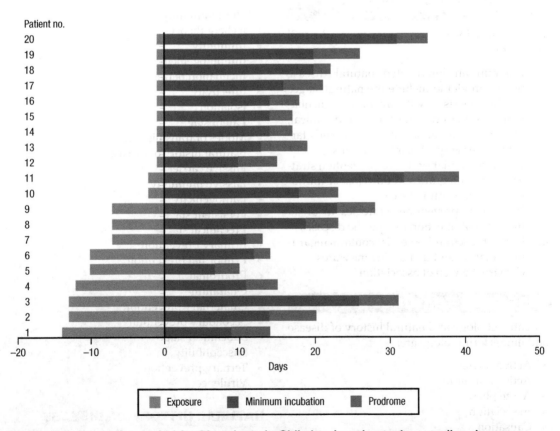

Figure 6.1 Incubation period for 20 patients in Chile in whom hantavirus cardiopulmonary syndrome caused by Andes virus developed after various periods of exposure. All patients progressed to the cardiopulmonary phase and were hospitalized at the end of the prodrome.

Source: Vial, P., Valdivieso, F., Mertz, G., Castillo, C., Belmar, E., Delgado, I., Tapia, M., & Ferrés, M. (2006). Incubation period of hantavirus cardiopulmonary syndrome. *Emerging Infectious Diseases, 12*(8), 1271–1273. https://doi .org/10.3201/eid1208.051127.

Table 6.1 Infectious Disease Terminology: Biologic Characteristics

Term	Definition
Infectivity	The ability of an agent to cause an infection in a susceptible host, the ability to invade the host, measured by the proportion of individuals who become infected (Number infected ÷ Number susceptible × 100)
Pathogenicity	The ability of the microorganism to induce disease, measured by the proportion of infected individuals who develop clinical disease (Number with clinical disease ÷ Number infected × 100)
Virulence	The severity of the disease after infection occurs, measured by the proportion of clinical cases that develop a severe form of the disease or die (Case fatality rate = Number of severe disease or deaths ÷ Number with disease (cases) × 100)
Immunoge-nicity	The ability of a microorganism to produce an immune response after the infection that results in future resistance

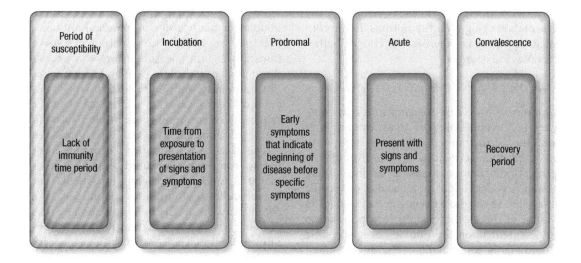

Figure 6.2 Stages of disease.

immune system reaction. The prodromal period consists of nonspecific symptoms that indicate a disease has occurred but is not specific at this time to differentiate the signs and symptoms. In the acute period, the individual presents with characteristic signs and symptoms. During the acute period, there is active replication of the pathogen. In the convalescence period, the individual begins to recover from the acute illness returning to a normal or healthy state.

Disease stages are also classified based on the clinical presentation (Figure 6.2). The clinical classification system for disease stages integrates the pathophysiological changes that correlate to the disease stage. The two broad clinical disease classifications are nonclinical (or inapparent)

and clinical. Nonclinical disease stages consist of four disease phases: preclinical, subclinical, persistent (chronic), and latent (Figure 6.3).

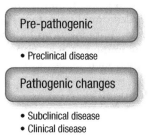

Figure 6.3 Disease stages by clinical and pathological changes.

The preclinical stage exists when the disease is not clinically apparent but is destined to progress to clinical disease. The subclinical stage exists when the disease is not clinically apparent and not destined to become clinically apparent. The preclinical stage can be determined by microscopic examination of cellular tissue and the subclinical stage can be determined by serologic antibody testing or organism cultures. Frequently, the preclinical and subclinical stages are considered one stage and known as the subclinical stage in which there is no pathogenesis evident. Persistent (chronic) stage exists when the disease persists for years or for the person's lifetime. Latent stage exists when there is no active multiplication of the infectious agent but only the existence of genetic material.

The clinical stage of disease is evident by the presentation of signs and symptoms. In the clinical stage of disease, there is evidence of pathophysiological changes.

IMMUNITY AND IMMUNOGENICITY

Immunity is a defense mechanism of the host factor in the epidemiologic triad. Immunity is the ability of the human immune system to resist an infectious organism or toxin from developing an infection or disease in an individual. Immunity is dependent on the action of specific antibodies or sensitized white blood cells. The amount of disease occurrence in a population is dependent upon the number of susceptible individuals in a population. The development of immunity breaks the chain of infection and interrupts the interaction of the epidemiologic triad to cause disease. Immunogenicity is an aspect of the agent that impacts the development of immunity. Immunogenicity is the ability of an organism to produce an immune response after an individual is infected. Immunogenicity impacts the ability of the individual to develop an antibody response that may result in the development of human immunity in the form of producing specific antibodies to resist future infection. Human immunity can be time limited, either lifelong immunity or a temporary protective immunity from disease.

Types of Immunity

There are several types of immunity that are capable of protecting individuals and populations. The types of immunity are active, passive, cocooning, and community or herd. Active immunity is the development of resistance by exposure to an infectious or disease-causing agent. Active immunity can develop from exposure to an actual organism or through vaccination. Vaccination exposes an individual to an antigen from an organism to stimulate the immune system to develop an immune response, resulting in the production of protective antibodies. A vaccine is considered antigenic but not pathogenic. That means the vaccine is capable of producing an antigenic immune response but does not result in the development of actual disease. Active immunity has the ability to produce long-term immunity through the production of immunologic memory. Passive immunity is immunity provided through indirect means such as providing an individual with immunoglobulin antibodies or the transfer of maternal antibodies. Maternal antibodies are capable of passively transferring immune protection to a newborn through placental circulation and breast milk.

Community immunity exists when those around them protect an individual. There are two types of community immunity: cocooning and herd immunity. Cocooning is considered a type of passive immunity. Cocooning is similar to community or herd immunity except that it is aimed at protecting a particular individual rather than an entire population in the community. An individual may not be capable of being given a vaccination for active immunity to develop, such as a child who may have a weakened immune system or engaged in active chemotherapy for the treatment of cancer. Therefore, cocooning would be ensuring that the entire family is immune to a disease such as measles to prevent at-risk child from developing a disease. Cocooning, as a passive immunity strategy, requires that everyone who comes into contact with the specific child is also immune to the condition such as measles. Cocooning is also sometimes referred to as indirect immunity.

Herd immunity is the resistance of a population from an attack by an infectious agent to which a large proportion of the population's members are immune (Figure 6.4). In herd immunity, if a large proportion of the population is immune either through previous infection or vaccination, then the disease is less likely to spread. Therefore, if a large number of individuals in a community or herd are vaccinated, they essentially provide protection to other members

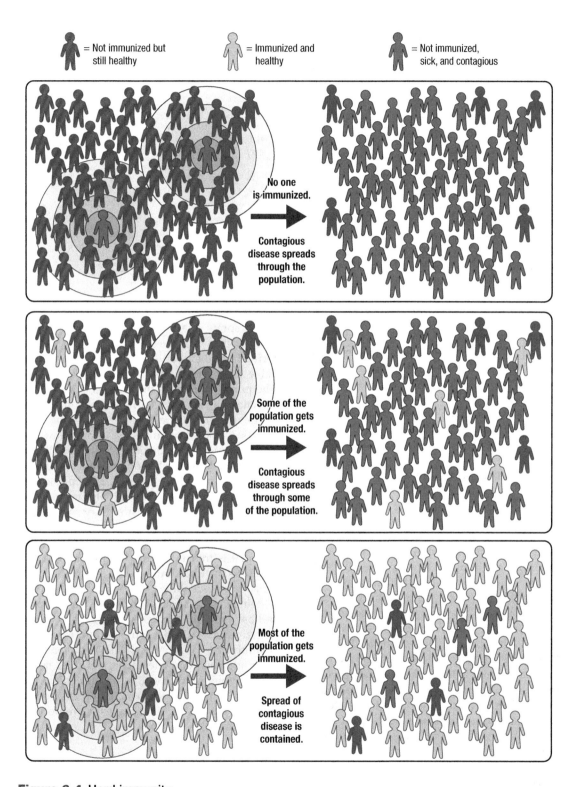

Figure 6.4 Herd immunity.

Source: National Institutes of Health (NIH).

who have not been vaccinated. Some necessary conditions for herd immunity are humans are the only reservoir, active exposure and infection produce immunity, and the infectious agent is restricted to one host species. A disease with a high infectivity rate requires a larger number of the population to have immunity for herd immunity to provide protection. Population level immunity changes over time resulting in a change in the level of herd immunity. For example, if vaccination levels for a disease are not maintained at a proportionately high enough level, then the level of herd immunity decreases in the population and the risk of exposure and infection increases. Therefore, it is necessary to continually monitor the level of herd immunity for infectious diseases in the population.

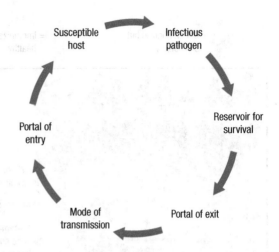

Figure 6.5 Chain of infection.

DISEASE TRANSMISSION

Disease transmission can occur from human to human, human to animal, animal to human, and animal to animal. In the last few years, we have experienced more zoonotic diseases that are infections transmitted between different species such as vertebrate animals to humans. A recent zoonotic disease is the novel coronavirus. Pathogenic organisms must have ecological competence to survive between temporal seasons with the fluctuations in the environment. Ecological competence is the ability of a pathogenic microorganism to survive and compete in a new habitat.

Infectious disease transmission occurs through a chain of infection. The chain of infection consists of six linkages. Prevention of infections can occur by breaking the interaction of any of the six linkages in this infection chain. The six linkages in the chain of infection are the infectious agent, reservoir, portal of exit, mode of transmission, portal of entry, and susceptible host (refer to the epidemiologic triad in Chapter 4). Figure 6.5 presents the chain of infection. The infectious agent is the pathogen that can cause the disease. The reservoir is the environmental place where the infectious agent or pathogen lives and thrives. Reservoirs can be people, animals, insects, soil, water, or medical equipment. Human reservoirs are also known as carriers (Table 6.2). Carriers can be active or passive.

The portal of exit is the site, manner, or way in which the infectious agent leaves its normal living environment to be transmitted to a susceptible host. Portals of exit are water contamination, open wounds, aerosols, splatter of blood or body fluids, coughing, sneezing, bites, and saliva spray. The mode of transmission is the manner in which the infectious agent is transferred from the reservoir to the susceptible host. Table 6.3 presents the modes of transmission. The portal of entry is the manner in which the infectious agent enters a new susceptible host. Portal of entry can be mucous membranes, broken skin or open wounds, respiratory tract, or insertion of medical devices. A susceptible host is an individual who has no resistance or immunity to the infectious agent. A susceptible host can be unvaccinated individuals or immunocompromised persons. In summary, the chain of infection is dependent on an agent being infectious that leaves its reservoir through a portal of exit that is transmitted to an environment that supports the infectious agent's survival and enters into a susceptible host to produce disease.

Humans can serve as the definitive reservoir or host for some infections. This host status can be characterized as definitive or intermediate. A definitive host is a preferred host and generally the pathogen completes a part of their sexual maturity within the host. An intermediate host is one in which the pathogen completes several immature stages of their life cycle or reproduces asexually within the host.

Mode of Transmission

The mode of transmission is the manner in which an infectious agent survives the transfer from a reservoir to a susceptible host. There are several categorizations for modes of transmission: direct or indirect, vertical or horizontal, or vehicle or vector (Table 6.3).

Table 6.2 Human Reservoir: Carrier

Carrier Type	Description
Active	Human host infected with pathogen who can be symptomatic or asymptomatic
Passive	Human host contaminated with the pathogen and can mechanically transmit the pathogen; for example, contaminated healthcare workers' hands

Table 6.3 Modes of Transmission

Mode	Description
Direct	Physical contact between persons, person-to-person contact (e.g., touching, kissing, droplet sprays, airborne, sexual, animal bites)
	Vertical: Transmitted from mother to child (pregnancy, birth, or breastfeeding)
	Horizontal: From infected person to susceptible person in community
Indirect	Common source transmission such as a vector or vehicle
	Vector (living intermediary): Mechanical (physically carry the agent from the reservoir to the host) or biological (the agent lives in the reservoir) transmission via an arthropod, insect
	Vehicle (non-living intermediary): Transmitted in water, food, air, soil, fomites

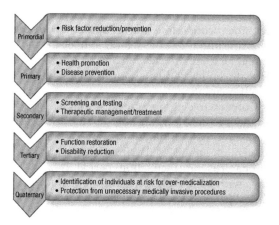

Figure 6.6 Prevention levels.

LEVELS OF PREVENTION

Prevention includes several public health interventions aimed at reducing risk factors, exposure, or threats to health. Levels of prevention typically refer to only three prevention levels: primary, secondary, and tertiary; however, five levels of prevention are proposed as essential to halting alterations in health (Figure 6.6). The five levels of prevention proposed are primordial, primary, secondary, tertiary, and quaternary. Primordial prevention is considered the earliest prevention intervention possible. Primordial prevention aims to target the underlying situations that may promote the exposure to at-risk conditions to promote disease onset. Primordial prevention measures strive to inhibit the future emergence of risk factors whether they are environmental, social, economic, behavioral, cultural, or lifestyle. Primary prevention interventions aim to prevent disease or injury before they occur. Primary prevention aims at preventing exposure to hazards that cause disease or injury, and generally consists of disease prevention and health promotion measures. Disease prevention strategies focus specifically at preventing the disease such as immunizations. Health promotion consists of strategies such as healthy diet and exercise that promote healthy living and lifestyle behaviors that are known to reduce disease risk factors. Secondary prevention interventions are aimed at reducing the impact of disease or injury and consist of early disease detection through screening measures and disease treatment. Some examples of secondary prevention are regular annual physical examinations, screening tests such as mammograms or colonoscopies, daily low-dose aspirin therapy, or antibiotic treatment for bacterial infections.

Tertiary prevention aims to prevent the long-term impact or disability of disease or injury. Some examples of tertiary prevention are cardiac, stroke, or pulmonary rehabilitation programs, and social support groups. Quaternary prevention is characterized as the actions taken to identify patients or patient populations at risk for over-medicalization to protect them from unnecessary risk exposure and medical treatment. Quaternary prevention has been associated with the ethical principle of "first, do no harm" (Pandve, 2014).

Prevention approaches have been characterized as existing in three buckets. The three buckets are traditional clinical preventive interventions, innovative preventive interventions outside of the clinical setting, and total population or community-wide interventions. The traditional clinical preventive interventions consist of the traditional care provided in the healthcare system such as childhood and seasonal vaccinations, diagnostic and screening test, and colonoscopies. Traditional clinical preventive interventions are the routine primary care interventions that occur in a one-to-one encounter. Within this bucket are the patient-oriented bucket of services based on evidence-based practice guidelines. The patient-oriented bucket targets health conditions and evidence-based practices that are known to improve the health of the patient population in the specific clinical practice or system. In the innovative preventive interventions outside the clinical setting, these interventions are similar to those in the traditional clinical preventive bucket in that they are clinical in nature and patient population focused. However, these interventions have not traditionally been delivered in the clinical setting possibly due to insurance coverage or not being paid for by fee-for-service. The innovative preventive interventions may be provided in the home or within community-based settings through grant or governmental contracts. The total population or community-wide interventions target an entire population or subpopulation identified typically by a geographical location. These interventions are targeting an entire population such as a neighborhood, city, county, or state (Auerbach, 2016). Total population or community-wide interventions could be smoking ban regulations, mass media health education campaigns, and cigarette or tobacco taxation.

Isolation and Quarantine

Humans can serve as both a host and reservoir for an infectious pathogen. Isolation and quarantine are public health interventions that target breaking the chain of infection through reducing or eliminating human-to-human contact. Isolation and quarantine are dependent upon reducing physical contact, segregation, and confinement of infected or exposed individuals. Isolation is a prevention strategy in which the infected person refrains from contact with others. Quarantine is a prevention strategy in which an exposure person refrains from contact with others.

Contact Tracing

Contact tracing is a public health prevention strategy. Contact tracing is considered an active surveillance method. During contact tracing, a public health provider interviews the infected individual to determine their recent contacts and points of community engagement. This is a prevention strategy to identify those potentially exposed individuals in order to provide them with notification of their potential exposure, to give them counseling and education about the exposure and infectious agent, to refer the individual for diagnostic testing or screening, and to educate the individual about the possible need to self-quarantine.

Contact tracing requires the public health provider to be knowledgeable about the disease incubation period, modes of transmission, and prevention strategies. For example, with novel coronavirus the incubation period is 2 to 14 days with an average of 5 days. The infectious period is considered to exist 48 hours prior to the first day of symptoms and at least 10 days after the onset of illness. However, novel coronavirus infectivity is considered until the individual has no fever for 72 hours (3 days) with improvement in symptoms (review the case in Box 6.1).

There are six steps to investigating cases and their contacts during contact tracing. It is important to ensure that the public health provider maintains confidentiality and never states to whom the individual was specifically exposed. The steps to conducting contact tracing are:

1. **Introduction:** Introduce yourself to the case, interview the case to determine their basic demographic information.

BOX 6.1. Contact Tracing Case

Mary presents with symptoms of COVID-19 on May 9, 2020. On May 11, 2020, it was confirmed through a nasopharyngeal swab that she was COVID-19 positive. Mary would be considered infectious from May 7, 2020 to May 19, 2020; provided on May 19, 2020 she has not had a fever greater than 101.1°F for the last 3 days and her symptoms are resolving. Mary should self-isolate for how many days? State the days that Mary should isolate?

As a clinician, you are assigned to conduct contact tracing on Mary. You call Veronica on May 12, 2020. Based on your call, you understand that Veronica and Mary were last together having lunch on May 8, 2020. Should you ask Veronica to self-isolate or self-quarantine? If so, for how many days? What is the final date in May you would recommend Veronica to self-isolate or self-quarantine?

---

2. **Inquire:** Question the case about their first day of symptoms, potential contact with an infected person or persons. Determine the case's infectious period.
3. **Identify contacts:** Ask the case about their contacts during the infectious period, nature of the contact, and length of time of contact.
4. **Isolate:** Educate the case on appropriate prevention strategies and self-isolation recommendations.
5. **Initiate contact tracing:** Contact all of the case's known contacts during the infectious period. Provide the contact with information about their potential exposure, inquire about symptoms, refer for testing as appropriate, and provide self-quarantine instructions.
6. **Regular check-in or follow-up:** Follow-up with both the case and contact during their self-isolation and self-quarantine phase.

ICEBERG THEORY

The iceberg theory is used as an analogy to understand and visualize what happens with the occurrence and presentation of a disease in the community and population. The iceberg theory analogy integrates the concepts of clinical disease presentation and pathogenesis into one model along with levels of prevention alignment. This is sometimes referred to as the "iceberg phenomenon of a disease." The phenomenon explains the progress of a disease from the prepathogenesis to pathogenesis stage along with the clinical presentation from subclinical to clinical presentation.

With an iceberg, only the tip is visible. This tip of the iceberg represents what the clinician or pathologist can detect with the disease. Therefore, the tip of the iceberg is analogous to the clinical and pathogenesis stage of the disease process. Below the water line is a large hidden part of the iceberg. This part of the iceberg that resides below the water line and is invisible is analogous to the subclinical and prepathogenesis stage of the disease (Figure 6.7). A goal with advancements in medical and basic science is to lower the water line to have more of the disease detected as soon as pathogenesis begins and before symptoms present. This would provide for the ability to detect disease early, preventing further development, or improving the cure rate or improving rehabilitation.

The iceberg theory analogy can also be aligned with the levels of prevention. Primary prevention should occur below the water line targeting the aspect of the iceberg that is not yet seen or detected. Secondary prevention is at the water line, detecting disease through screening for pathogenic changes or signs that are right below the water line or detecting the early presentation of symptoms that indicate a disease is present or in the early stages of development. Tertiary prevention focuses on the visible aspect of the disease iceberg.

ASSOCIATION AND CAUSATION

An aim of epidemiology is to determine the etiology or causes of diseases. The case for causation is built upon the association of a risk factor and the presence of disease. An association is the relationship between two variables, such as a risk factor and a disease outcome. Causation is determined using the Bradford Hill criteria. The Bradford Hill criteria provide an epidemiologic framework from which to determine a causal relationship between an etiologic agent exposure and the disease condition. The following are the Bradford Hill criteria used to determine if an observed association is likely to be considered causal:

1. **Strength of association:** The stronger the association or magnitude of the relationship between a risk factor and the disease outcome, the more likely the association is likely to be considered causal.

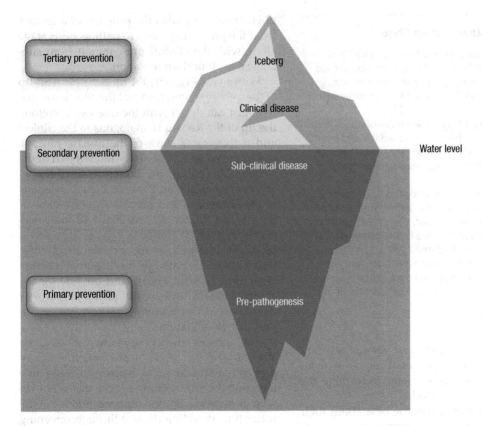

Figure 6.7 Iceberg theory.

2. **Consistency:** Consistency is the extent to which the associated findings are observed among different populations using different study designs and methods over different time periods.
3. **Specificity:** Specificity exists if there is a one-to-one relationship between the risk factor and the disease outcomes. Specificity is the extent to which this risk factor is only associated to one specific disease.
4. **Temporal sequence:** Temporal sequence indicates that the risk factor or exposure must precede the development of the disease outcome.
5. **Biological gradient:** Biological gradient is also known as dose-response relationship. This indicates that the intensity of exposure to the risk factor results in a change in the severity or risk of developing the disease.
6. **Coherence:** Coherence is the associated findings consistent with existing and current knowledge about the natural history of the disease or consistent with the known biological changes or pathophysiology of the disease.

7. **Biological plausibility:** Biological plausibility is the extent to which there is a known biological explanation of the risk factor and disease outcome.
8. **Experiment:** Experiment indicates that if the risk factor or exposure is removed, the frequency of the outcomes is negatively impacted.
9. **Analogy:** Analogy indicates that the relationship identified is consistent with other established cause-and-effect relationships (Hill, 1965).

The epidemiologist must make a judgment decision regarding the statistical association and the cause-and-effect relationship based on the extent to which the associated risk factor and disease outcome meet the Bradford Hill criteria. Many epidemiologists, rather than determining or stating there is a direct and exclusive cause-and-effect relationship, will state there is a strong association from which causation can be inferred. This is known as causal inference.

BEINGS Model of Causation

The BEINGS acronym indicates the model of disease causation and postulates that human disease and the resulting consequences are a result of multicausal factors. This model purports that there are nine different factors that cause disease through complex interaction:

- **B**iological factors that are innate to the specific individual;
- **B**ehavioral factors associated with the specific individual's lifestyle;
- **E**nvironmental factors such as physical, chemical, and biological aspects of the environment;
- **I**mmunological factors;
- **N**utritional factors;
- **G**enetic factors;
- **S**ocial factors;
- **S**piritual factors; and
- **S**ervice factors related to various aspects of health care such as access.

Wheel Theory of Causation

The Wheel Theory of Causation presents a visual model of causative factors. Human disease is depicted in the form of a wheel (Figure 6.8). The wheel's center hub represents the individual human genetic components associated with disease causation. The outer aspects of the wheel represent the environmental components that are generally expressed as three spokes. The three spokes represent the environmental components of disease causation to include biological, social, and physical environmental components.

Web of Association

The web of association is a tool that can be constructed to explore the epidemiologic determinants of a disease. The web of association is constructed to study the disease determinants that can be characterized as risk factors, antecedents, or etiologic factors. It is considered a web since this epidemiologic tool is used to consider as many predisposing factors and their interrelationships as possible. From this visual display, the interrelations of disease determinants can be explored through an epidemiologic investigation or research study.

The web is constructed by first identifying the disease under investigation. This is placed in a box, such as human immunodeficiency virus (HIV) infection. Then, the question is asked, "What is known or suspected to cause HIV infection?" For example, exposure to infected blood and body fluids, unsafe sexual intercourse, and unsafe contaminated needle usage. Next the question is asked, "What is known or suspected to cause or lead an individual to exposure to infected blood and body fluids, unsafe sexual intercourse, and unsafe contaminated needle usage?" This continues until the epidemiologist is satisfied with the level of disease determinants identified. The result of the web of causation is a visual depiction of potential or known disease determinants interacting relationship identified in a visual web. Each determinant factor has its own relative importance in the causation of the disease, as well as interacting with other determinants to modify the effects of each other. From this web of association, the epidemiologist can further explore and expand the knowledge and scientific basis for the disease determinants.

Prognostics

Association and causation are also inferred through prognostics. Prognostics is the prediction of a disease outcome or the course of a disease following risk factor exposure and the development of pathological changes. Prognostics assist with clinical decision-making regarding disease presence and causation. Screening and diagnostic tests assist with an epidemiologist or clinician's prognostic judgments.

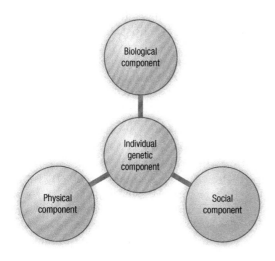

Figure 6.8 Wheel theory.

END-OF-CHAPTER RESOURCES

SUMMARY POINTS

- The natural history of disease consists of five stages of disease—susceptibility, incubation, prodromal, acute, and convalescence.
- Disease stages are also classified based on the clinical presentation.
- The two broad clinical disease classifications are nonclinical (or inapparent) and clinical.
- Immunity is a defense mechanism of the host factor in the epidemiologic triad.
- The development of immunity breaks the chain of infection and interrupts the interaction of the epidemiologic triad to cause disease.
- The types of immunity are active, passive, cocooning, and community or herd.
- Disease transmission can occur from human to human, human to animal, animal to human, and animal to animal.
- Pathogenic organisms must have ecological competence to survive between temporal seasons with the fluctuations in the environment.
- The six linkages in the chain of infection are the infectious agent, reservoir, portal of exit, mode of transmission, portal of entry, and susceptible host.
- The mode of transmission is the manner in which an infectious agent survives the transfer from a reservoir to a susceptible host.
- There are several categorizations for modes of transmission—direct or indirect, vertical or horizontal, or vehicle or vector.
- The five levels of prevention proposed are primordial, primary, secondary, tertiary, and quaternary.
- The three prevention buckets are traditional clinical preventive interventions, innovative preventive interventions outside of the clinical setting, and total population or community-wide interventions.
- Isolation and quarantine are public health interventions that target breaking the chain of infection through reducing or eliminating human-to-human contact.
- Isolation and quarantine are dependent upon reducing physical contact, segregation, and confinement of infected or exposed individuals.
- Contact tracing is considered an active surveillance method.
- During contact tracing, a public health provider interviews the infected individual to determine their recent contacts and points of community engagement.
- The iceberg theory is used as an analogy to understand and visualize what is occurring with the occurrence and presentation of a disease in the community and population.
- The iceberg theory analogy integrates the concepts of clinical disease presentation and pathogenesis into one model along with levels of prevention alignment.
- The Bradford Hill criteria provide an epidemiologic framework from which to determine a causal relationship between an etiologic agent exposure and the disease condition.
- Bradford Hill criteria consist of strength of association, consistency, specificity, temporal sequence, biological gradient, coherence, biological plausibility, experiment, and analogy.
- The epidemiologist must make a judgment decision regarding the statistical association and the cause-and-effect relationship based on the extent to which the associated risk factor and disease outcome meet the Bradford Hill criteria.
- The BEINGS model consists of biological factors, behavioral factors, environmental factors, immunological factors, nutritional factors, genetic factors, social factors, spiritual factors, and healthcare service factors.
- Wheel theory consists of genetic, biological, social, and physical environmental components.
- The web of association is a tool that can be constructed to explore the epidemiologic determinants of a disease.

EPIDEMIOLOGY CRITICAL REASONING QUESTIONS

1. Select a disease outbreak—H1N1, Middle East respiratory syndrome (MERS), novel coronavirus (COVID-19), Ebola virus, measles, yellow fever, or cholera. Develop a narrative epidemiologic case summary that outlines the stages of the disease, etiologic agent characteristics, modes of transmission, chain of infection, types of prevention strategies to be implemented, contact

tracing strategies, and isolation and quarantine recommendations. Draw a web of association for the disease.

2. John has been diagnosed with novel coronavirus infection on May 13, 2020. The incubation period for novel coronavirus infection is from 2 to 14 days with an average of 5 days. As a preventive strategy, contact tracing of John's contacts has been instituted. Eric has been identified as a contact of John's on May 14, 2020. Should Eric be ordered to isolate or quarantine? What should be the length of time in days that Eric should isolate or quarantine?

ADDITIONAL RESOURCES

 SPRINGER PUBLISHING **CONNECT™** | A robust set of instructor resources designed to supplement this text is located at http://connect. springerpub.com/content/book/978-0-8261-8514-3. Qualifying instructors may request access by emailing textbook@springerpub.com.

REFERENCES

Auerbach, J. (2016). The 3 buckets of prevention. *Journal of Public Health Management Practice, 22*(3), 215–218. https://doi.org/10.1097/PHH.0000000000000381

Hill, A. (1965). The environment and disease: Association or causation? *Proceedings of the Royal Society of Medicine, 58,* 295–300.

Pandve, H. (2014). Quaternary prevention: Need of the hour. *Journal of Family Medicine Primary Care, 3*(4), 309–310.

Chapter 7

DISEASE OCCURRENCE: MORBIDITY AND MORTALITY

Demetrius J. Porche

The goal is to turn data into information, and information into insight.
—Carly Fiorina

CHAPTER COMPETENCIES

At the conclusion of this chapter, the reader will be able to:

1. Calculate morbidity statistics
2. Calculate mortality statistics
3. Utilize morbidity and mortality data to describe the distribution and determinants of disease within specific populations
4. Differentiate the population surveillance system methods used to generate epidemiologic data
5. Determine essential elements of population surveillance systems to prevent and control outbreaks, epidemics, and pandemics

ESSENTIAL TERMINOLOGY

Essential morbidity and mortality terminology are:

- Active surveillance
- Case definition
- Case-fatality rate
- Common source outbreak
- Continuous common source outbreak
- Crude rate
- Direct age adjustment
- Endemic
- Epidemic
- Hyperendemic disease
- Incidence
- Indirect age adjustment
- Mortality
- Notifiable diseases
- Outbreak investigation
- Outbreak science
- Pandemic
- Passive surveillance
- Point prevalence
- Prevalence
- Propagated outbreak
- Quality of life
- R-naught
- Sporadic endemic
- Surveillance
- Years of potential life lost
- Intermittent common source outbreak
- Morbidity

Epidemiologic tools consist of counts, rates, ratios, and proportions. The tools of epidemiology present data about health conditions with consideration to person, place, and time. At the core of epidemiology is the desire to understand the distribution of illness (morbidity) and death (mortality), and the determinants of morbidity and mortality within a population. Measures of disease occurrence provide essential data to understand the dynamics of morbidity and mortality in a population in order to develop population-based measures of control and prevention.

The patient's healthcare record is a primary source of epidemiologic data. Epidemiologic data are dependent upon the nurse and other

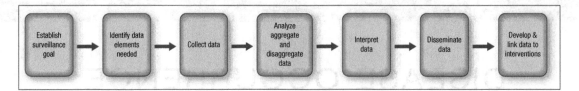

Figure 7.1 Surveillance process.

healthcare providers' documentation of signs, symptoms, and chronological history of events surrounding the development of a "case." In addition, the documentation of healthcare interventions is another source of primary data collection in an epidemiologic investigation or in the determining of the progression of an epidemic within a community or population.

POPULATION SURVEILLANCE

Surveillance is an important epidemiologic tool to facilitate the identification and monitoring of health and health alterations in a population. A goal of population surveillance is to provide information that can be used to guide actions by public health professionals, government leaders, and the general public to guide public health policy and programs. The Centers for Disease Control and Prevention (CDC) defines surveillance as the "ongoing, systematic collection, analysis, and interpretation of data that is then disseminated to those responsible for preventing diseases and other health conditions" (CDC, 2012). Similarly, the World Health Organization (WHO) defines public health surveillance as "an ongoing, systematic collection, analysis and interpretation of health-related data essential to the planning, implementation, and evaluation of public health practice" (WHO, 2020). Surveillance serves as an early alert system to identify emerging public health problems or emergencies, informs the effectiveness of disease prevention and control measures, and guides public health policy. The data produced from surveillance activities provide the information used to understand and monitor the epidemiology of a health condition or public health problem. Other uses of surveillance data are to identify patients and their contacts (contact tracing) for interventions, detect epidemics and outbreaks, estimate the magnitude and scope of a health problem, measure and characterize health trends, monitor changes in infectious and environmental agents, assess control program measures, and generate hypotheses that stimulate research.

BOX 7.1. Surveillance data sources
- Health records—paper and electronic
- Vital statistic records
- Disease registries
- Health assessments and surveys

Surveillance should be guided by a specific data collection goal. Figure 7.1 outlines the surveillance process. Data sources used for surveillance will depend on the surveillance goal and health condition under surveillance. Box 7.1 outlines potential surveillance data sources.

Surveillance data should be generated from a coordinated and integrated system. The essential functions of an effective surveillance system are outlined in Figure 7.2 (WHO, 2020). Effective surveillance systems result in epidemiologic information that guides public health interventions.

A key aspect of surveillance is the cycle of detecting, responding to, and preventing health problems. Ongoing surveillance is accomplished through active, passive, or hybrid surveillance methods. In active surveillance, the public health provider actively seeks out the identification of cases. Active surveillance attempts to identify every case in a comprehensive manner and requires a commitment of significant human and financial resources for implementation. In passive surveillance, the public health providers depend on the healthcare providers and established healthcare system's operational procedures and processes to report surveillance information regarding health conditions and reportable conditions. A passive surveillance system is a dependent system and has the potential to miss cases due to a lack of consistent reporting and integrated health systems. A passive surveillance system requires less human and financial resources. In several local and state healthcare systems, a hybrid method is used to conduct ongoing surveillance. A hybrid system uses a combination of both passive and active surveillance methods

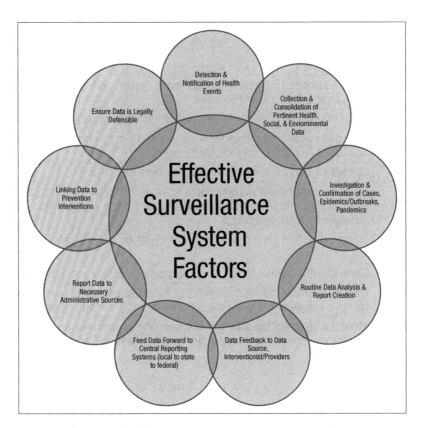

Figure 7.2 Effective surveillance system functions.
Source: Data from the World Health Organization. (2020). *Public health surveillance.*

where the public health professional depends on notifiable condition to be reported into the public health system; however, should there be an increase in the number of cases or should a potential outbreak occur, public health professionals would engage in active surveillance to identify cases and conduct contact tracing. Contact tracing is an active surveillance strategy to identify actual and potential contacts or persons in close proximity to a known case with a notifiable condition.

Sentinel surveillance is a type of surveillance conducted by a single or small number of healthcare facilities that are responsible for collecting data on cases using a specific case definition. Sentinel surveillance provides data on data trends within one or number of healthcare facilities.

Table 7.1 outlines other types of disease surveillance methods (Murray & Cohen, 2017).

According to the CDC, a well-conducted surveillance system has the following characteristics:

- **Acceptability:** Persons and organizations are willing to participate in the surveillance

process by either submitting or completing reports.
- **Flexibility:** The surveillance methods can accommodate changes as the conditions dictate the necessity for change.
- **Predictive value positive:** The proportion of cases reported are truly cases.
- **Quality:** Data used in the surveillance system are accurate and valid with little to no missing data.
- **Representativeness:** The surveillance data accurately portrays the population by person, place, and time.
- **Sensitivity:** The screening and testing measure detects the condition it was intended to detect.
- **Simplicity:** The surveillance system is easy to operationalize.
- **Stability:** Data remain reliable over time.
- **Timeliness:** Surveillance data are capable of being reported in a timely manner to inform public health authorities and others for timely decision-making.
- **Validity:** Data are sensitive and valid with strong predictive value positive data (CDC, 2012).

Table 7.1 Surveillance Methods

Surveillance Method	Description
Community based	Captures cases beyond the healthcare system, conducts screenings within the community to identify cases
Population based	Case identification in a defined population (geographical or high risk)
Aggregate	Includes number of cases for a region and time period, lacks detailed specific information on individual cases
Case based	Collects individual level case-based information
Syndromic (clinical)	Collects data based on presentation of a collection of signs and symptoms, lacks diagnostic testing, provides for rapid case identification, used in emergency alert systems
Laboratory confirmed	Cases identified based on confirmatory laboratory results
Zoonotic	Case identification of zoonotic infection in animals and humans
Serosurveillance	Cases identified through analysis of blood specimens, uses diagnostic testing, can determine burden of disease or immunity gaps in population
Adverse events	Identifies unintended adverse consequences from healthcare services (such as medical errors) or therapeutic treatments (such as immunization reactions)

NOTIFIABLE CONDITIONS

Notifiable conditions are sometimes referred to as reportable diseases or health conditions. Notifiable conditions are required through local, state, territorial, or national laws to be reported to the public health system. Surveillance is dependent upon diseases or health conditions being reported in a timely manner. The notification of reportable diseases is necessary to alert healthcare providers regarding actual or potential health threats.

Internationally notifiable conditions require each country to report specific diseases to WHO. The internationally notifiable conditions are smallpox, poliomyelitis (wild type), human influenza caused by a new subtype, and severe acute respiratory syndrome (SARS). Each country establishes a list of nationally reportable diseases that at a minimum must include WHO internationally notifiable conditions. In the United States, the CDC along with the Council of State and Territorial Epidemiologist (CSTE) determine which health conditions are nationally notifiable. Each respective state, through public health law or sanitary code, determine what conditions are notifiable at the state level. At a minimum, each state must include the nationally notifiable conditions required by the CDC and CSTE. Figure 7.3 shows the notifiable disease reporting structure.

Case Definition

Notifiable conditions use case definitions as a measure of valid reporting (Murray & Cohen, 2017). A case definition determines what an epidemiologist counts as a case (CDC, 2021). Three essential components of case definitions are person, place, and time. Case definitions generally consist of clinical signs and symptoms, laboratory, or confirmatory data, and contact or exposure information along with a time period. Time limitations are more likely to be included during an outbreak or epidemic. Case definitions are modified over time as diagnostic testing advances, or the clinical presentation of the health condition changes over time.

Case definitions vary in sensitivity and specificity. It is best for case definitions to be as sensitive and specific as possible. Sensitive case definitions are more inclusive and have the potential to incorrectly identify patients who do not have the disease or health condition (false positive). Specific case definitions have stricter criteria and tend to exclude more patients that do not have the disease or health condition. Specific case definitions have the potential to miss mild or atypical presentations of the health condition (Murray & Cohen, 2017).

There are three types of case definitions: probable, suspected, and confirmed. A suspected case may have clinical signs and symptoms that are associated with the condition but may not be

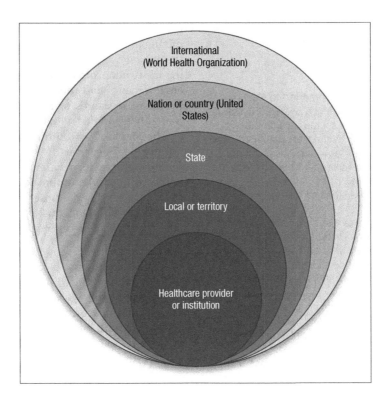

Figure 7.3   International, national, and state notifiable disease structure.

specific enough to differentiate one health condition from another. During an outbreak, a case may be classified as suspected if the individual presents with the characteristic clinical presentation of the health condition. A probable case generally has the clinical signs and symptoms along with some type of epidemiologic link such as recent contact with a confirmed case or other supportive laboratory tests. A confirmed case meets all the expected standard criteria for the case definition. A confirmed case generally has the clinical signs and symptoms, an epidemiologic linkage to a confirmed case, and confirmatory diagnostic test results (CDC, 2020). Exhibit 7.1 presents the typical format for a case definition.

OUTBREAK SCIENCE

An outbreak is an indication of the amount of disease occurrence within a population. An outbreak is considered when more cases of a condition than expected present in a specific location over a specific period of time, and frequently it may also be within a specific population. Outbreak is sometime used synonymously with cluster. However, a cluster is generally referred to as an unusual increase in the number of cases in a very narrowly defined location or population. A cluster can also be a single, unexpected

EXHIBIT 7.1. Case Definition Example—Measles

Measles (revised 9/96) clinical case definition
An illness characterized by all of the following:
- A generalized rash lasting ≥3 days
- A temperature ≥101.0°F (≥38.3°C)
- Cough, coryza, or conjunctivitis

Laboratory criteria for diagnosis
- Positive serologic test for measles immunoglobulin M antibody, or
- Significant rise in measles antibody level by any standard serologic assay, or
- Isolation of measles virus from a clinical specimen

Case classification
Suspected: Any febrile illness accompanied by rash
   Probable: A case that meets the clinical case definition, has noncontributory or no serologic or virologic testing, and is not epidemiologically linked to a confirmed case
   Confirmed: A case that is laboratory confirmed or that meets the clinical case definition and is epidemiologically linked to a confirmed case. A laboratory-confirmed case does not need to meet the clinical case definition.

(continued)

EXHIBIT 7.1. Case Definition Example—Measles (*continued*)

Comment
Confirmed cases should be reported to National Notifiable Diseases Surveillance System (NNDSS). An imported case has its source outside the country or state. Rash onset occurs within 18 days after entering the jurisdiction, and illness cannot be linked to local transmission. Imported cases should be classified as:

- International: A case that is imported from another country
- Out-of-State: A case that is imported from another state in the United States. The possibility that a patient was exposed within their state of residence should be excluded; therefore, the patient either must have been out of state continuously for the entire period of possible exposure (at least 7–18 days before onset of rash) or have had one of the following types of exposure while out of state: (a) face-to-face contact with a person who had either a probable or confirmed case or (b) attendance in the same institution as a person who had a case of measles (e.g., in a school, classroom, or day care center).

An *indigenous case* is defined as a case of measles that is not imported. Cases that are linked to imported cases should be classified as indigenous if the exposure to the imported case occurred in the reporting state. Any case that cannot be proved to be imported should be classified as indigenous.

Source: From Centers for Disease Control and Prevention. (1997). Case definitions for infectious conditions under public health surveillance. *MMWR. Recommendations and Reports, 46*(RR-10), 23–24.

presentation of a condition. Outbreak science is a body of knowledge and methods that guide the investigation of an outbreak of a health condition or disease (Houlihan & Whitworth, 2019).

OUTBREAK INVESTIGATION

An outbreak investigation consists of several steps that integrate surveillance strategies with measures of disease occurrence. An outbreak investigation is both a deductive (reasoning from previous theories, propositions, or hypotheses) and inductive (reasoning from fact to arrive at general conclusions or hypotheses) reasoning process. The multiplicative purposes of an outbreak investigation consist of determining the

extent of the population at risk or affected; determining the measure of disease spread; identifying the etiologic agent and/or reservoir; characterizing the relationship between the agent, host, and environment; and determining preventive or treatment measures to limit the morbidity and mortality associated with the respective outbreak.

The steps of an outbreak investigation are not always linear but frequently consist of an iterative process as new information is gathered and confirmed. An outbreak investigation does occur in a rigid serial order; frequently several steps occur simultaneously. The following outlines the steps of an outbreak investigation:

1. *Preparation*
    a.   If the disease is known, research information regarding clinical presentation, etiologic agent, screening or diagnostic measures, modes of transmission, natural history of disease, incubation period, infectivity information, case definitions, and control measures
2. *Outbreak establishment and surveillance*
    a.   Establish there is an outbreak
    b.   Define the numerator (cases) for the disease occurrence measurement
    c.   Define the denominator or the population at risk or susceptible to developing the health condition or disease
    d.   Determine that the number of cases exceeds the expected number of cases
    e.   Calculate attack rates
    f.   Examine the distribution of cases according to person, place, and time. Characterize the possible outbreak using who, when, where, and how
    g.   Develop surveillance procedures to investigate contacts
3. *Formulate or confirm a case definition*
    a.   The presentation of the health condition could be nonspecific or very specific and a characteristic presentation of a disease process; use this information to assist with case definition development
    b.   Utilize existing symptomatology, knowledge regarding the potential exposure, and host characteristics to formulate a broad-based case definition. If these findings are associated with a known condition with a diagnostic or screening test, use the accepted case definition to classify suspected cases. If not, develop a tentative case definition

4. *Verify the diagnosis*
   a. Conduct screening or diagnostic measures to confirm cases
   b. If there is a known screening or diagnostic test, confirm that suspected cases investigated are actual cases
   c. Surveillance continues to occur to identify new or associated cases
5. *Characterize the outbreak.*
   a. Use descriptive epidemiology to focus on person, place, and time. Characterize the personal characteristics of the cases, changes in disease occurrence over time, and difference in disease frequency based on location
   b. Develop a line listing of all cases
      i. Personal information
      ii. Signs and symptoms
      iii. Laboratory test results
      iv. Relevant exposures
   c. Construct epidemic curves
   d. Determine potential source of outbreak
      i. Point source
      ii. Continuous common source
      iii. Propagated
6. *Hypothesis development*
   a. Develop hypotheses about the existing knowledge of the health condition
   b. Possible etiology and mode of transmission
   c. Consider the following with the cases
      i. **Differences:** Frequency in which cases vary in location or circumstances
      ii. **Similarities:** Frequency by which cases have a common factor
      iii. **Correlations:** Frequency of the relationship between a factor and presentation of the factor with host cases
7. *Evaluate hypotheses*
   a. Conduct an analytic epidemiologic study; cohort or case-control study
   b. Refine hypothesis as new information is learned
8. *Control and prevention*
   a. Implement control measures for the outbreak
   b. Implement preventive measures to reduce further transmission or outbreaks
9. *Communicate findings*
   a. Write a report of the outbreak investigation

DISEASE OCCURRENCE LEVEL

Health and disease states vary within a population at different levels during different periods of time. The amount of a disease that is usually present in a population or what is sometimes considered the baseline level of disease is known as endemic. Endemic is sometimes used to refer to the constant presence or usual prevalence of a disease. The endemic level does not mean that this is the desired level of a disease or health condition but simply the amount of the respective disease or health condition that generally exists within the specific population at that time. The desired level could be zero. Diseases can be considered sporadic or hyperendemic. A sporadic endemic condition occurs at infrequent and irregular periods of time. A hyperendemic disease refers to a persistent, high level of disease occurrence.

If the amount of a disease increases in a population above the expected level, this is referred to as an epidemic. An epidemic is an increase or sudden rise in the number of cases above the expected endemic rate within the population at that time. As mentioned earlier, outbreak and cluster are terms also used along with epidemic. An outbreak is generally considered an increase in the number of cases above the expected or usual number of cases within a limited geographic area. A cluster is generally an increase in the number of cases above the endemic or expected rate within a smaller aggregate population in the same place/location and time period. A pandemic describes an epidemic that has spread over several countries and continents, affecting a large number of persons.

OUTBREAK OR EPIDEMIC PATTERNS

An epidemic cure provides clues about the possible source of an outbreak. An outbreak or epidemic is characterized according to the manner in which the disease is spread or transmitted throughout the community or population. A common source outbreak/epidemic is one in which all the affected individuals/cases are exposed to one agent or host. All cases originate from one source agent or host. A point source outbreak/epidemic is the term used to refer to an outbreak or epidemic that originates from a focal source that affects a number of individuals during a limited period of time. For example, a cook in a restaurant has subclinical, asymptomatic hepatitis A infection. The cook sheds the virus for weeks. In this point source outbreak/ epidemic, the number of cases occur during a specific span of time that is equal to the incubation period for hepatitis A. Some outbreaks occur where individuals are exposed over a period of day, weeks, months, or longer. In this case the source is prolonged over an extended period of time and there is the presentation of cases over more than one incubation period. This is known as a continuous common source outbreak or epidemic. In a continuous common source outbreak or epidemic, the incubation periods on the epidemic curve tend to flatten and widen the peaks of the curve. An intermittent common source outbreak or epidemic occurs when the source does not consistently affect others creating the presence of disease. A propagated outbreak or epidemic presents as an initial cluster of cases in which the initial cluster of cases serves as the source for later cases. The propagated outbreak or epidemic results from person-to-person transmission over a period of time. Propagated outbreaks occur when the mode of transmission is generally person-to-person contact. Lastly, mixed outbreaks or epidemics occur when there is a combination of the outbreak/epidemic patterns occurring during the same time period.

BASIC DISEASE OCCURRENCE EXPLORATION—WHO, WHEN, AND WHERE

A basic approach to disease exploration consists of the who, when, and where model. Three basic questions provide the foundation for this basic exploration of disease:

- Who was affected by the disease?
- When did the disease occur?
- Where are the cases of the disease occurring?

Who Was Affected by the Disease?

This question is best answered using demographic information to characterize the individuals affected by the disease. Common demographic variables are age, race, and sex. Other factors that can be used to characterize who is affected by disease consist of behavioral or lifestyle factors such as smoking, alcohol consumption, and diet. Figure 7.4 presents crude annual candidemia incidence rates by race in the United States from 2012 to 2016. Figure 7.5 presents crude annual candidemia incidence rates by sex in the United States from 2012 to 2016.

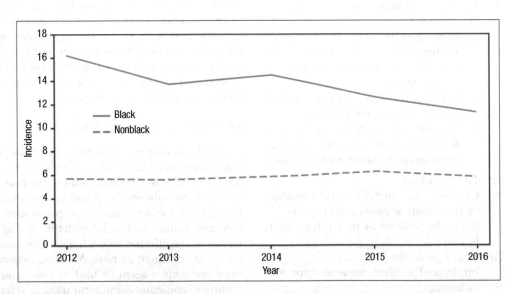

Figure 7.4 Crude annual candidemia incidence (per 100,000 population, calculated from the U.S. Census Bureau population and housing unit estimates for the corresponding years), by race—four sites (Georgia, Maryland, Oregon, and Tennessee), United States, 2012–2016.

Source: Toda, M, Williams, S. R., Berkow, E. L, Farley, M. M., Harrison, L. H., Bonner, L., Marceaux, K. M., Hollick, R., Zhang, A. Y., Schaffner, W., Lockhart, S. L., Jackson, B. R., & Vallabhaneni, S. (2019). Population-based active surveillance for culture-confirmed candidemia—Four sites, United States, 2012–2016. *MMWR Surveillance Summaries, 68*(SS-8), 1–15. http://doi.org/10.15585/mmwr.ss6808a1.

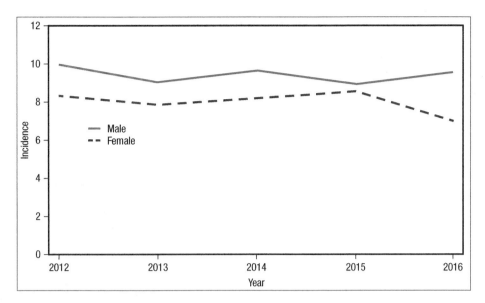

Figure 7.5 Crude annual candidemia incidence (per 100,000 population, calculated from the U.S. Census Bureau population and housing unit estimates for the corresponding years), by sex—four sites (Georgia, Maryland, Oregon, and Tennessee), United States, 2012—2016.

Source: Toda, M, Williams, S. R., Berkow, E. L, Farley, M. M., Harrison, L. H., Bonner, L., Marceaux, K. M., Hollick, R., Zhang, A. Y., Schaffner, W., Lockhart, S. L., Jackson, B. R., & Vallabhaneni, S. (2019). Population-based active surveillance for culture-confirmed candidemia—Four sites, United States, 2012–2016. *MMWR Surveillance Summaries, 68*(SS-8), 1–15. http://doi.org/10.15585/mmwr.ss6808a1.

When Did the Disease Occur?

This refers to the time period in which the disease happened. Some diseases are seasonal with an increased incidence within certain months of the year such as influenza occurring more during the winter months. This question of "when" is answered by examining trends in the disease incidence overtime. Figure 7.6 demonstrates that the number of malaria cases by *Plasmodium* species had an increase in the number of imported cases during the months of about May to November in 2015 and 2016.

Where Are the Diseases Occurring?

This question examines the location of the cases within a specific period of timee and provides the geographic distribution of the number of cases within the population during a period of time. "Where" can be analyzed in the smallest of geographic measures, such as local city block, to larger geopolitical areas such as counties, or larger measures such as states or countries. Figure 7.7 presents the rates of reported chlamydia cases by county in the United States in 2018.

DISEASE OCCURRENCE: MORBIDITY

Morbidity disease occurrence can be expressed as a rate or proportion. The two primary measures of morbidity disease occurrence rates are incidence and prevalence. Incidence and prevalence are expressed as rates. Rates provide information about how fast a disease or condition is occurring within a population in a specific period of time. A proportion provides information on the fraction of the population that is affected by the disease or condition.

Incidence

The incidence rate of a disease is defined as the number of new cases of a disease or condition occurring within a specific period of time in a population at risk for the disease or condition. The numerator in the incidence rate consists of the number of "new" cases of a disease or condition during the specific time period. The denominator in an incidence rate consists of all individuals at risk for the disease or condition during the specific time period. In an incidence rate, those persons in the numerator should be represented also in the denominator. The incidence rate calculation is expressed as a factor

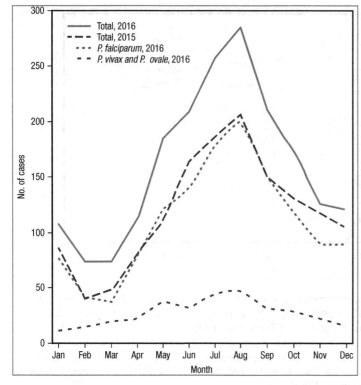

Figure 7.6 Total number of imported malaria cases, by *Plasmodium* species and month of symptom onset—United States, 2016: Total number of cases for 2016 was 1,935, which includes the following: 279 *P. malariae*, mixed, and unknown species determination; 1,325 infections with *P. falciparum*; and 331 infections with *P. vivax* and *P. ovale*. Total number of cases for 2015 was 1,419 infections with all species.

Source: Mace, K. E., Arguin, P. M., Lucchi, N. W., & Tan, K. R. (2019). Malaria surveillance—United States, 2016. *MMWR Surveillance Summaries, 68*(SS-5):1–35. http://doi.org/10.15585/mmwr.ss6805a1.

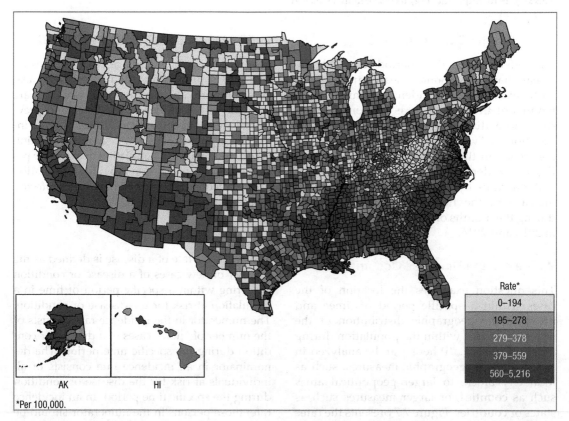

Figure 7.7 Chlamydia—rates of reported cases by county, United States, 2018. *Per 100,000.

Source: Centers for Disease Control and Prevention. (2019). *Sexually transmitted disease surveillance 2018.* U.S. Department of Health and Human Services. https://doi.org/10.15620/cdc.79370.

(10^n) to provide the population measurement perspective. If the 10^n is 1,000 then the incidence rate calculated will be expressed as per 1,000 persons and if it is 10,000, then it would be expressed as per 10,000 persons. The formula for an incidence rate is:

$$\frac{\text{Number of new cases of a disease in an at-risk population during a specific period of time}}{\text{Number of persons at-risk of developing the disease during the specific period of time}} \times 10^n$$

For example, if the total at-risk population for a disease is 3,000 in 2019 and the number of new cases of the disease in 2019 was 338 and the multiplier is 1,000, then, the incidence rate is:

$$\frac{338}{3,000} \times 1,000 = 112.6 \text{ per 1,000 persons.}$$

It is critical to remember that incidence rates indicate only the number of new cases of an event (disease or condition). Incidence rates can be specific by several variables such as age, race, and sex. These are respectively known as age-specific incidence rates, race-specific incidence rates, and sex-specific incidence rates. To adjust a rate by a specific variable, the numerator and denominator must only represent the number of new cases and at-risk population of that respective variable. For example, if a male specific incidence rate is calculated for a disease, then the formula would be:

$$\frac{\text{Number of men with new disease or condition during the specific time period}}{\text{Total number of men at-risk for disease or condition during the specific time period}} \times 10^n$$

Prevalence

The prevalence rate is defined as the number of persons in the population within a specific period of time affected with the disease or condition. The prevalence rate represents both "new and old" cases of a disease or condition. In contrast to the incidence rate, the prevalence rate numerator has both the number of new cases and old or existing cases of a disease or condition within the specific time period. Prevalence data provide a picture of the disease in the population at a specific point in time. Prevalence data provide information for long-term planning for healthcare service utilization. It is also considered a measure of the disease burden within the population. Prevalence data consider individuals with the disease or condition at different stages of the disease process. In contrast, incidence rate represents only the "newly identified" cases of the disease or condition within the specific time period. The formula for a prevalence rate is:

$$\frac{\text{Number of cases of disease present (new and old cases) in an at-risk population during a specific period of time}}{\text{Number of persons at-risk of developing the disease during the specific period of time}} \times 10^n$$

For example, if the at-risk population consist of 3,000 persons during 2019 and the number of newly diagnosed individuals in 2019 was 213 but there were already a total of 1,115 persons living with the disease in 2019, and the multiplier is 1,000. Then, the prevalence rate is:

$$\frac{213 \text{ new cases} + 1,115 \text{ existing cases during time period}}{3,000 \text{ persons at-risk during time period}} \times 1,000 = 442.6 \text{ per 1,000.}$$

Prevalence rate data can be collected and utilized via two methods, point and period prevalence. Point prevalence is the number of new and old cases (total cases) at a certain point of time. The typical question that elicits point prevalence data is "Do you currently have X disease or condition?" Period prevalence is the number of new and old cases (total cases) during a specific time period such as 3 months, a calendar year, or a 5-year period of time. The typical questions that elicit period prevalence data are "Have you had X disease or condition during the last 3 months? Have you had X disease or condition during the last year from January 1 to December 31? Or have you had X disease or condition during the last 5 years (from January 1, 2015 to December 31, 2019)?"

Incidence and Prevalence Dynamic Relationship

There is a dynamic interdependent relationship between incidence and prevalence rates in a population (Figure 7.8). Incidence rates increase as the number of new cases increases. The prevalence rate can be impacted by the incidence rate, mortality rate, and cure rate of a disease or condition. A cure rate for a disease is the number of individuals with a disease who are cured (numerator) divided by the number of persons who have the disease in the specific time period.

As stated earlier, prevalence is a good measure of disease burden in a population. If the incidence of a disease in a population increases, then the prevalence in the population also increases if the mortality rate and cure rates remain unchanged. If the incidence rate in a population remains constant and the mortality rate or the cure rate in a population increases in a specific period of time, then the prevalence rate decreases. If the

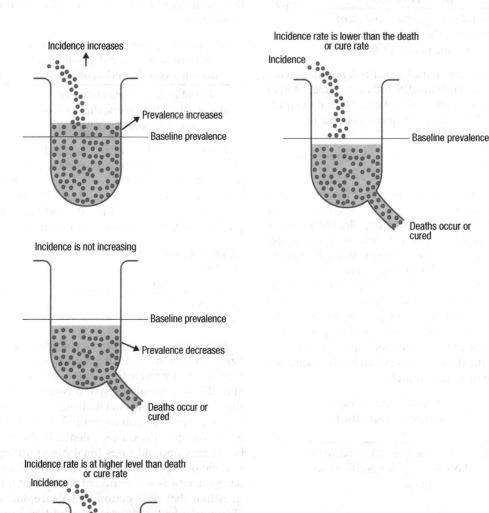

Figure 7.8 Incidence and prevalence dynamic relationships.

BOX 7.2. Morbidity Data Sources
- Disease registries
- Communicable or notifiable disease data
- Healthcare facility generated data
- Occupational data; absenteeism records
- Educational data; absenteeism data
- Contact tracing data
- Military records
- Morbidity surveys: national, regional, or local
- Insurance data
  - ☐ Hospital insurance plans
  - ☐ Medicare/Medicaid
  - ☐ Long-term disability
  - ☐ Accident insurance

---

incidence rate and mortality rate or cure rate of a disease in a population within a specific time period are the same rate, then the prevalence rate remains stable or unchanged in the population within that time period.

Prevalence is impacted by the duration of an illness. If there is a limited number of new cases but there is a low cure rate for a disease and the disease has a long chronic period, then the prevalence rate will increase over time. This relationship between incidence and prevalence is also impacted by the amount of in-migration and out-migration within a population. If there is a steady state of in-migration and out-migration, then prevalence rate can be calculated as:

Prevalence = Incidence × Duration of disease.

Morbidity Data Sources

Morbidity data are generated from multiple sources. Morbidity data can be either primary or secondary data. Primary data are data collected by the epidemiologist for morbidity analysis. In contrast, secondary data are data collected and compiled by another individual and used by the epidemiologist to calculate morbidity statistics. Box 7.2 outlines several sources used by epidemiologist for morbidity statistics.

R-Naught (R_0)

R-naught is a value calculated that represents on average the number of individuals to whom a single infected individual can be expected to transmit an infection. R-naught is represented by the symbol R_0 and provides essential information to understand the potential of an infectious disease to spread within a population. It is frequently referred to as the "average spreadability" of an infection or the "reproduction number." R_0 calculation is specific to the infectious agent.

R-naught is calculated using three data elements: infectious period of the disease, mode of transmission, and contact rate. The infectious period is the duration of time that an individual is infected and able to transmit the infection to another individual. The longer the infectious period of a disease, the higher the average R_0 value. The efficiency of the infectious agent to spread from individual to individual impacts the R_0. The easier it is for an infectious agent to be transmitted via a mode of transmission, the higher the R_0 value. The contact rate is the number of individuals an infected person can be expected to be in contact with during the infectious period. The contact rate is frequently impacted by measures to control an infectious outbreak such as isolation, quarantine, or travel restriction. These three factors are specific to the context of the infectious agent and disease process to produce a R_0 that is specific to the outbreak.

The R_0 value has three potential meanings. The R_0 meanings are:

- If R_0 is less than 1, each existing infected individual can transmit the infection to less than one new individual. With a R_0 less than 1, the disease can likely decline and eventually dissipate.
- If R_0 equals is 1, each existing infected individual can transmit the infection to one other individual. With a R_0 of 1, the disease is likely to remain stable for a while but most likely will not produce an outbreak or epidemic.
- If R_0 is greater than 1, each existing infected individual can transmit the infection to more than one person (or the R_0 number); for example, an R_0 of 3 indicates each existing infected individual can transmit the infection to three other individuals.

R-naught characterizes the intensity of an infectious disease outbreak or epidemic. The situation-dependent R_0 is affected by host characteristics. An immune host will not transmit the infection; however, a host that is immunocompromised or highly susceptible can impact the R_0. Other factors that can impact the R_0 are environmental factors such as climate, population density, life expectancy, socioeconomics, and comorbidities. Figure 7.9 presents an estimation of the reproductive number changes over time based on different growth rates and intervals.

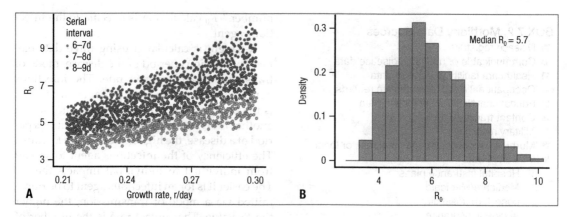

Figure 7.9 Estimation of reproductive number with growth rates and serial intervals. Estimation of the basic reproductive number (R_0), derived by integrating uncertainties in parameter values, during the coronavirus disease outbreak in China. (A) Changes in R_0 based on different growth rates and serial intervals. Each dot represents a calculation with mean latent period (range 2.2–6 days) and mean infectious periods (range 4–14 days). Only those estimates falling within the range of serial intervals of interests were plotted. (B) Histogram summarizing the estimated R_0 of all dots in panel A (i.e., serial interval ranges of 6–9 days). The median R_0 is 5.7 (95% CI 3.8–8.9).

Source: Sanche, S., Lin, Y., Xu, C., Romero-Severson, E., Hengartner, N., & Ke, R. (2020). High contagiousness and rapid spread of severe acute respiratory syndrome coronavirus 2. *Emerging Infectious Diseases, 26*(7), 1470–1477. https://doi.org/10.3201/eid2607.200282

DISEASE OCCURRENCE MORTALITY

Death within a population can be expressed as mortality rates. Mortality rates provide information that differentiates the causes, associated risk factors, demographic, and geographical differences in death occurrence by disease. The absolute number of individuals dying from a specific disease can be expressed graphically by case count and year of occurrence. The presentation of mortality data by case count and year of occurrence provides an indication if the number of cases is increasing or decreasing over time but does not provide a measure by rate, since the data do not include the population at risk (denominator).

Mortality Rate

Mortality rates can be crude or specific. For the mortality rate, the numerator includes all the deaths of the entire population (crude) or from a specific disease (specific) that occurred in a population during a specific period of time.

Crude and Specific Mortality Rates

Crude rates provide a measure for the experience of the entire population. The numerator for a crude mortality rate includes all the deaths from all the causes or all of the deaths from a single cause. The formula would be:

$$\frac{\text{Number of deaths from all causes in the year}}{\text{Number of individuals in the population at midyear}} \times 100,000$$

The midyear population is used as the denominator since the population dynamics within the geographical area fluctuate during the entire year.

For example, the crude death rate from a cerebrovascular incidence (CVI) in Louisiana in 2018 would include all CVI deaths in Louisiana during 2018. The respective formula would be:

$$\frac{\text{Number of deaths from CVI in Louisiana in 2018}}{\text{Total population of Louisiana in 2018 at midyear}} \times 100,000$$

In contrast, a specific rate provides data on a subpopulation of the total population. Specific rates can be calculated by cause, age, race, sex, or any variable for which there is total and subpopulation data. The mortality rate can be specifically calculated for a cause, known as a cause-specific mortality rate. The cause-specific annual mortality rate for colon cancer formula would be:

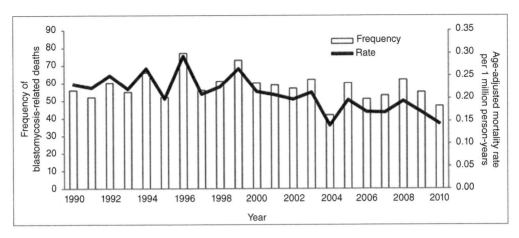

Figure 7.10 Mortality rates: blastomycosis related. Number of blastomycosis-related deaths and age-adjusted mortality rates per 1 million person-years, by year, United States, 1990–2010.

Source: Khuu, D., Shafir, S., Bristow, B., & Sorvillo, F. J. (2014). Blastomycosis mortality rates, United States, 1990–2010. *Emerging Infectious Diseases, 20*(11), 1789–1794. https://doi.org/10.3201/eid2011.131175

$$\frac{\text{Number of deaths from colon cancer in the year}}{\text{Number of individuals in the population at mid-year}} \times 1,000$$

In addition to calculating the mortality rate for all causes of death (crude), we may also be interested in the causes of all deaths for only a specific age group in the population, this would be an age-adjusted or age-specific mortality rate. The formula for the annual age-adjusted mortality rate of all causes is:

$$\frac{\text{Number of deaths from all causes in children aged 1 to 10 years}}{\text{Number of children in the population at mid-year aged 1 to 10 years}} \times 1,000$$

Mortality rates can be calculated for more than one specific characteristic at the same time, such as gender and cause. For example a female cause-specific mortality rate for CVI in 2018 would be calculated with the following formula:

$$\frac{\text{Number of females who died from CVI in Louisiana during 2018}}{\text{Total female population in Lousiana in 2018}} \times 100,000$$

Figure 7.10 presents mortality per 1 million of the blastomycosis-related deaths from 1990 to 2010.

Case-Fatality Rate

The case-fatality rate provides data on the number of individuals who die from a certain disease within a certain time period. The case-fatality rate is expressed as a percentage (%) of all cases. In a case-fatality rate, a case is someone who has died from the disease after the disease onset or disease diagnosis. The case-fatality rate differs from the mortality rate in the denominator. In a mortality rate calculation, the denominator is the entire population at risk of dying from a disease. In a case-fatality rate, the denominator consists only of those who have the specific disease (those who died and those who remain alive). In a case-fatality rate, the numerator consists of all individuals who have died from the specific disease. The formula for the case-fatality rate is:

$$\frac{\text{Number of individuals who died from a specific disease after diagnosis or disease onset in a specific time period}}{\text{Number of individuals with the specific disease during the specific time period}} \times 100 = \_\_\_\%.$$

Proportionate Mortality

The proportionate mortality represents all the deaths that have occurred within the time period and what proportion of the deaths were the result of a specific type of cause or disease. For example, of all the deaths that have occurred in the United States in 2019, what proportion of the deaths were from colon cancer? Proportionate mortality rates can also be calculated by specific demographic variables such as age, race, and sex. The formula for proportionate mortality rate is:

$$\frac{\text{Number of deaths from (specific disease)}}{\text{in the (geographic location) in (year)}}{\text{Total deaths in (geographic location) in}} \times 100$$
$$\text{(year)}$$

Years of Potential Life Lost

Years of potential life lost (YPLL) is considered a mortality index. The YPLL is used to establish health priorities. Years of productive life is a measure of premature death. It indicates that death at a younger population involves a greater amount of lost productive years of life. In the United States, the predetermined "standard" age is 75 years. The calculation of YPLL involves two steps. Step one involves, for each case, the deceased individual's age at death subtracted from the predetermined age at death for the respective country. Therefore, in step one, if an individual dies from prostate cancer at age 45, then the YPLL is $75 - 45 = 30$ years of life lost. In the second step, the YPLL for each individual is added together to calculate the total YPLL for a specific cause of death. Table 7.2 presents annual death estimates and YPLL from smoking-attributable mortality.

Mortality Data Comparison: Different Populations

Mortality data can be compared in two or more populations or one population over different time periods using either a direct or indirect age adjustment. Direct age adjustment uses a hypothetical standard population to apply age-specific mortality rates from two time periods. A direct age adjustment mortality rate permits the elimination of age between two or more populations compared. This is known as the age adjusted death rate (ADR).

If the age is not known, then an indirect age adjustment can be calculated. This is known as the standardized mortality ratio (SMR). SMR is frequently used to study occupational exposure in specific populations leading to death. SMR is the ratio of total deaths actually observed to the total number of deaths expected. The formula for SMR is:

$$\text{SMR} = \frac{\text{Observed number of deaths per year}}{\text{Expected number of deaths per year}}$$

Sources of Mortality Data

The primary source of mortality data is derived from the death certificate. Deaths are coded according to the underlying cause. An underlying cause of death is defined as the disease, injury, or precipitating event that initiated the cascade of events leading directly or indirectly to the death or the circumstances surrounding the fatal injury such as violence or accident (National Center for Health Statistics, 1983). Exhibit 7.2 presents a standard U.S. Certificate of Death.

There are several problems encountered with the accuracy of certificate of death information. Some problems are the underlying cause of death listed may not accurately represent the immediate cause of death and other contributing causes of death. The cause of death should be listed with an approximated time interval to the onset of the death. However, this information is sometimes missing from the Certificate of Death. Missing information is a problem with using Certificate of Death as a source of mortality data. Additionally, the causes of death should be coded according to the latest version of the International Classification of Diseases (ICD). Some clinicians do not accurately code the cause of death using the ICD system. Additionally, as the ICD system changes codes with each revision, this impacts the ability to compare causes of death coded over time when the coding system changes.

Alternative Measures of Disease Impact: Quality of Life

Diseases or health alterations have an impact on a person's quality of life prior to death. The quality of life measures the extent to which a disease or health condition causes alterations in an individual's daily life and ability to participate in and contribute to society. Quality of life impact can also impact an individual's productivity and image within society. Some indicators used to determine impact on quality of life are access to clean air and water, soil quality, exposure to natural conditions and hazards, shelter quality, access to and quality of nutrition, education, economic conditions, security and safety, and ability to participate in desired social and leisure activities. The ability to remain actively engaged as a member of society in a productive manner impacts quality of life. Some tools used to measure quality of life are the Quality of Life Scale (QOL), Health-Related Quality of Life (HRQOL), McGill Quality of Life Questionnaire (MQOL), and World Health Organization Quality of Life Scale (WHOQOL-BREF).

Table 7.2 Annual Deaths and Estimates[a] of Smoking-Attributable Mortality (SAM), Years of Potential Life Lost (YPLL), and Productivity Losses, by Sex and Cause of Death—United States, 2000–2004

Causes of Death (ICD-10 Code[b])	Male				Female			
	Deaths	SAM	YPLL	Productivity Losses (in Thousands) ($)	Deaths	SAM	YPLL	Productivity Losses (in Thousands) ($)
Malignant Neoplasm								
Lip, oral cavity, pharynx (C00–C14)	5,126	3,749	65,336	1,613,319	2,494	1,144	19,047	354,635
Esophagus (C15)	9,707	6,961	108,847	2,464,063	2,926	1,631	25,382	43,273
Stomach (C16)	7,056	1,900	27,602	600,702	5,024	584	8,971	157,891
Pancreas (C25)	14,845	3,147	50,201	1,162,577	15,481	3,536	53,334	884,761
Larynx (C32)	2,984	2,446	38,012	853,914	778	563	9,914	186,317
Tracheal/lung/bronchus (C33–C34)	90,025	78,680	1,118,359	23,189,096	66,874	46,842	770,655	13,597,333
Cervix uteri (C53)	0	0	0	0	3,774	447	11,918	307,412
Kidney and renal pelvis (C64–C65)	7,469	2,827	43,898	997,062	4,527	216	3,722	70,680
Urinary bladder (C67)	8,508	3,907	44,166	742,898	3,951	1,076	13,245	174,529
Acute myeloid leukemia (C92.0)	3,889	855	12,527	272,429	3,189	337	5,496	99,772
Subtotal	**149,609**	**104,472**	**1,508,948**	**31,896,060**	**109,018**	**56,376**	**921,684**	**16,266,603**
Cardiovascular Diseases								
Ischemic heart disease (I20–I25)	248,506	50,884	804,551	19,019,062	238,845	29,191	389,974	6,068,242
Other heart disease (I00–I09, I26–I51)	72,312	12,944	55,62	1,134,588	95,304	8,060	31,745	428,084
Cerebrovascular disease (I60–I69)	61,616	7,896	127,280	3,075,304	97,681	8,026	140,894	2,878,017
Atherosclerosis (I70–I71)	5,000	1,282	11,814	155,198	8,430	611	5,475	40,423
Aortic aneurysm (I71)	8,861	5,628	70,512	1,339,220	5,862	2,791	34,192	445,625

(continued)

Table 7.2 Annual Deaths and Estimates[a] of Smoking-Attributable Mortality (SAM), Years of Potential Life Lost (YPLL), and Productivity Losses, by Sex and Cause of Death—United States, 2000–2004 *(continued)*

Cause of Death								
Other circulatory diseases (I72–I79)	4,238	505	6,636	134,357	5,715	749	9,386	133,702
Subtotal	**85,612**	**53,795**	**494,391**	**7,463,057**	**95,277**	**49,543**	**527,255**	**6,350,527**
Respiratory Diseases								
Pneumonia, influenza (J10–J18)	27,517	6,042	29,828	448,507	35,008	4,381	23,438	273,061
Bronchitis, emphysema (J40–J42, J43)	8,321	7,536	42,842	708,007	7,941	6,391	40,844	532,162
Chronic airways obstruction (J44)	49,774	40,217	421,721	6,306,543	52,328	38,771	462,973	5,545,304
Subtotal	**85,612**	**53,795**	**494,391**	**7,463,057**	**95,277**	**49,543**	**527,255**	**6,350,527**
Perinatal Conditions								
Short gestation/low birth weight (P07)	2,557	219	16,315	–	2,030	174	13,898	–
Respiratory distress syndrome (P22)	550	18	1,358	–	382	13	1,007	–
Other respiratory (newborn) (P23–P28)	786	35	2,611	–	556	25	1,983	–
Sudden infant death syndrome (R95)	1,357	173	12,878	–	935	119	9,531	–
Subtotal	**5,250**	**445**	**33,161**	–	**3,903**	**331**	**26,419**	–
Residential Fire	**1,600**	**416**	–	–	**1,270**	**320**	–	–
Secondhand Smoke								
Lung cancer	–	2,131	–	–	–	1,269	–	–
Ischemic heart disease	–	29,256	–	–	–	16,744	–	–
Subtotal	–	**31,388**	–	–	–	**18,012**	–	–
Total	**269,655**		**3,112,914**	**64,216,846**		**173,94**	**2,087,024**	**32,611,223**

[a]CDC estimates from 2000 to 2004 National Health Interview Survey responses and 2000–2004 National Center for Health Statistics death certificate data; smoking-attributable residential fire-related death estimates from 2002 to 2005 data, productivity losses in 2004 dollars.

[b]*International classification of diseases and health conditions, 10th revision.* http://www.who.int/classifications/app/icd/icd10online

Source: From https://www.cdc.gov/mmwr/PDF/wk/mm5745.pdf.

EXHIBIT 7.2. U.S. Standard Certificate of Death

U.S. STANDARD CERTIFICATE OF DEATH

LOCAL FILE NO.　　　　　　　　　　　　　　　　　　　　　　　　　STATE FILE NO.

NAME OF DECEDENT
For use by physician or institution

1. DECEDENT'S LEGAL NAME (Include AKA's if any) (First, Middle, Last)	2. SEX	3. SOCIAL SECURITY NUMBER

To Be Completed/Verified By: FUNERAL DIRECTOR:

4a. AGE-Last Birthday (Years)	4b. UNDER 1 YEAR		4c. UNDER 1 DAY		5. DATE OF BIRTH (Mo/Day/Yr)	6. BIRTHPLACE (City and State or Foreign Country)
	Months	Days	Hours	Minutes		

7a. RESIDENCE-STATE	7b. COUNTY	7c. CITY OR TOWN

7d. STREET AND NUMBER	7e. APT. NO.	7f. ZIP CODE	7g. INSIDE CITY LIMITS? ☐ Yes ☐ No

8. EVER IN US ARMED FORCES? ☐ Yes ☐ No	9. MARITAL STATUS AT TIME OF DEATH ☐ Married ☐ Married, but separated ☐ Widowed ☐ Divorced ☐ Never Married ☐ Unknown	10. SURVIVING SPOUSE'S NAME (If wife, give name prior to first marriage)

11. FATHER'S NAME (First, Middle, Last)	12. MOTHER'S NAME PRIOR TO FIRST MARRIAGE (First, Middle, Last)

13a. INFORMANT'S NAME	13b. RELATIONSHIP TO DECEDENT	13c. MAILING ADDRESS (Street and Number, City, State, Zip Code)

14. PLACE OF DEATH (Check only one: see instructions)

IF DEATH OCCURRED IN A HOSPITAL: ☐ Inpatient ☐ Emergency Room/Outpatient ☐ Dead on Arrival	IF DEATH OCCURRED SOMEWHERE OTHER THAN A HOSPITAL: ☐ Hospice facility ☐ Nursing home/Long term care facility ☐ Decedent's home ☐ Other (Specify):

15. FACILITY NAME (If not institution, give street & number)	16. CITY OR TOWN , STATE, AND ZIP CODE	17. COUNTY OF DEATH

18. METHOD OF DISPOSITION: ☐ Burial ☐ Cremation ☐ Donation ☐ Entombment ☐ Removal from State ☐ Other (Specify):	19. PLACE OF DISPOSITION (Name of cemetery, crematory, other place)

20. LOCATION-CITY, TOWN, AND STATE	21. NAME AND COMPLETE ADDRESS OF FUNERAL FACILITY

22. SIGNATURE OF FUNERAL SERVICE LICENSEE OR OTHER AGENT	23. LICENSE NUMBER (Of Licensee)

ITEMS 24-28 MUST BE COMPLETED BY PERSON WHO PRONOUNCES OR CERTIFIES DEATH

	24. DATE PRONOUNCED DEAD (Mo/Day/Yr)	25. TIME PRONOUNCED DEAD

26. SIGNATURE OF PERSON PRONOUNCING DEATH (Only when applicable)	27. LICENSE NUMBER	28. DATE SIGNED (Mo/Day/Yr)

29. ACTUAL OR PRESUMED DATE OF DEATH (Mo/Day/Yr) (Spell Month)	30. ACTUAL OR PRESUMED TIME OF DEATH	31. WAS MEDICAL EXAMINER OR CORONER CONTACTED? ☐ Yes ☐ No

CAUSE OF DEATH (See instructions and examples)

Approximate interval: Onset to death

32. PART I. Enter the chain of events--diseases, injuries, or complications--that directly caused the death. DO NOT enter terminal events such as cardiac arrest, respiratory arrest, or ventricular fibrillation without showing the etiology. DO NOT ABBREVIATE. Enter only one cause on a line. Add additional lines if necessary.

IMMEDIATE CAUSE (Final disease or condition ⟶ resulting in death)　a._____

Due to (or as a consequence of):_____

Sequentially list conditions, if any, leading to the cause listed on line a. Enter the **UNDERLYING CAUSE** (disease or injury that initiated the events resulting in death) **LAST**
　b._____

Due to (or as a consequence of):_____

　c._____

Due to (or as a consequence of):_____

　d._____

PART II. Enter other significant conditions contributing to death but not resulting in the underlying cause given in PART I	33. WAS AN AUTOPSY PERFORMED? ☐ Yes ☐ No
	34. WERE AUTOPSY FINDINGS AVAILABLE TO COMPLETE THE CAUSE OF DEATH? ☐ Yes ☐ No

To Be Completed By: MEDICAL CERTIFIER

35. DID TOBACCO USE CONTRIBUTE TO DEATH? ☐ Yes ☐ Probably ☐ No ☐ Unknown	36. IF FEMALE: ☐ Not pregnant within past year ☐ Pregnant at time of death ☐ Not pregnant, but pregnant within 42 days of death ☐ Not pregnant, but pregnant 43 days to 1 year before death ☐ Unknown if pregnant within the past year	37. MANNER OF DEATH ☐ Natural ☐ Homicide ☐ Accident ☐ Pending Investigation ☐ Suicide ☐ Could not be determined

38. DATE OF INJURY (Mo/Day/Yr) (Spell Month)	39. TIME OF INJURY	40. PLACE OF INJURY (e.g., Decedent's home; construction site; restaurant; wooded area)	41. INJURY AT WORK? ☐ Yes ☐ No

42. LOCATION OF INJURY: State:		City or Town:
Street & Number:	Apartment No.:	Zip Code:

43. DESCRIBE HOW INJURY OCCURRED:	44. IF TRANSPORTATION INJURY, SPECIFY: ☐ Driver/Operator ☐ Passenger ☐ Pedestrian ☐ Other (Specify)

45. CERTIFIER (Check only one):
☐ Certifying physician-To the best of my knowledge, death occurred due to the cause(s) and manner stated.
☐ Pronouncing & Certifying physician-To the best of my knowledge, death occurred at the time, date, and place, and due to the cause(s) and manner stated.
☐ Medical Examiner/Coroner-On the basis of examination, and/or investigation, in my opinion, death occurred at the time, date, and place, and due to the cause(s) and manner stated.

Signature of certifier:_____

46. NAME, ADDRESS, AND ZIP CODE OF PERSON COMPLETING CAUSE OF DEATH (Item 32)

47. TITLE OF CERTIFIER	48. LICENSE NUMBER	49. DATE CERTIFIED (Mo/Day/Yr)	50. FOR REGISTRAR ONLY- DATE FILED (Mo/Day/Yr)

To Be Completed By: FUNERAL DIRECTOR

51. DECEDENT'S EDUCATION-Check the box that best describes the highest degree or level of school completed at the time of death.	52. DECEDENT OF HISPANIC ORIGIN? Check the box that best describes whether the decedent is Spanish/Hispanic/Latino. Check the "No" box if decedent is not Spanish/Hispanic/Latino.	53. DECEDENT'S RACE (Check one or more races to indicate what the decedent considered himself or herself to be)
☐ 8th grade or less		☐ White
☐ 9th - 12th grade; no diploma	☐ No, not Spanish/Hispanic/Latino	☐ Black or African American
☐ High school graduate or GED completed	☐ Yes, Mexican, Mexican American, Chicano	☐ American Indian or Alaska Native (Name of the enrolled or principal tribe) _____
☐ Some college credit, but no degree		☐ Asian Indian
☐ Associate degree (e.g., AA, AS)	☐ Yes, Puerto Rican	☐ Chinese / ☐ Filipino / ☐ Japanese
☐ Bachelor's degree (e.g., BA, AB, BS)	☐ Yes, Cuban	☐ Korean / ☐ Vietnamese / ☐ Other Asian (Specify)_____
☐ Master's degree (e.g., MA, MS, MEng, MEd, MSW, MBA)	☐ Yes, other Spanish/Hispanic/Latino (Specify) _____	☐ Native Hawaiian / ☐ Guamanian or Chamorro / ☐ Samoan / ☐ Other Pacific Islander (Specify)_____
☐ Doctorate (e.g., PhD, EdD) or Professional degree (e.g., MD, DDS, DVM, LLB, JD)		☐ Other (Specify)_____

54. DECEDENT'S USUAL OCCUPATION (Indicate type of work done during most of working life. DO NOT USE RETIRED).

55. KIND OF BUSINESS/INDUSTRY

REV. 11/2003

END-OF-CHAPTER RESOURCES

SUMMARY POINTS

- Surveillance is an important epidemiologic tool to facilitate the identification and monitoring of health and health alterations in a population.
- Surveillance is defined as the "ongoing, systematic collection, analysis, and interpretation of data that is then disseminated to those responsible for preventing diseases and other health conditions."
- Ongoing surveillance is accomplished through active, passive, or hybrid surveillance methods.
- Active surveillance is when the public health provider actively seeks out the identification of cases.
- Passive surveillance is when the public health provider depends on the healthcare providers and established healthcare system operational procedures and processes to report surveillance information regarding health conditions and reportable conditions.
- A hybrid system uses a combination of both passive and active surveillance methods.
- Sentinel surveillance is a type of surveillance conducted by a single or small number of healthcare facilities that are responsible for collecting data on cases using a specific case definition.
- Notifiable conditions are sometimes referred to as reportable diseases or health conditions.
- Notifiable conditions are required through local, state, territorial, or national laws to be reported to the public health system.
- A case definition is a set of standard criteria for classifying whether an individual has a disease, syndrome, or other health condition.
- There are three types of case definitions—probable, suspected, and confirmed.
- A suspected case may have clinical signs and symptoms that are associated with the condition but may not be specific enough to differentiate one health condition from another.
- A probable case generally has the clinical signs and symptoms along with some type of epidemiologic link such as recent contact with a confirmed case or other supportive laboratory tests.

- A confirmed case meets all the expected standard criteria for the case definition.
- A confirmed case generally has the clinical signs and symptoms, an epidemiologic linkage to a confirmed case, and confirmatory diagnostic test results.
- Outbreak is considered as more cases of a condition than expected occur in a specific location over a specific period of time and frequently may also be within a specific population.
- The multiplicative purposes of an outbreak investigation consist of determining the extent of the population at risk or affected; determining the measure of disease spread; identifying the etiologic agent and/or reservoir; characterizing the relationship between the agent, host, and environment; and determining preventive or treatment measures to limit the morbidity and mortality associated with the respective outbreak.
- Endemic is sometimes referred to as the constant presence or usual prevalence of a disease.
- A hyperendemic disease refers to a persistent, high level of disease occurrence.
- An epidemic is an increase or sudden rise in the number of cases above the expected endemic rate within the population at that time.
- A pandemic describes an epidemic that has spread over several countries and continents, affecting a large number of persons.
- A common source outbreak/epidemic is one in which all the affected individuals/cases are exposed to one agent or host.
- A point source outbreak/epidemic is the term used to refer to an outbreak or epidemic that originates from a focal source that affects a number of individuals during a limited period of time.
- A propagated outbreak or epidemic presents as an initial cluster of cases in which the initial cluster of cases serves as the source for later cases.
- Epidemiologic tools consist of counts, rates, ratios, and proportions.
- Epidemiology is the desire to understand the distribution of illness (morbidity) and death

(mortality) and the determinants of illness (morbidity) and death (mortality) within a population.

- A basic approach to disease exploration consists of the who, when, and where model.
- Morbidity disease occurrence can be expressed as a rate or proportion.
- The two primary measures of morbidity disease occurrence rates are incidence and prevalence.
- The incidence rate of a disease is defined as the number of new cases of a disease or condition occurring within a specific period of time in a population at risk for the disease or condition.
- The prevalence rate is defined as the number of persons in the population within a specific period of time who are affected with the disease or condition.
- The prevalence rate represents both "new and old" cases of a disease or condition.
- Point prevalence is the number of new and old cases (total cases) at a certain point of time.
- Period prevalence is the number of new and old cases (total cases) during a specific time period.
- The prevalence rate can be impacted by the incidence rate, mortality rate, and cure rate of a disease or condition.
- A cure rate for a disease is the number of individuals with a disease who are cured (numerator) divided by the number of persons who have the disease in the specific time period.
- Prevalence is a good measure of disease burden in a population.
- Prevalence is impacted by the duration of an illness.
- Primary data are data collected by the epidemiologist for morbidity analysis.
- Secondary data are data collected and compiled by another individual and used by the epidemiologist to calculate morbidity statistics.
- R_0 provides essential information to understand the potential of an infectious disease to spread within a population.

- R-naught is calculated using three data elements—infectious period of the disease, mode of transmission, and contact rate.
- Death within a population can be expressed as mortality rates.
- The absolute number of individuals dying from a specific disease can be expressed graphically by case count and year of occurrence.
- Crude rates provide a measure for the experience of the entire population.
- Specific rates can be calculated by cause, age, race, sex, or any variable for which there is total and subpopulation data.
- The case-fatality rate provides data on the number of individuals who die from a certain disease within a certain time period.
- The proportionate mortality represents all the deaths that have occurred within the time period and what proportion of the deaths were the result of a specific type of cause or disease.
- Years of productive life lost is a measure of premature death.

EPIDEMIOLOGY CRITICAL REASONING QUESTIONS

1. A new emerging infectious disease has been introduced into the United States. Describe the steps that would be utilized to ensure adequate surveillance and reporting of this disease as it impacts the population's health.
2. Explain the significance of a case definition. What differentiates a probable, presumptive, and confirmed case?
3. Differentiate between incidence rate and prevalence rate.
4. Describe the dynamic relationship between incidence rate, prevalence rate, cure rate, and mortality rate.
5. Explain the potential impact of quarantine and isolation on an infectious disease with a R_0 of 5.
6. Differentiate between a crude and disease-specific mortality rate.
7. What is the difference between a case-fatality rate and a proportionate mortality rate?

ADDITIONAL RESOURCES

	A robust set of instructor resources designed to supplement this text is located at http://connect. springerpub.com/content/book/978-0-8261-8514-3. Qualifying instructors may request access by emailing textbook@springerpub.com.

REFERENCES

CDC. (2021). *Surveillance case definition for current and historical conditions.* https://ndc .services.cdc.gov

Centers for Disease Control and Prevention. (2012). *Principles of epidemiology in public health practice.* Author.

Houlihan, C. & Whiworth, J. (2019). Outbreak science: recent progress in the detection and response to outbreaks of infectious diseases. *Clinical Medicine, 19*(2):140–144. https://doi .org/10.7861/clinicalmedicine.19-2-140.

Murray, J., & Cohen, A. (2017). *Infectious disease surveillance. International Encyclopedia of Public Health* (2nd ed., Vol. 4). World Health Organization.

National Center for Health Statistics. (1983). *Instructions for classifying the underlying cause of death.* Author.

World Health Organization. (2020). *Public health surveillance.* https://www.who.int/ immunization/monitoring_surveillance/ burden/vpd/en/

Chapter 8

DIAGNOSTIC AND SCREENING TESTS: VALIDITY AND RELIABILITY

Demetrius J. Porche

Diagnosis is not the end, but the beginning of practice.
–Martin H. Fischer

CHAPTER COMPETENCIES

At the conclusion of this chapter, the reader will be able to:

1. Differentiate between screening and diagnostic testing
2. Calculate sensitivity and specificity rate
3. Calculate predictive value positive and predictive value negative measures
4. Differentiate the types of reliability measures

ESSENTIAL TERMINOLOGY

- Diagnostic test
- Differential diagnosis
- High-risk screening
- Mass screening
- Predictive value negative
- Predictive value positive
- Reliability
- Screening test
- Sensitivity
- Specificity
- Validity

Testing consists of screening and diagnostic testing, both of which are secondary prevention measures. The actual test used for screening and diagnostic testing is often the same. However, the differentiation is the context and purpose for which the test is conducted. Screening and diagnostic testing are essential components of surveillance systems.

Screening has several meanings. Screening is testing in an asymptomatic population for the presence of a disease or health condition. Screening is also the presumptive identification of an unrecognized disease or health condition in a population by the application of a test, examination, or other procedure. Some common screening tests are blood pressure measurements, skin assessments for melanoma presence, hearing or vision test, annual tuberculosis test, amniocentesis, or capillary blood glucose test. Screening tests target a population without the intent of diagnosis but rather identifying the presence of a disease process. Frequently individuals with a positive finding on a screening test must undergo further testing for differential diagnosing (Centers for Disease Control and Prevention [CDC], 2012) and disease confirmation. Nurses are actively involved in both the implementation of screening tests, screening tests education, and counseling.

Differential diagnosis is the diagnostic process that typically includes administering a diagnostic test to differentiate what conditions are present or not. As a clinician assesses an individual's history and symptoms, the clinician generates multiple possible diagnoses. As the clinician conducts a physical examination and diagnostic test, health conditions are ruled in or out based on the diagnostic test administered. In contrast to screening tests, diagnostic testing is conducted on a specific individual with the intent of confirming the presence of a disease or health condition based on symptomatology or sometimes confirming the presence of a disease or health condition in an asymptomatic individual. Advanced practice nurses are involved in the determination of the most appropriate diagnostic test to facilitate discerning the differential diagnosis that supports the individual's medical history and physical examination.

A screening test can be conducted to assess an entire population. This type of screening test is typically referred to as mass screening. Another approach is to focus the screening test on individuals who are suspected of being at risk for the disease or health condition. This latter approach is known as a high-risk screening approach (CDC, 2012). The recent COVID-19 pandemic has demonstrated the extent to which nursing has planned, implemented, and evaluated mass screening tests for entire communities.

SCREENING PROGRAM CRITERIA

The administration of a screening test has the potential for legal and ethical issues. Testing raises concerns around confidentiality and privacy of the test results. The presence of some diseases and health conditions carries societal stigma. The actual administration of a screening test could pose some potential psychological and physical harm. Good screening programs are developed in a manner in which the individual has autonomy over participation with consideration given to the potential legal and ethical issues. Physical and psychological risk are also minimized. Screening programs must conduct an individual risk versus benefit assessment both at individual, population, and societal levels. The following are considered essential criteria for a screening program; this could be considered the litmus test for nurses determining the appropriateness of developing a screening program:

- High sensitivity and specificity
- High positive predictive value

- The disease that is the focus of the screening test is sufficiently serious as evident in incidence, case fatality, disability, discomfort, and financial cost
- The screening provides evidence of the condition at an early stage of the natural history of the disease (i.e., close to the pre-clinical phase)
- Simply administered and interpreted
- Safe to administer
- Acceptable to the patient in terms of comfort, physical and psychological risk, and pain/ concerns
- Follow-up diagnostic and treatment services are available for referral (Porche, 2004).

TESTING VALIDITY

A valid test has the ability to detect the disease or health condition that it is meant to measure. The validity of the test distinguishes between those individuals who have and those who do not have the disease. There are two components to validity measurement: sensitivity and specificity.

Sensitivity

Sensitivity of a test is the ability to correctly identify those individuals with the disease. A sensitive test correctly detects the presence of a disease in those individuals who actually have the disease. In other words, sensitivity is the proportion of true positives (those who test positive and actually have the disease) among all those who have the disease (true positives and those who test negative but actually have the disease otherwise known as false negatives; Celentano & Szkio, 2018). Table 8.1 defines sensitivity and specificity in terms of true or false positives and true or false negatives. Exhibit 8.1 presents a 2 × 2 contingency table of disease characteristics and screening test results. The formula for sensitivity is:

Table 8.1 Sensitivity and Specificity Terminology

Term	Definition
True positive	Test result is positive and individual actually has disease
False positive	Test result is positive but the individual does not have the disease
True negative	Test result is negative and the individual actually does not have the disease
False negative	Test result is negative and the individual actually has the disease

Sensitivity =

$$\frac{\text{True positives}}{\text{True positives + False negatives}} \times 100$$

A sensitivity exemplar explanation is described in Exhibit 8.2. A screening test was administered to a population of 1,000 individuals. Of these 1,000 individuals, 120 individuals have the disease. Of these 120 individuals with the disease, 80 tested positive and actually had the disease present (true positive). However, 40 individuals tested negative but actually had the disease (false negative). Therefore, the sensitivity of this test was 66.6%. Table 8.1 presents a summary of important terms.

A test with 90% sensitivity means that 90% of the individuals screened by the test will have a "true positive" result with 10% having a "false negative" result.

Specificity

Specificity of a test is the ability to correctly identify those who do not have the disease. A specific test correctly does not detect the presence of a disease in those individuals who actually do not have the disease. In other words, sensitivity is the proportion of true negatives (those who test negative and do not have the disease) among all those who do not have the disease (true negatives and those who test positive but actually do not have the disease otherwise known as false positives; Celentano & Szkio, 2018). Exhibit 8.1 presents a 2 × 2 contingency table of disease characteristics and screening test results. The formula for specificity is:

Specificity =

$$\frac{\text{True negatives}}{\text{True negatives + False positives}} \times 100$$

A specificity exemplar is presented in Exhibit 8.2. A population of 1,000 individuals

---

EXHIBIT 8.1. 2 × 2 Contingency Table of Disease Characteristics and Screening Test Results

	True Disease Characteristics in the Population	
Results of Screening Test	Disease Present	Disease Not Present
Positive	True positive (a)	False positive (b)
Negative	False negative (c)	True negative (d)

Sensitivity = True positives ÷ True positives + False negatives

Or

Sensitivity = $a \div a + c$

Specificity = True negatives ÷ True negatives + False positives

Or

Specificity = $d \div d + b$

EXHIBIT 8.2. Sensitivity and Specificity Exemplar

	True Disease Characteristic in the Population		
Results of Screening	Disease Present	Disease Not Present	Totals
Positive	80	220	300
Negative	40	660	700
Totals	120	880	1,000

Sensitivity:

80 ÷ 120 = 66.6%

Specificity:

660 ÷ 880 = 75%

Table 8.2 Sensitivity and Specificity Dynamics

Screening Test Result	True Diagnosis		
	Disease Present	Disease Not Present	Total
Positive	True positives	False positives	True positives + False positives
Negative	False negatives	True negatives	False negatives + True negatives
Total	True positives + False negatives	False positives + True negatives	True positives + False positives + False negatives + True negatives

were tested. Of these 1,000 individuals, 880 do not have the disease. Of these 880 individuals without the disease, 660 tested negative (true negative). However, 220 individuals tested positive but do not have the disease (false positive). Therefore, the specificity of the test is 75%.

A 90% specificity means that 90% of the persons without the disease will have a "true negative" result and 10% of those without the disease will have a "false positive" and be wrongly diagnosed with the disease.

Table 8.2 presents a summary of the dynamics of sensitivity and specificity occurring within a population. A summary of the population-based formulas for sensitivity and specificity are presented.

POSITIVE PREDICTIVE VALUE

Whereas the sensitivity is a measure of whether the test is positive in an individual who actually has the disease, the positive predictive value (PPV) is a measure of the frequency in which the test results represent the correct identification of the disease among those individuals screened—a population measurement, not an individual measurement. The PPV is the proportion of those individuals who tested positive who have the disease among those screened. The PPV is dependent upon the prevalence of a disease within a population. The higher the prevalence of a disease, the higher the PPV. As the prevalence of disease in a population decreases, the PPV will decrease (Celentano & Szkio, 2018). The formula for PPV is:

$$\text{Positive predictive value } (\text{PPV}) = \frac{\text{True positives}}{\text{True positives + False positives}} \times 100$$

NEGATIVE PREDICTIVE VALUE

Negative predictive value (NPV) of a test is the proportion of individuals of those screened who test negative who do not have the disease. As the prevalence of a disease decreases in a population the negative predictive value will increase (Celentano & Szkio, 2018). The formula for NPV of disease is:

$$\text{Negative predictive value } (\text{NPV}) = \frac{\text{True negative}}{\text{True negative + False negative}} \times 100$$

Exhibit 8.3 presents a 2 × 2 contingency table for predictive values. Exhibit 8.4 presents an exemplar for PPV and NPV calculations.

Nurses must be familiar with each screening and diagnostic test sensitivity, specificity, PPV and PVN values. This information is used to educate and counsel the patient and community regarding the performance of the test in measuring the presence of the disease or health condition at the individual level and how well the test performs at the population level.

POSITIVITY RATE

The positivity rate is the number of positive test results out of the total number of tests administered. The formula for positivity rate is:

$$\text{Positivity} = \frac{\text{Number of positive test results}}{\text{Total number of tests conducted}} \times 100$$

For example, there were 1,000 tests conducted to detect a novel coronavirus. Of those 1,000 tests conducted, 825 test results were positive.

EXHIBIT 8.3. 2 × 2 Contingency Table for Predictive Values

True Disease Characteristic in the Population

Results of Screening Test	Disease Present	Disease Not Present
Positive	True positive (a)	False positive (b)
Negative	False negative (c)	True negative (d)

Predictive value positive = True positive ÷ True positive + False positive

Or

Predictive value positive = $a ÷ a + b$
Predictive value negative = True negative ÷ True negative + False negative

Or

Predictive value negative = $d ÷ d + c$

EXHIBIT 8.4. Predictive Value Positive and Predictive Value Negative Calculations Exemplar

True Disease Characteristic in the Population

Results of Screening Test	Disease Present	Disease Not Present	
Positive	800 (a)	4,000 (b)	12,000
Negative	200 (c)	95,000 (d)	95,200
	1,000	99,000	

Predictive value positive = True positive ÷ True positive + False positive

Or

Predictive value positive = 800 ÷ 800 + 4,000 × 100 or 800/12,000 × 100 = 6.66%
Predictive value negative = True negative ÷ True negative + False negative

Or

Predictive value negative = 95,000 ÷ 95,000 + 200 × 100 or 95,000/95,200 × 100 = 99.7%

Table 8.3 Sensitivity, Specificity, and Predictive Value: Zika Virus Infection, Singapore August 26 to September 5, 2016

Performance of case definitions for diagnosing Zika virus infection in a human cohort during an outbreak, Singapore, August 26 to September 5, 2016

Case Definition	Sensitivity, %	Specificity, %	PPV, %	NPV, %	LR+ (95% CI)	LR– (95% CI)
United States	100	2	42	100	1.02 (1.00–1.04)	0
WHO	38	70	47	61	1.3 (0.9–1.7)	0.9 (0.8–1.0)
PAHO	49	76	59	68	2.1 (1.5–2.8)	0.7 (0.6–0.8)
ECDC	56	74	60	70	2.1 (1.6–2.8)	0.6 (0.5–0.7)
Singapore MOH	54	76	61	70	2.2 (1.7–3.0)	0.6 (0.5–0.7)

ECDC, European Centre for Disease Prevention and Control; LR, likelihood ratio; MOH, Ministry of Health; NPV, negative predictive value; PAHO, Pan American Health Organization; PPV, positive predictive value; WHO, World Health Organization; +, positive; –, negative.

Source: From Chow, A., Ho, H. J., Win, M., & Leo, Y. (2017). Assessing sensitivity and specificity of surveillance case definitions for Zika virus disease. *Emerging Infectious Diseases*, 23(4), 677–679. https://dx.doi.org/10.3201/eid2304.161716

Therefore, the novel coronavirus positivity rate is 825/1,000 × 100 = 82.5%. This means that 82.5% of all tests conducted were positive for the novel coronavirus. Table 8.3 summarizes the impact of case definitions on the reporting of sensitivity, specificity, and predictive value rates. The actual test along with the case definition impacts the reported test sensitivity, specificity, and predictive value calculations. It is important to know the case definition used to identify or diagnose a case before solely relying on the sensitivity, specificity, and predictive value data to determine the effectiveness of a screening or diagnostic test.

TESTING INTERPRETATION

Screening and diagnostic tests can be binary or continuous. A test that produces either a positive or negative result is considered a binary or dichotomous test result. A continuous test measures a continuous variable that varies over time. Examples of continuous tests are blood pressure, heart rate, or blood glucose levels. For a continuous test, there are no "positive" or "negative" test results or binary/dichotomous test labeling.

For continuous test results, a decision point must be established as a cut-off level from which to interpret the test result as characteristic or not characteristic of the disease presence. This cut-off level forms the basis of interpreting the test as positive or negative for the disease.

Sometimes interpretation of the test relies upon use of multiple tests. These multiple tests can be administered at the same time (simultaneously) or one after the other (sequentially). Typically, a combination of tests is used as a means of enhancing the test sensitivity.

Simultaneous Testing

Simultaneous testing uses two tests for a disease at the same time. The goal of using the two simultaneous test methods is to increase the net sensitivity and specificity to the maximum potential. In simultaneous testing, there is a net gain in sensitivity but a net loss in specificity compared with either test administered alone.

Net Sensitivity With Simultaneous Testing

The net sensitivity with simultaneous administration of two tests at the same time is calculated with those individuals who test positive with both tests (Exhibit 8.5 and Figure 8.1). The net sensitivity with simultaneous testing is calculated by first determining the sensitivity for both screening tests separately, Novel Test A and Novel Test B, for this hypothetical exemplar. To

---

EXHIBIT 8.5. Net Sensitivity and Specificity

Novel Test A	Novel Test B
Sensitivity = 75%	Sensitivity = 88%
Specificity = 63%	Specificity = 94%

Screening Test 1 (Novel Test A)

Test Results	Disease Present	Disease Absent	Total
Positive	150	300	450
Negative	50	500	550
Total	200	800	1,000

Sensitivity = $a \div a + c$ OR $150 \div 150 + 50 = 75\%$
Specificity = $d \div d + b$ OR $500 \div 500 + 300 = 62.5\%$ or 63%

Screening Test 2 (Novel Test B)

Test Results	Disease Present	Disease Absent	Total
Positive	175	50	225
Negative	25	750	775
Total	200	800	1,000

Sensitivity = $a \div a + c$ OR $175 \div 175 + 25 = 87.5\%$ or 88%
Specificity = $d \div d + b$ OR $750 \div 750 + 50 = 93.75\%$ or 94%

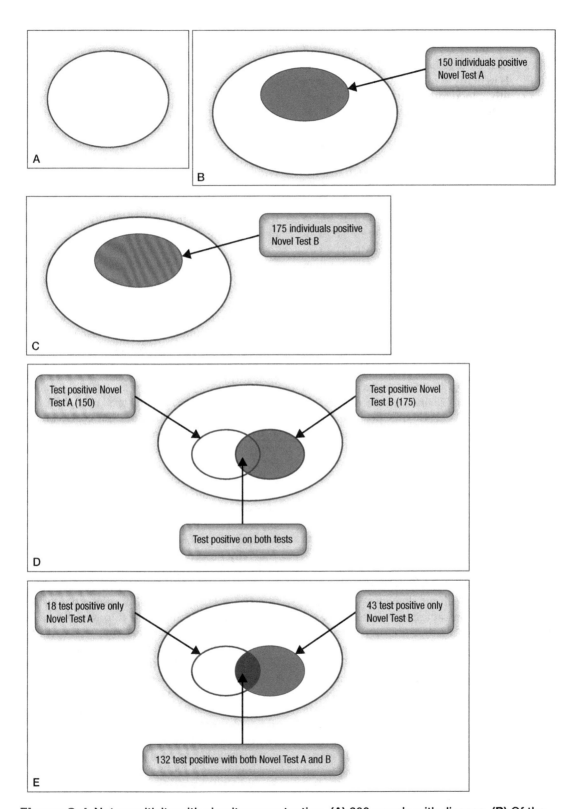

Figure 8.1 Net sensitivity with simultaneous testing. **(A)** 200 people with disease. **(B)** Of the 200 with disease, 150 test positive for Novel Test A. **(C)** Of the 200 people with disease, 175 test positive for Novel Test B. **(D)** Testing positive on both tests. **(E)** Breakdown of the 200 with disease. Net sensitivity = 18 + 132 + 43 / 200 or 96.5% or 97%.

calculate the net sensitivity for Novel Test A and Novel Test B, the sensitivity for both tests cannot simply be added together, since there are some individuals in both Novel Test A and B that have tested positive; therefore, adding the two sensitivities together would count the individuals who tested positive on both tests twice.

To calculate the net sensitivity for both Novel Test A and Novel Test B, we must identify those individuals who tested positive by each test exclusively. Novel Test A has a sensitivity of 75%, identifying 75% of the 200 individuals with the disease (150 individuals). Novel Test B has a sensitivity of 88%; therefore, it identified 88% of the same 150 individuals who were identified by Novel Test A (132 individuals). Therefore, when Novel Test A and B are used simultaneously, 132 individuals are correctly identified as positive by both tests.

As stated earlier, Novel Test A identified 150 individuals as positive who have the disease. Since 132 individuals were identified by both tests, then Novel Test A correctly identified only 150 minus 132 or 18 individuals. Novel Test B correctly identified 175 individuals of the 200 individuals with the disease as positive. Since 132 individuals were identified by both tests, 175 minus 132, or 43 individuals were correctly identified as having only Novel Test B. Thus, the net sensitivity is 97%; refer to the following formula.

$$\text{Net sensitivity} = \frac{18+132+43}{200}$$

$$= \frac{193}{200} = 96.5\% \text{ or } 97\%$$

Net Specificity With Simultaneous Testing

The net specificity with simultaneous administration of two tests at the same time is calculated with those individuals who test negative with both tests (Exhibit 8.5 and Figure 8.2). The net specificity with simultaneous testing is calculated by first determining the specificity for both screening tests separately, that is, Novel Test A and Novel Test B, for this hypothetical exemplar. To calculate the net specificity for Novel Test A and Novel Test B, the specificity for both tests cannot simply be added together, since there are some individuals in both Novel Test A and Novel Test B that tested negative; therefore, adding the two specificities together would count these individuals twice.

To calculate the net specificity for both Novel Test A and Novel Test B, we must identify those individuals who tested negative by each test. Novel Test A has a specificity of 63%, identifying 63% of the 800 individuals without the disease (500 individuals). Novel Test B has a specificity of 94%; therefore, it identified 94% of the same 800 individuals who do not have the disease (750 individuals). To be considered negative in simultaneous testing, only those who test negative on both tests are considered negative results. Novel Test B identified as negative 94% of the same 500 individuals identified as negative with Novel Test A (470 individuals). Thus, when Novel Test A and B are used simultaneously, 470 individuals are identified as negative by both tests. Therefore, the net specificity for simultaneous testing is:

$$\text{Net specificity} = \frac{470}{800} = 58.7\% \text{ or } 59\%$$

In this hypothetical exemplar, there is a net loss in specificity compared to each test used alone (Novel Test A = 63% and Novel Test B = 94%).

Sequential Testing

Sequential testing administers two tests, one after the other. Sequential testing is also known as two-stage testing. Frequently, the first test administered is less invasive, less expensive, more comfortable (less invasive), and easy to interpret. Those individuals who screen positive on the first test are recalled for the administration of a second test. The second test may be more expensive, more invasive, and more uncomfortable. The second test in the sequential test generally has greater sensitivity and specificity than the first test administered in the sequence. Sequential testing is developed to reduce the number of false positives. In sequential testing, there is generally a net loss in sensitivity but a net gain in specificity as compared with the results of either test alone (Celentano & Szkio, 2018). Exhibit 8.6 describes the gain and loss of net sensitivity and specificity with a hypothetical test administered sequentially.

In this hypothetical scenario, of the 10,000 individuals tested with both Novel Test A and B, 31 people of the 500 actual diseased individuals were correctly identified as positive, a 63% net sensitivity (loss). Of the 9,500 who never had the disease, 7,600 were correctly classified as negative by the first test and were not tested with the second test. However, an additional 1,710 of those 9,500 individuals were correctly classified as negative by the second test. Therefore, 7,600 + 1,710 / 9,500 × 100 results in a 98% specificity gain.

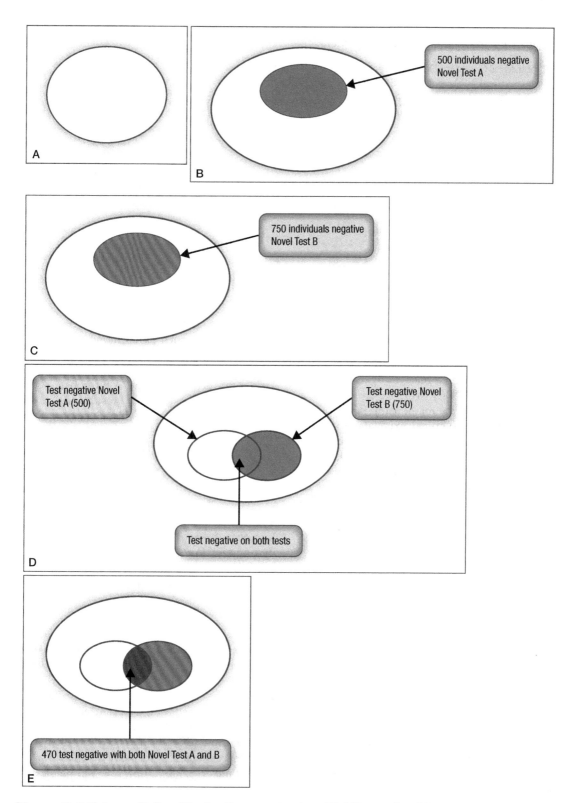

Figure 8.2 Net specificity with simultaneous testing. **(A)** 800 people without disease. **(B)** Of the 800 people without disease, 500 test negative for Novel Test A. **(C)** Of the 800 people without disease, 750 test negative for Novel Test B. **(D)** Testing negative on both tests. **(E)** Breakdown of the 800 people without disease. Net specificity = 470 / 800 = 58.7% or 58%.

EXHIBIT 8.6. Sequential (Two Stage) Testing

Hypothetical Scenario: Disease Prevalence Is 5%, Population Size Is 10,000
Screening Test 1 (Novel Test A) Sensitivity = 70%, Specificity = 80%

Test Results	Disease Present	Disease Absent	Total
Positive	350	1,900	2,250
Negative	150	7,600	7,750
Total	500	9,500	10,000

Screening Test 2 (Novel Test B) Sensitivity = 90%, Specificity = 90%

Test Results	Disease Present	Disease Absent	Total
Positive	315	190	2,250
Negative	35	1,710	7,750
Total	350	1,900	10,000

Receiver-Operating Characteristic Curve

The most precise method to determine a cut-score for a disease is using a receiver-operating characteristic curve (ROC). The ROC curve is a graphic display of the relationship between the true positive rate (vertical axis) and the false positive rate (horizontal axis). A ROC curve is used to determine the critical cut-off value for the presence or absence of a disease. Figures 8.3 and 8.4 present ROC for anthrax. These figures demonstrate the impact of cut-off score determination on the interpretation of test results as positive or negative.

TEST RELIABILITY

Reliability is the consistency with which a test accurately measures a characteristic over time. Reliability of test results is dependent upon consistent procedures for test administration and specific criteria for test interpretation. Variations in test administration and interpretation can negatively impact the reliability of a test result. Table 8.4 presents the different types of reliability measures that can impact screening and diagnostic test reliability.

Reliability is also influenced by intrasubject variability. Some characteristics measured in humans vary over time and some biological indicator measures have temporal variations during the day such as hormone secretion. In addition, many physiological measures such as heart rate and blood pressure vary over time and with environmental conditions. Therefore, the interpretation of all test results should factor into consideration intrasubject variability and other factors that can influence interpretation such as test administration and test interpretation.

Percent Agreement: Interobserver Agreement

Interobserver variation can impact the reliability of a test. Percent agreement is a measure of reliability among multiple observers. Exhibit 8.7 presents the formula for percent agreement.

Kappa Statistic

The Kappa statistic is used to evaluate interobserver reliability. It is a measure of interobserver agreement compared to the expected level of agreement by chance alone. The Kappa statistic measures the extent to which the observed agreement exceeds the expected agreement by chance alone. The Kappa quantifies the extent to which two different observer agreements exceed the expected agreement by chance alone (Celentano & Szkio, 2018). The Kappa statistic formula is:

$$Kappa = \frac{(Percent\ agreement\ observed) - (Percent\ agreement\ expected\ by\ chance\ alone)}{100\% - (Percent\ agreement\ expected\ by\ chance\ alone)}$$

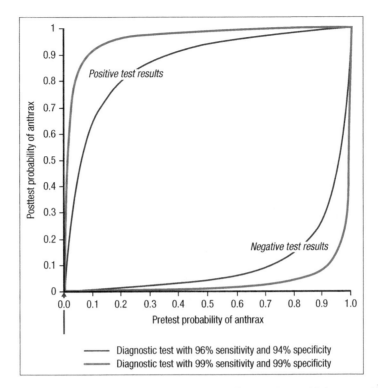

Figure 8.3 Receiver-operating curve (ROC): Anthrax. Effect of sensitivity, specificity, and pretest probability on posttest probability of anthrax being present. Upper curves show the posttest probability of anthrax being present after a positive detection or diagnostic test result. Lower curves show the posttest probability of anthrax being present after a negative detection or diagnostic test result. Separate curves are drawn for two diagnostic tests described in the text: one with 99% sensitivity and 99% specificity (blue line) and another with 96% sensitivity and 94% specificity (black line). The arrow marks a pretest probability of disease of 0.0014, which relates to the example described in the text.

Source: From Bravata, D. M., Sundaram, V., McDonald, K. M., Smith, W. M., Szeto, H., Schleinitz, M. D., & Owens, D. K. (2004). Evaluating detection and diagnostic decision support systems for bioterrorism response. *Emerging Infectious Diseases*, *10*(1), 100–108. https://dx.doi.org/10.3201/eid1001.030243

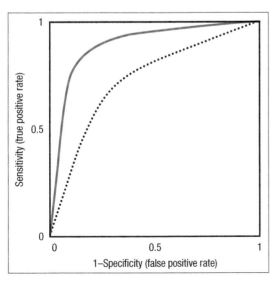

Figure 8.4 Receiver-operating curves (ROC) test interpretation impact on sensitivity and specificity. Each point along an ROC represents the trade-off in sensitivity and specificity, depending on the threshold for an abnormal test. Here, two hypothetical diagnostic tests are compared. The diagnostic test represented by the unbroken ROC curve is a better test than that represented by the broken ROC curve, as demonstrated by its greater sensitivity for any given specificity (and thus, greater area under the curve).

Source: From Bravata, D. M., Sundaram, V., McDonald, K. M., Smith, W. M., Szeto, H., Schleinitz, M. D., & Owens, D. K. (2004). Evaluating detection and diagnostic decision support systems for bioterrorism response. *Emerging Infectious Diseases*, *10*(1), 100–108. https://dx.doi.org/10.3201/eid1001.030243

Table 8.4 Types of Reliability

Type	Definition
Test–retest reliability	Consistent correlation of two test results on the same sample at two different time periods
Interrater reliability	Consistent correlation of two test results completed by two or more individuals on the same sample
Intrarater reliability	Consistent correlation of two test results completed by the same individual at two different time periods
Internal reliability	Consistency of results across several items within a test
External reliability	Consistency of a test result from one use to another use
Parallel forms reliability	Consistent correlation of test results between two tests constructed to measure the same domain or disease that are constructed and administered in a similar manner
Split half reliability	Items on a test are divided into two sets, the test is administered to the sample population in the same manner. The consistent correlation of the total score of the two sets of items are the split half reliability
Item to total reliability	An internal measure of reliability, the extent to which each item on the test consistently correlates to the total test score

EXHIBIT 8.7. Percent Agreement: Two Observers and Formula

Observer 1

	Positive	Negative
Observer 2		

Positive	A	B
Negative	C	D

$$\text{Percent Agreement} = \frac{A + D}{A + B + C + D} \times 100$$

Table 8.5 presents guidelines for Kappa statistic interpretation.

Table 8.5 Kappa Interpretation

Kappa Value	Agreement Interpretation
<0	Less than chance agreement
0.01–0.20	Slight agreement
0.21–0.40	Fair agreement
0.41–0.60	Moderate agreement
0.61–0.80	Substantial agreement
0.81–0.99	Almost perfect agreement
1	Perfect agreement

Source: From Viera, A., & Garrett, J. (2005). Understanding interobserver agreement: The Kappa statistic. *Family Medicine, 37*(5) 360–363.

END-OF-CHAPTER RESOURCES

SUMMARY POINTS

- Testing consists of screening and diagnostic testing.
- Screening is referred to as testing in an asymptomatic population for the presence of a disease or health condition.
- Differential diagnosis is the diagnostic process that typically includes administering a diagnostic test to differentiate what conditions are present or not.
- Diagnostic testing is conducted on a specific individual with the intent of confirming the presence of a disease or health condition based on symptomatology or sometimes confirming the presence of a disease or health condition in an asymptomatic individual.
- Mass screening is conducted to assess an entire population.
- High-risk screening tests individuals who are suspected of being at risk for a disease.
- Good screening programs are developed in a manner in which the individual has autonomy over participation with consideration given to the potential legal and ethical issues.
- A valid test has the ability to detect the disease or health condition that it is meant to measure.
- The validity of the test distinguishes between those individuals who have and those who do not have the disease.
- Sensitivity of a test is the ability to correctly identify those individuals with the disease.
- Specificity of a test is the ability to correctly identify those who do not have the disease.
- The positive predictive value (PPV) is a measure of the frequency which the test results represent the correct identification of the disease among those individuals screened – a population, not individual measurement.
- The higher the prevalence of a disease, the higher the PPV.
- As the prevalence of disease in a population decreases, the PPV will decrease.
- Negative predictive value (NPV) of a test is the proportion of individuals of those screened who test negative who do not have the disease.

- As the prevalence of a disease decreases in a population, the NPV will increase
- The positivity rate is the number of positive test results out of the total number of tests administered.
- Reliability is the consistency with which a test accurately measures a characteristic over time.
- Reliability of a test result is dependent upon consistent procedures for test administration and specific criteria for test interpretation.

EPIDEMIOLOGY CRITICAL REASONING QUESTIONS

1. Describe the characteristics of a good screening test.
2. Differentiate test validity and reliability.
3. Calculate the sensitivity and specificity of the test results in Table 8.6:

Table 8.6 Sensitivity and Specificity Calculation

Results of Screening	True Disease Characteristic in the Population		
	Disease Present	Disease Not Present	Totals
Positive	70	400	470
Negative	30	500	530
Totals	100	900	1,000

4. Calculate the predictive value positive and PVN using the information provided in Table 8.7:

Table 8.7 Predictive Value Calculation

Results of Screening Test	True Disease Characteristic in the Population		
	Disease Present	Disease Not Present	
Positive	300	3,500	3,800
Negative	700	95,500	96,200
	1,000	99,000	

5. Using the information provided in Exhibit 8.8, calculate the net sensitivity and net specificity of a Novel Test A and B.

EXHIBIT 8.8

Novel Test A	Novel Test B
Sensitivity = 80%	Sensitivity = 90%
Specificity = 60%	Specificity = 90%

Screening Test 1 (Novel Test A)

Test Results	Disease Present	Disease Absent	Total
Positive	160	320	480
Negative	40	480	520
Total	200	800	1,000

Screening Test 2 (Novel Test B)

Test Results	Disease Present	Disease Absent	Total
Positive	180	80	260
Negative	20	720	740
Total	200	800	1,000

ADDITIONAL RESOURCES

 A robust set of instructor resources designed to supplement this text is located at http://connect. springerpub.com/content/book/978-0-8261-8514-3. Qualifying instructors may request access by emailing textbook@springerpub.com.

REFERENCES

Celentano, D., & Szkio, M. (2018). *Gordis epidemiology* (6th ed.). Elsevier.

Centers for Disease Control and Prevention. (2012). *Principles of epidemiology in public health practice*. CDC.

Porche, D. (2004). *Community and public health nursing practice: A population-based approach*. Sage.

Chapter 9

RISK ASSESSMENT AND ESTIMATION

Demetrius J. Porche

CHAPTER COMPETENCIES

At the conclusion of this chapter, the reader will be able to:

1. Describe the steps of a risk assessment
2. Calculate a relative risk
3. Calculate an odds ratio
4. Calculate an attributable risk

ESSENTIAL TERMINOLOGY

- Attributable risk
- Ecological risk assessment
- Human health risk assessment
- Modifiable risk factor
- Nonmodifiable risk factor
- Odds ratio
- Prognosis
- Risk
- Risk analysis
- Risk assessment
- Risk assessment matrix
- Risk communication
- Relative risk
- Risk factor
- Risk management

Epidemiologic investigations provide evidence regarding the linkage between an exposure and the occurrence of a disease or health condition. This epidemiologic investigation also provides evidence as to the magnitude of risk associated with the exposure as compared to the extent to which the exposure's relationship to the disease or health condition occurred by chance alone. Risk can be defined as the probability or likelihood that an adverse health event will occur in an individual or population. Nurses, as healthcare providers, educate patients on the risk associated with lifestyle behaviors and exposures to various disease-causing agents. During the

nursing assessment, various types of risks can be further investigated and explored to determine an individual level risk profile.

Risk analysis is an overall term used for risk science. Risk science consists of four elements: risk assessment or risk evaluation, risk communication, risk perception, and risk management. Risk assessment or risk evaluation is the understanding of the health effects of a risk agent on humans. Risk assessment consists of the four steps described in the following. This chapter focuses on risk, risk assessment, and epidemiologic risk measurement.

Risk analysis or risk assessment attempts to determine the risk factors and magnitude of risk that exist. Risk factors are the characteristics or events that are associated with an increased probability or likelihood of an adverse health event occurring. Risk factors may be related to or associated with an adverse health event without being directly the cause of the adverse health event. Common risk factor categories are biologic, behavioral or lifestyle, stressors, or environmental exposures. Risk factors are also categorized as modifiable and nonmodifiable. Modifiable risk factors are those that can be altered such as behavior or lifestyle (e.g., cigarette smoking, lack of exercise). Nonmodifiable risk factors are age, race/ethnicity, and biological sex (this can also be considered modifiable in some populations). Nursing education is generally focused on modifiable risk factors.

A related but different concept to risk is prognosis. Prognosis is considered the prediction of the future course of a disease after disease onset. Prognosis is a frequently asked question of healthcare providers. Prognosis is assessed through cohort studies. A distinction between risk and prognosis is that risk increases the propensity of developing a disease, whereas prognostic factors indicate the course that the disease takes once it has already developed. Prognostic factors are associated with the disease outcome. For risk, the event being measured epidemiologically is the occurrence of disease. For prognosis, epidemiologists measure the consequences of having a disease over time. Figure 9.1 distinguishes risk and prognosis.

RISK ASSESSMENTS/EVALUATION

Risk assessments are conducted in various settings to determine the risk factors associated with an exposure and the potential impact of an exposure to a disease or health condition occurrence. Nurses are active in the risk assessment and evaluation process. The risk assessment attempts to characterize the nature and magnitude of the health risk to humans associated with a risk agent. Three factors that impact the risk assessment findings are the amount of the risk agent present, the extent of exposure to the risk agent, and the toxicity or infectiousness of the risk agent. Risk assessments are categorized as human health or ecological. A human risk assessment attempts to determine the potential risk of a "risk agent" to cause a health concern in humans. An ecological risk assessment is more expansive, measuring the potential risk posed by a risk agent to humans and all living organisms in the environment.

Most risk assessments are of a quantitative nature. The risk assessment process involves four steps: hazard identification, exposure assessment, dose–response assessment, and risk characterization. These steps are described in the following and presented in Figure 9.2. Nurminen et al. (1999) propose that these four steps of risk assessment are related to four epidemiologic strategies to influence the risks: descriptive epidemiology, molecular epidemiology, analytic epidemiology, and intervention epidemiology.

Epidemiologists develop a risk assessment matrix to measure the size and scope of the risk, to determine appropriate epidemiologic preventive and control measures to minimize the risk, and to determine methods to triage or prioritize risks. A risk assessment matrix can be used as a communication tool to advance the understanding of potential risk (Burns et al., 2019). A risk assessment matrix can be developed by identifying the risk universe (identify all potential risk in the setting or population), determining the risk criteria, assessing the risks, and prioritizing the risks. In the identification of the risk universe, the epidemiologist examines the full scope of risks present within the setting or population. The determination of risk criteria characterizes the risk along two main criteria, likelihood (level of possibility) and consequence (level of impact) of the risk agent exposure to cause an adverse occurrence. Once the risk criteria have been determined, the next step is to assess the risk of each potential risk agent. After the risk agents are assessed, the levels of risk are prioritized for the possibility of occurrence, potential impact, and importance of risk. The risk assessment matrix facilitates the decision-making around risk mitigation interventions. The typical decisions are to accept the risk as tolerable; to reduce the risk; to share the risk to reduce impact on specific individuals, groups, or settings; to avoid the risk; or to attempt risk elimination.

Human Health Risk Assessment

The human risk assessment process utilizes the four risk assessment steps identified: hazard identification, exposure assessment, dose–response assessment, and risk characterization.

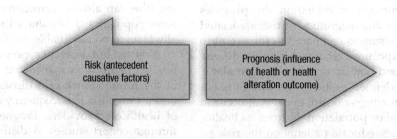

Figure 9.1 Risk and prognosis distinguished.

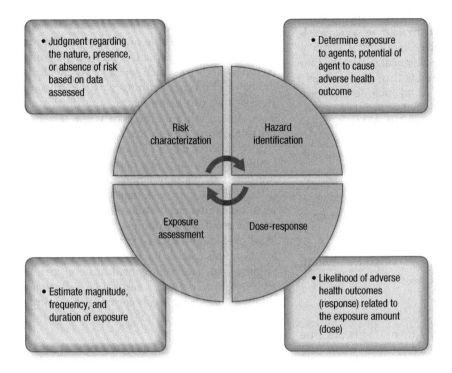

Figure 9.2 Risk assessment process.

The epidemiologist specifically attempts to determine the following:

1. Who, what, and where is the risk? Individual level, population level, segment of the population at risk, age groups at risk?
2. What is the "risk agent" or hazard of concern? Physical, mental, chemical, or biological?
3. What is the origin of the risk agent or hazard? Is there a point source, propagated source?
4. What is/are the route(s) of exposure? Mode of transmission, portal of entry?
5. What is the physiological response to risk agent exposure? Is the agent absorbed, distributed throughout the body, or localized or concentrated in specific tissue, metabolized, or excreted?
6. What are the pathophysiological changes?
7. What amount of the agent is required to initiate pathophysiological changes?
8. What is the minimum time period for the agent to cause a toxic effect or signs/symptoms? (Environmental Protection Agency [EPA], 2017a)

Ecological Risk Assessment

The ecological risk assessment encompasses the human health risk assessment questions. In addition, the ecological risk assessment explores the following additional information:

1. What other living species are impacted? Where are these living species impacted?
2. What ecological effects are impacting the species' mortality rates, reproductive rates?
3. What extent has the risk impacted the ecological life cycle? (EPA, 2016)

Workplace Risk Assessment

A workplace risk assessment can be conducted in five easy steps. The workplace risk assessment steps are:

1. Determine the identification of potential workplace hazards. Workplace hazards can be categorized as physical, mental, chemical, and biological. In the workplace, the physical hazards could be noise, dust exposure, awkward working postures, physical environmental dangers such as wet

surfaces. Mental hazards could be the work culture, excessive workload or long work hours, and workplace incivility. Chemical hazards can be any chemical substance that the worker is exposed to during their work. Biological hazards could include exposure to environmental biological agents or exposure to individuals with active infections for healthcare workers.

2. Determine epidemiologically who is at risk for harm and the route of potential harm.
3. Assess the level of risk and implement necessary actions.
4. Document workplace risk assessment findings and outcomes.
5. Conduct a postmortem on the risk assessment to determine areas for quality improvement.

Superfund Risk Assessment

A superfund risk assessment evaluates the threatening nature of a hazardous waste site to humans and the environment. The purpose of the superfund risk assessment is to determine a safe level for each potentially dangerous contaminant present at the superfund site. A superfund risk assessment includes both a human health risk assessment and ecological risk assessment (EPA, 2018). More information on conducting a superfund risk assessment can be accessed at: https://www.epa.gov/risk/superfund-risk-assessment#:~:text=%20Superfund%20Risk%20Assessment%20%20 1%20Basic%20Superfund,provides%20technical %20information%20and%20addresses%20 ecological...%20More%20.

RISK COMMUNICATION

Risk communication informs individuals about the potential hazard of exposure to their person, property, or community. Risk communication generally occurs in a high stress and high concern situational context, especially if there has been a recent environmental or accidental exposure to an agent. Risk communication engages all forms of communication—written, verbal, and visual. The risk communicator is challenged to place the particular risk within a situational context while providing comparative information to gauge an individual's level of risk. The risk communicator may also be challenged with providing risk reduction information to the population.

RISK MANAGEMENT

Risk management is the process of determining how to protect the public. Risk management includes decisions such as determining levels of chemical discharged into water supply; substances that can be stored at hazardous waste sites; determining the need of waste site clean up; establishing permit levels for discharge, storage, or transportation of chemicals; establishing ambient air quality standards; and determining levels of contamination in drinking water (EPA, 2017b). These risk management decisions must take into consideration the scientific information available; economic factors; laws and legal precedents; social factors such as income level, ethnic/racial backgrounds, community values, land use, zoning, healthcare access, life styles, technological factors, political climate, public values, and psychological impact on the population.

RELATIVE AND ATTRIBUTABLE RISK

Association measures quantify the relationship between an exposure and a disease or health occurrence. Measures of association compare the occurrence of a disease or health condition to another group.

In risk assessment, it is important to remember that incidence rate is also a measure of risk. The absolute risk of disease occurrence is the incidence rate. Relative and attributable risks are measures of the association between an exposure and the risk of developing an adverse health outcome.

Relative risk is the ratio of the incidence of a group with the exposure to the incidence of the group without the exposure. Relative risk is also known as risk ratio (RR). Relative risk reflects the strength of an association between an exposure and the health outcome. Relative risk is useful in the study of disease etiology. The relative risk is determined using prospective cohort study findings as this study design generates incidence rates. Relative risk is measured using the following formula:

$$\text{Relative risk} = \frac{\text{Incidence rate among exposed}}{\text{Incidence rate among nonexposed}}$$

The relative risk provides information regarding the extent to which an individual with an exposure may experience the health condition. A relative risk or RR of 1.0 indicates an identical risk is present among both the exposed and nonexposed group. A relative risk or RR greater than 1.0 indicates an increased risk for the group in the numerator (exposed) as compared to the denominator (nonexposed) group. A relative risk or RR less than 1.0 indicates a decreased risk for the numerator (exposed) group as compared to the denominator (nonexposed) group.

The attributable risk is the preventive fraction among those exposed. Attributable risk or risk difference is the portion of the incidence of a disease in the exposed population that is associated with an exposure. The attributable risk is the disease incidence in the exposed group that would be eliminated if the exposure was eliminated. Attributable risk is also referred to as the "excess risk." Simply stated, the population attributable risk (PAR) is the portion of the incidence of the disease in the population (exposed plus nonexposed) that is a result of the exposure. It is the incidence of the disease that could be eliminated if the exposure was eliminated. Attributable risk is used more commonly in planning health programs targeting the risk factors or etiology. Attributable risk is measured using the following formula:

$$\text{Attributable risk} = \frac{\text{Incidence rate among exposed} - \text{incidence rate among nonexposed}}{\text{Incidence rate among exposed}} \times 100$$

The attributable risk for a population is similar. The PAR is:

$$\text{PAR} = \frac{\text{Risk in total population} - \text{Risk in unexposed population}}{\text{Risk in total population}}$$

The rate ratio can be calculated using a measure of the incidence rates, person–time rates, or mortality rates of two groups of interest. Similar to the relative risk or RR, the two groups are differentiated by some characteristic such as demographic variables or exposure to a risk agent. The rate for the group of primary interest is divided by the rate of the comparison group. This is a general risk formula that can be used to measure risk among groups of interest. The rate ratio formula is:

$$\text{Rate ratio} = \frac{\text{Rate for primary interest group}}{\text{Rate for comparison group}}$$

The interpretation of the rate ratio is similar to the relative risk or RR. A rate ratio of 1.0 indicates equal rates among the groups. A rate ratio greater than 1.0 indicates an increased risk for the numerator (primary interest group). A rate ratio less than 1.0 indicates a decreased risk for the numerator (primary interest group) (Centers for Disease Control and Prevention [CDC], 2012).

ODDS RATIO

The odds ratio is generated from case–control study designs. Case–control studies generate epidemiologic data as displayed in Table 9.1. An odds ratio is a measure of association that quantified the relationship between two exposure categories and a disease or health outcome. The odds ratio is also sometimes referred to as a cross-product ratio since the value in cell a is multiplied by the value in cell d for the numerator and for the denominator, cell b is multiplied by cell c. An odds ratio is calculated using the formula:

$$\text{Odds ratio} = \frac{a \times d}{b \times c} \text{ (refer to Table 9.1)}$$

The odds ratio can be calculated and interpreted as an approximation of the RR.

Table 9.1 Case–Control Odds Ratio Formula Data

Disease Status			
Exposure Status	Disease Present	Disease Absent	Total
Exposed	(Disease and exposure) a	(No disease and exposure) b	$a + b$
Nonexposed	(Disease and no exposure) c	(No disease and no exposure) d	$c + d$
Total	$a + b$	$b + d$	$a + b + c + d$

INTEGRATED RISK INFORMATION SYSTEM

The Integrated Risk Information System (IRIS) supports the Environmental Protection Agency's (EPA) mission to protect human and environmental health by identifying and characterizing health hazards of chemicals found in the environment (EPA, 2020). IRIS is located within the EPA's Center for Public Health and Environmental Assessment and provides toxicity values for health effects resulting from chemical exposures. The toxicity values are reference concentration (RfC) and reference dose (RfD). Reference concentration is an estimate of the continuous human population inhalation exposure likely without an appreciable risk of deleterious effects during a lifetime. The RfD is an estimate of a daily human population oral exposure likely without a risk of deleterious effects during a lifetime.

IRIS also provides cancer descriptors for chemical agents. The chemical cancer descriptors are carcinogenic to humans, likely to be carcinogenic to humans, suggestive evidence of carcinogenic potential, inadequate information to assess carcinogenic potential, and not likely to be carcinogenic to humans. In addition, IRIS also provides two other risk estimates for cancer, oral slope factor (OSF) and inhalation unit risk (IUR). The OSF is an estimate of the increased cancer risk from oral exposure to the agent at a dose of 1 mg/g/day for a lifetime. The IUR is an estimate of the increased cancer risk from inhalation exposure to the agent at a dose of 1 $\mu g/m^3$ for a lifetime (EPA, 2020). This information provided by IRIS is essential in the two steps of the risk assessment process, hazard identification and dose–response assessment.

END-OF-CHAPTER RESOURCES

SUMMARY POINTS

- Epidemiologic investigations provide evidence regarding the linkage between an exposure and the incidence of a disease or health condition.
- Risk science consists of four elements: risk assessment or risk evaluation, risk communication, risk perception, and risk management.
- Common risk factor categories are biologic, behavioral or lifestyle, stressors, or environmental exposures.
- Modifiable risk factors are those that can be altered such as behavior or lifestyle.
- Prognosis is considered the prediction of the future course of a disease after disease onset.
- Three factors that impact the risk assessment findings are the amount of the risk agent present, the extent of exposure to the risk agent, and the toxicity or infectiousness of the risk agent.
- Risk assessments are categorized into human health or ecological.
- A human risk assessment attempts to determine the potential risk of a "risk agent" to cause a health concern in humans.
- An ecological risk assessment is more expansive in that an ecological risk assessment measures the potential risk posed by a risk agent to humans and all living organisms in the environment.
- The risk assessment process involves four steps: hazard identification, exposure assessment, dose–response assessment, and risk characterization.
- Epidemiologists develop a risk assessment matrix to measure the size and scope of the risk, to determine appropriate epidemiologica preventive and control measures to minimize the risk, and to determine methods to triage or prioritize risks.
- The human risk assessment process utilizes the four risk assessment steps: hazard identification, exposure assessment, dose–response assessment, and risk characterization.
- A superfund risk assessment evaluates the threatening nature of a hazardous waste site to humans and the environment.
- Risk communication informs individuals about the potential hazard exposure to their person, property, or community.

- Risk management is the process of determining how to protect the public.
- Relative risk is the ratio of the disease incidence of a group with the exposure to the incidence of the group without the exposure.
- Relative risk is also known as risk ratio (RR).
- The attributable risk is the preventive fraction among those exposed.
- The Integrated Risk Information System (IRIS) provides toxicity values for health effects resulting from chemical exposures.

EPIDEMIOLOGY CRITICAL REASONING QUESTIONS

1. What is the use of attributable risk factor for a healthcare provider in relation to a prevention program?
2. What does absolute risk measure? When can it be used?
3. What is the relative risk of developing colon cancer for female cigarette smokers compared with female nonsmokers?

Colon Cancer Rate per 100,000 Females	
Smoker	48.0
Nonsmoker	25.4

    a. 48.0
    b. 48 − 25.4 = 22.6 per 100,000
    c. 48/25.4 = 1.89*
    d. 48 − 25.4/48
4. What is the attributable risk of colon cancer with cigarette smoking in female smokers:
    a. 48/25.4 = 1.89
    b. 48 − 25.4 − 22.6 per 100,000*
    c. 48
    d. 48/100,000 = 0.00048
5. What epidemiologic measure would be most useful to select risk factors for an intervention to impact a population's overall health?
    a. Incidence rate among those exposed
    b. Attributable risk*
    c. Prevalence rate among those exposed
    d. Relative risk
6. What is the best epidemiologic measure to determine the strength of an exposure to a disease?
    a. Incidence rate among those exposed
    b. Attributable risk
    c. Relative risk*
    d. Proportionate mortality

ADDITIONAL RESOURCES

A robust set of instructor resources designed to supplement this text is located at http://connect. springerpub.com/content/book/978-0-8261-8514-3. Qualifying instructors may request access by emailing textbook@springerpub.com.

REFERENCES

Burns, C., LaKind, J., Mattison, E., Alcala, C., Branch, F., Castillo, J., Clark, A., Clougherty, J., Darney, S., Erickson, H., Goodman, M., Greiner, M., Jurek, A., Miller, A., Rooney, A., & Zidek, A. (2019). A matrix for bridging the epidemiology and risk assessment gap. *Global Epidemiology*, 1–6. https://doi.org/10.1016/j.gloepi.2019.100005

Centers for Disease Control and Prevention. (2012). *Principles of epidemiology in public health practice*. Author.

Environmental Protection Agency. (2016). *Conducting an ecological assessment*. https://www.epa.gov/risk/conducting-ecological-risk-assessment

Environmental Protection Agency. (2017a). *Conducting a human health risk assessment*. https://www.epa.gov/risk/conducting-human-health-risk-assessment

Environmental Protection Agency. (2017b). *Risk management* https://www.epa.gov/risk/risk-management

Environmental Protection Agency. (2018). *Superfund risk assessment*. https://www.epa.gov/risk/superfund-risk-assessment

Environmental Protection Agency. (2020). *Basic information about integrated risk information system*. https://www.epa.gov/iris/basic-information-about-integrated-risk-infomration-system

Nurminen, M., Nurminen, T., & Corvalan, C. (1999). Methodological issues in epidemiologic risk assessment. *Epidemiology*, 10(5), 585–593. https://www.who.int/quantifying-ehimpacts/methods/en/nurminen1.pdf

Section III: Tools and Epidemiologic Study Designs

OBSERVATIONAL EPIDEMIOLOGIC RESEARCH: INTRODUCTION TO OBSERVATIONAL RESEARCH— DESCRIPTIVE, CASE STUDIES, CASE SERIES, ECOLOGICAL, AND CROSS-SECTIONAL

Demetrius J. Porche

The only true wisdom is knowing you know nothing.

–Socrates

The important thing is not to stop questioning. Curiosity has its own reason for existence. One cannot help but be in awe when he contemplates the mysteries of eternity, of life, of the marvelous structure of reality. It is enough if one tries merely to comprehend a little of this mystery each day.

–Albert Einstein

CHAPTER COMPETENCIES

At the conclusion of this chapter, the reader will be able to:

1. Differentiate observational research designs
2. Differentiate sampling methods
3. Describe the components of a research proposal
4. Describe the components of a research report
5. Differentiate descriptive, case study, case series, and cross-sectional study designs
6. Contrast Type I and Type II errors

ESSENTIAL TERMINOLOGY

The essential observational epidemiological research terminology is:

- Case series
- Case series design
- Case study
- Case study design
- Cluster sampling
- Convenient sampling
- Cross-sectional design
- Descriptive study design
- Ecological design

- External validity
- Internal validity
- Network sampling
- Nonprobability sampling
- Probability sampling
- Purposive sampling
- Quota sampling
- Research design
- Research proposal
- Research report
- Sample
- Sampling method
- Simple random sampling
- Statistical conclusion validity
- Stratified random sampling
- Systematic random sampling
- Type I error
- Type II error

Epidemiologic research studies are conducted to describe the burden of disease in a population, the presence of risk factors, health behaviors, or other characteristics of a population that influence health alterations or disease processes. Epidemiologic studies can determine risk factors associated with disease, causal inferences, and effectiveness of health-related interventions. Epidemiologic research relies on primary and secondary data collection methods. Primary data collection is when the epidemiologist collects the data, such as from medical examinations and direct observations. Secondary data collection is when the data have been collected by others such

as data from medical records, census data, and vital statistic data. Based on the research question and data required, the epidemiologist develops a research design. Nurse epidemiologists or nurses who engage in epidemiologic research use both primary and secondary data sources to answer the proposed research question.

RESEARCH DESIGN

A research design is the "blueprint" from which to conduct a study. Research design is also considered the framework or set of methods and procedures employed to collect, analyze, and summarize the data generated from the variables under investigation for a particular research problem (Ranganathan & Aggarwal, 2018). A study's research design is dictated by the nature of the research question, goal of the research question, resources available, current state of science, and study context (Figure 10.1). There are four basic research design elements to consider. These research design elements are time, intervention or treatment implementation, observations or measurements, and individual or group sampling. Other factors impacting the epidemiologic study design are the exposure of interest, outcomes of interest, and ethical issues. A solid detailed research design facilitates nurses or epidemiologists in the replication of the study. It is considered essential to detail the research design to the point that anyone can follow the design and carry out the study.

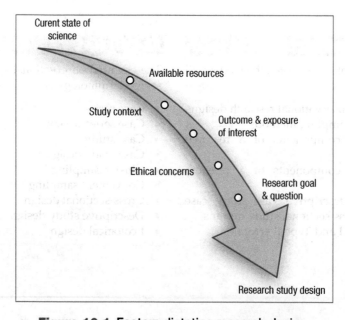

Figure 10.1 Factors dictating research design.

Research studies are designed to measure variables. Variables are measurable attributes of a phenomenon that vary over units or time. In research studies, variables are measured to determine if one variable is associated with or responsible for a change in the value of the other variable. Variables are considered independent or dependent. An independent variable is also known as predictor, exposure, intervention, or risk factor variable in epidemiology. The dependent variable is also known as the outcome or predicted variable. The dependent variable is the consequence of a risk factor, intervention, or exposure under investigation (Ranganathan & Aggarwal, 2018). In addition to discerning the dependent and independent variables, some research variables will need to have both a theoretical and operational definition. The theoretical definition conceptually defines the variable from the philosophical and theoretical perspective. The operational variable clearly details how the variable is measured. Operationalization of research variables is dependent on the principles of reliability and validity.

Four important characteristics of a "good" research design are:

- Provides for maximum strength of evidence regarding the relationship between two variables.
- Ensures that the strength of the evidence between the independent variables rather than other factors caused the outcome.
- Facilitates the application of findings about observed relationships are generalizable across populations, settings, and time.
- Captures adequately the theoretical constructs underlying the research variables.

A good research design attends to three types of validity: statistical conclusion, internal, and external. Statistical conclusion validity ensures that the statistical tests support the inferences between the empirical relationships of the independent and dependent research variables. Statistical power facilitates statistical conclusion validity to detect true relationships among variables. The ability of the researcher to maximize differences between groups increases the statistical conclusion validity. In addition, intervention fidelity enhances the power of the intervention and promotes statistical conclusion validity.

Internal validity is the extent to which the researcher can make an inference that the independent variable is truly associated with or causally influences the dependent variable. There are several threats to internal validity that the epidemiologic researcher must attend to when designing a research study. The internal threats to validity are:

- **Selection:** Bias results from pre-existing differences between groups; this occurs when there is a lack of random assignment or non-equivalent group comparison.
- **History:** Events occur concurrently with the independent variable that affects the dependent variable.
- **Testing:** Did the pretest measurement affect the posttest measurement score?
- **Design contamination:** Did the control and experimental groups interact; did the researcher contaminate the design?
- **Maturation:** This is not developmental changes, but changes that occur as a result of the passage of time.
- **Mortality:** Loss of subjects due to different forms of attrition.

External validity is the extent to which the observed relationships can be held true for different individuals, populations, conditions, or settings. External validity is the extent to which the findings of a study are generalizable. Some common threats to external validity are:

- Selection bias
- Setting effect on data collection and sampling
- History effect
- Subject knowledge of experiment
- Pygmalion or Rosenthal effect—a phenomenon in which the greater the expectation placed on people, then the better they perform

Research Design Notation

The structure of a research study is noted using symbols to understand the research design. The following are common symbols used to explain the research structure design. Observations or measures are symbolized with a "O" in the design notation. An "O" can refer to a single measure, a single instrument with multiple items, a complex multi-part instrument or survey, or a battery of tests or measures. If there needs to be a distinction between the specific observations or measures at different points in time, a subscript is used with the O; for example, O, O_1, O_2, and so on.

The treatment or intervention is noted with an "X" symbol in the design notation. "X" can refer to a single intervention or a complex bundle of interventions. If there is no treatment or if a comparison group is used, there is no symbol used in the design notation. Other design notations used are R for random assignment and N for nonequivalent group. When using these design notations to explain a research study design, each group in the design is provided a line in the design structure notation. Research design notations will be used to explain research designs in the chapters that follow. Figure 10.2 provides an exemplar.

STUDY DESIGN CLASSIFICATION

Epidemiologic study designs are classified as observational or experimental. Observational study designs document naturally occurring relationships between exposures and the outcome under investigation. In an observational study design, the epidemiologist does not intervene to affect the outcome. Observational studies can be descriptive (nonanalytical) or analytical (inferential). Figure 10.3 presents a diagram of

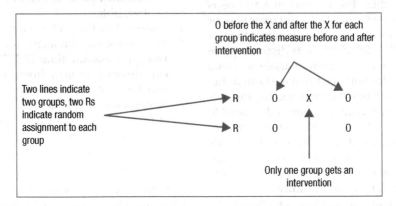

Figure 10.2 Research design notation exemplar.

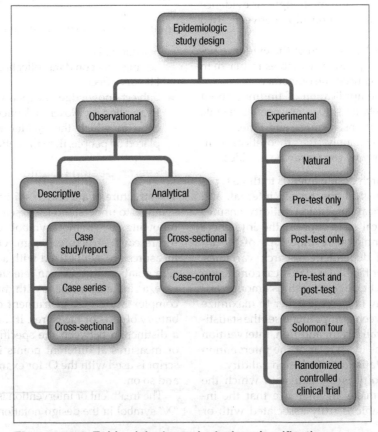

Figure 10.3 Epidemiologic study design classification.

epidemiologic study designs. Analytical studies test hypotheses about exposure and outcome relationships. Analytical study designs include a comparison group. It is important to note that nurse researchers use similar terminology to classify research study designs.

Descriptive or nonanalytical observational study designs describe the data of one or more characteristics of a group of individuals or a sample. Descriptive nonanalytical study designs do not answer questions or establish the existence of relationships between variables. Several descriptive nonanalytical study designs will be presented in this chapter—case study, case series, case reports, and cross-sectional studies. It is important to note that cross-sectional studies can be descriptive nonanalytical or analytical. A cross-sectional study can be classified as analytical if a relationship is determined between an exposure and an outcome (Omair, 2015).

Descriptive analytical observational study designs attempt to establish relationships between variables or test hypothesis. Analytical studies can be observational and also interventional (Ranganathan & Aggarwal, 2018). Analytical studies answer the how and why questions.

Each study design presents a different level and type of data based on the research question and methodological characteristics that limit the internal and external validity threats. Figure 10.4 presents the hierarchy of evidence generated from research studies based on the research design. Knowledge of the levels of evidence hierarchy assists with evidence synthesis and translation of epidemiologic data into population-based public health practice.

SAMPLING METHODS

The first step in sampling by an epidemiologist is to identify the population of interest. The population is the entire set of subjects, objects, events, or other elements being investigated (Fain, 2017). This population should possess specific characteristics of interest to the investigation. It is not feasible or plausible to sample the entire population; therefore, the epidemiologist selects a representative subset of the population, known as the sample. The better the sample represents the population, the more generalizable the findings of the epidemiologic research findings. The target population is that representative sample

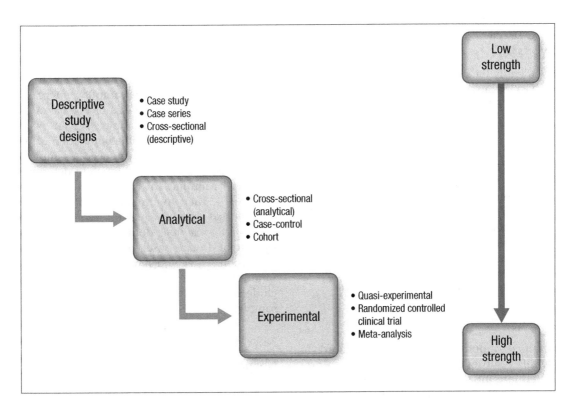

Figure 10.4 Epidemiologic study design evidence hierarchy.

to which the epidemiologist would like to make an inference and that contains the elements of the population of origin (2017).

Sampling is the process of selecting individuals from the population for participation in a research study. The two main sampling methods are probability and nonprobability. Probability sampling is the sampling method that provides an equal chance, or probability, of being selected. In a nonprobability sampling method, the sample is not selected randomly and there is less of an equal chance of being selected (Fain, 2017). In sampling, it is important to distinguish between random selection and random assignment. Random selection is the equal and independent chance of being selected from the population into the sample. Random assignment is the allocation of a subject from the sample into a subset or group of the sample such as an experimental or control group (2017).

The probability sampling methods are simple random sample, stratified random sample, cluster or multi-stage sample, and systematic sample.

Simple Random Sampling

Simple random sampling provides each subject an equal and independent opportunity (chance) to be selected. The simple random sampling process is:

1. Identify the population.
2. Determine sample size.
3. List all members of the accessible population.
4. Assign all members of the accessible population a consecutive number from 1 to the required number for the sample size.
5. Select an arbitrary number from the table of random numbers.
6. If the number selected corresponds with the assigned number of an individual in your accessible population, then that individual is included in your sample.
7. Then go to the next number in the table of random numbers and repeat step 6.

Stratified Random Sampling

Stratified random sampling selects a sample to identify a subset of the population to be represented into the sample. This process attempts to ensure that specific subset or subgroup characteristics are represented into the sample. This can be done proportionally or disproportionally. Proportionate stratified random sampling would randomly select from the population into a sample; then, from the sample, assign the same number of individuals into each strata or group based on the specific characteristic under investigation. Disproportionate stratified random sampling selects subjects from the population, then assigns them to groups based on the specific characteristic under investigation, but the groups are not of equal size (Fain, 2017)

Cluster Sampling

Cluster sampling is also known as multistage sampling. In cluster sampling, groups rather than individuals are randomly selected. Then individuals are randomly sampled from the identified clusters into the sample (Fain, 2017). As an example, the sampling of an entire state can used cluster sampling by clustering different cities within the state into a cluster based on cluster selection criteria. These city clusters could be based on geographical regions or demographic parameters such as population density.

Systematic Random Sampling

Systematic random sampling individuals are selected from the population via a list by taking every kth individual. The "kth" refers to the sampling interval. The sampling interval is determined based on the size of the accessible population and desired sample size. For example, if you have an accessible population of 100 infected individuals, and you need a sample of 25 subjects, you divide 100 by 25 to determine the kth or sampling interval. For this example, the kth is 4. Then you randomly list each of the 100 infected persons to ensure the list is truly random; for example, do not list alphabetically, by date of disease onset, or by date of hospital admission. After you have the 100 listed, you randomly select a first name on the list, then include every 4th individual, until you have your sample size (Fain, 2017).

Nonprobability Sampling

Nonprobability sampling has the opportunity for chance to play a role in sample selection. There are several nonprobability sampling methods such as convenience, purposive, snowball, network, and quota.

Convenience Sampling

Convenience sampling is also known as nonrandom sampling or accidental sampling. The sample in convenience sampling is truly one of convenience for the epidemiologist. Convenience sampling is the selection of subject, events, or objects from those that are "readily available and accessible to the researcher" and meet the established inclusion criteria. This form of sampling is easy, inexpensive, and convenient; however, it lacks generalizability (Fain, 2017).

Purposive Sampling

Purposive sampling is also known as judgmental or theoretical sampling. In purposive sampling, the epidemiologist intentionally selects certain individuals or cases to be included in the study. These individuals are intentionally selected based on current knowledge or the fact that they represent the phenomenon of interest being studied. In purposive sampling, there are specific intentional characteristics included in the sample inclusion criteria from which the research intentionally selects research subjects (Fain, 2017).

Snowball Sampling Technique

Snowball sampling is more a technique than a true sampling method. The snowball sampling technique is beneficial for sampling rare events or characteristics and difficult-to-find or -identify populations. The snowball sampling technique is useful for researching sensitive characteristics such as gender identity or sexual orientation, where privacy and confidentially is of concern and there is not an established list of population members. Snowball sampling technique uses index cases or subjects selected or identified to assist with the identification, location, and potential invitation of other population members to participate in the research study (Fain, 2017).

Network Sampling

Network sampling is similar to but different from snowball sampling. In network sampling, there may be established groups or lists of networks that exist. The epidemiologist uses these existing networks of individuals who generally have some association with the characteristic under investigation. Once the epidemiologist accesses the network, then the snowball sampling technique may also be employed to select research subjects (Fain, 2017).

Quota Sampling

Quota sampling identifies strata of a population based on a specific characteristic, similar to stratified random sampling. For quota sampling, the number of individuals needed in each strata to meet the sample size is determined. Then individuals are selected from the population strata using a nonprobability sampling method such as convenience or snowball sampling (Fain, 2017).

TYPE I AND TYPE II ERROR

The decision of an epidemiologist to accept the findings and reject the hypothesis can result in a type of research error. This error is generally known as a Type I or Type II error. If the epidemiologist decides there is a difference but in reality, there is no difference, then a Type I error has occurred. A Type I error is also known as a false positive that occurs when the epidemiologist incorrectly rejects a true null hypothesis. In a Type I error, this means the epidemiologist considers the findings significant when the findings have mostly likely occurred by chance.

In contrast, if the epidemiologist concludes that there is not a difference, when in reality there was a difference that was not detected, then a Type II error has occurred. A Type II error is also known as a false negative and occurs when an epidemiologist fails to reject a null hypothesis which is truly false. In Type II error, the epidemiologist concludes there is not a significant difference or effect, when there actually is a significant difference.

Figures 10.5 and 10.6 outline Type I and Type II errors. The probability of making a Type I error is known as alpha (α). Typically, the alpha is established at 0.05. With an alpha of 0.05, we would reject a null hypothesis (deciding there is no difference) if the statistical test yields a "p" value less than the alpha. The probability of making a Type II error is known as (β). The probability of not making a Type II error is known as the statistical power of a test and equals $1 - \beta$. Power is directly impacted by sample size. The larger the sample size, the larger the power (Chatburn, 2017). Table 10.1 summarizes error terminology (Celentano & Szklo, 2018).

		Reality	
		No difference exists	**Difference exists**
Decision	**No difference**	Correct decision	*Type II error (false negative)*
	Difference	*Type I error (false positive)*	Correct decision

Figure 10.5 Types of error in decision-making.

		Reality	
		No difference exists	**Difference exists**
Decision	**No difference**	Probability 1−α (>0.95)	Probability β (<0.20)
	Difference	Probability α (<0.05)	Probability 1−β (>0.80) Power

α = A rejection for decision making
β = Probability of observed results

Figure 10.6 Probability associated with Type I and Type II errors.

Table 10.1 Error Terminology Summary

Error Term	Definition
Alpha (α)	• Probability of a Type I error • The probability that the conclusion is that there is a difference between treatments when in reality there is not a difference between treatments
Beta (β)	• Probability of Type II error • The probability that the conclusion is that there is no difference between treatments when in reality there is a difference between treatments
Power	• Formula is 1 − probability of making a Type II error OR $1 - \beta$ • Probability of making the correct conclusion about the differences in the treatment effect • Probability of detecting a difference between the treatments when in reality there is a difference between treatments

Source: From Celentano, D., & Szkio, M. (2018). *Gordis epidemiology* (6th ed.). Elsevier.

RESEARCH PROPOSAL AND RESEARCH REPORT

A research proposal is a written plan that outlines the major elements of a research study design. The components of a research proposal are outlined in Box 10.1. A research proposal assists the epidemiologist in the clarification process to design a methodologically rigorous study. The written research proposal is a formal method of communicating the research design to secure approval to conduct the study or secure funding (Gray & Grove, 2020). Refer to Appendix D.

BOX 10.1. Quantitative Research Proposal Components

I. Introduction
   a. Background of problem, issue, phenomenon
   b. Problem statement
   c. Purpose statement
   d. Research question
   e. Formulated objectives/aims or hypotheses
   f. Study assumptions
   g. Rationale
   h. Significance

II. Review of literature (Relevant)
   a. Review theoretical literature
   b. Review clinical literature
   c. Review quality improvement literature
   d. Review research literature
   e. Synthesize review of literature into a summary

III. Theoretical or Conceptual Framework
   a. Introduce and describe the theoretical or conceptual framework
   b. Propose the theoretical or conceptual framework or model
   c. Define relevant concepts

IV. Methods
   a. Describe the research design
   b. Identify the population
   c. Describe the sampling method—sample size, power analysis conducted, sampling criteria (inclusion and exclusion), sampling process
   d. Describe setting characteristics and selection method
   e. Describe human subjects protection and other ethical considerations
   f. **Measurement methods:** Instruments used, reading level, instrument psychometrics (reliability and validity), scoring methods, level of measurement generated from instrument, calibration methods proposed for accuracy
   g. Data collection plan

   h. Data management plan
   i. Data analysis plan
   j. Study limitations and strengths
   k. Discussion of findings within the current state of knowledge/science
   l. Proposed budget
   m. Research team role and responsibilities
   n. Research study implementation timeline

The research proposal is written prior to the implementation of a research study and the research report is written after the research study is completed. A research report is the formal method of communicating what occurred during the implementation of the research study and the study findings. Research reports can be submitted to human subject protection boards, funding agencies, approval bodies, or as a means of scholarly dissemination. Box 10.2 outlines the typical format of a research report (Gray & Grove, 2020) for a scholarly journal. The general format for a journal research report is IMRAD (introduction, method, results, and discussion).

Nurses and epidemiologists typically write the proposal to secure approval and funding for the respective epidemiologic study. Simply stated, the research reports document the manner in which the epidemiologic study was conducted and concludes with presentation of the epidemiologic study findings and recommendations.

DESCRIPTIVE DESIGNS

A descriptive study design describes the characteristics of an attribute or the distribution of one or more variables, without determining relationships (Box 10.3). Descriptive study designs promote the development of exploratory studies and hypothesis generation. Simply, a descriptive study design describes the characteristics of the sample under investigation. From an epidemiologic perspective, descriptive study designs examine patterns of characteristics according to person, place, and time, much like an outbreak investigation. Descriptive studies answer the what, who, where, and when questions. Hypotheses are generated about the exposures and determinants of a health condition in terms of person, place, and time with the goal of determining differences and similarities.

BOX 10.2. Quantitative Research Report Format (IMRAD)

I. Study title
II. Abstract
III. Introduction (I)
  a. Present research problem, issue, or phenomenon
  b. Significance
  c. Problem statement
  d. Literature summary
  e. Theoretical or conceptual framework
  f. Research questions, objectives/aims, hypothesis
  g. Operational and theoretical definitions
IV. Methods (M)
  a. State research design
  b. Variables under investigation
  c. Intervention description and protocol (if applicable)
  d. **Describe sample:** Size, power analysis, selection criteria, acceptance rate, response rate, sample attrition or retention rate
  e. Describe setting
  f. Describe measurement methods and data collection procedures
V. Results (R)
  a. Describe data analysis procedures
  b. Present findings (use summary tables and figures to support narrative)
VI. Discussion (D)
  a. Summarize major findings in context of existing literature
  b. Identify limitations
  c. Identify strengths
  d. Identify implications for practice
  e. Provide recommendations for policy, programs, research, and future epidemiologic investigations

Source: From Gray, J., & Grove, S. (2020). *Burns and Grove's the practice of nursing research: Appraisal, synthesis, and generation of evidence* (9th ed.). Saunders.

BOX 10.3. Descriptive Epidemiology of Classic Swine Fever Outbreaks in the Period 2013–2018 in Colombia

Summary: The purpose of this descriptive epidemiological study was to characterize the herds affected by classic swine flu from the years 2013 to 2018 in Colombia. Each outbreak's information was obtained by the veterinarians of the official veterinary services via the use of two questionnaires. Upon notification of the suspicion of the outbreak, the first questionnaire was completed. The second questionnaire was completed during the follow-up of the outbreak. Information included in the questionnaires related to disease notification date, farm characteristics, vaccination information, affected animals by groups, clinical signs, and movements of animals and people. If the infection affected different backyard areas sharing an environment and management practices, the small village was considered one epidemiologic unit defined as a single outbreak. The identification of clusters of high risk of infection with classic swine flu virus (CSFV) aids in strengthening and redirecting the health strategies of surveillance, vaccination, and biosecurity, especially in backyard piggeries of these areas, in order to reduce the number of susceptible animals that can become infected and decrease the viral circulation of CSFV on the Atlantic Coast. The classic swine flu epidemic was mainly related with the backyard production system. The affected region has an extremely high proportion of premises based on the subsistence economy. Despite the efforts of the veterinary services, there are no registers of an unknown number of backyards. Therefore, these are not covered by the vaccination campaigns or the surveillance network. It is important to increase efforts to record as many premises as possible and to develop education campaigns including basic biosecurity measures, especially those related with animal movements.

Source: Pineda, P., Deluque, A., Peña, M., Diaz, O. L., Allepuz, A., & Casal, J. (2020). Descriptive epidemiology of classical swine fever outbreaks in the period 2013–2018 in Colombia. *PLoS One, 15*(6). https://doi.org/10.1371/journal.pone.0234490

Characteristics under investigation for the person factor are demographic information, personal characteristics of the individual (age, sex, race/ethnicity, occupation), and behavioral characteristics specific to the health condition or disease under investigation. Place characteristics examine information regarding the geographic extent of the problem with attention to clustering or patterns associated with geographical locations (residence, work, hospital). The time characteristics generally focus on the date of onset of a health condition or disease plotted over time with the development of cases to produce an epidemic curve (also includes time of

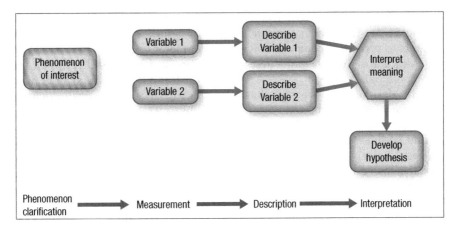

Figure 10.7 Descriptive study design.

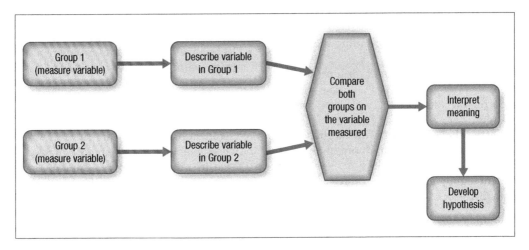

Figure 10.8 Comparative descriptive design.

diagnosis, reporting, and screening test). The epidemic curve is used in descriptive studies to demonstrate the frequency of new cases over time based on the time of disease or health condition onset. The shape of the epidemic curve facilitates the understanding of the disease transmission patterns as discussed in Chapter 7. Figure 10.7 presents a representation of a descriptive design.

Comparative Descriptive Design

A comparative descriptive design describes a phenomenon in two groups or more and describes these differences in the variables in two or more groups in one setting. There is no treatment or intervention in a comparative design. Figure 10.8 presents a representation of a comparative descriptive design.

Case Study Design

A case study design provides descriptive information that can be used as evidence and support the generation of hypotheses. Case study design can be used as a triangulation design to provide context and additional information to support quantitative methods. The case study design is an intensive exploration of a single unit of study, which could be an individual person, family, incident such as an outbreak, community, small population of individuals, or institution (Gray et al., 2016). The case study design examines the single unit "case" within a broader context of a "real-life" environment or situation. The intense depth of analysis in a case study design provides the epidemiologist with the ability to gather information using a variety of information sources with different data collection methods employed for a detailed analysis of a single case. The primary objective of a case design is to provide a comprehensive and detailed description of the case under investigation (Celentano & Szkio, 2018).

In a case study design, the researcher must establish the parameters and boundaries of what defines a "case." A case should be specific, unique, and bounded (Tappen, 2015). The design of the case study is dictated by the circumstances of the case under investigation. A defining element of the case study design, like many epidemiologic studies, is the element of time. Some purposes of a case study are:

- Explore the situation surrounding the implementation of an intervention that does not have a clearly defined intervention outcome and metric identified.
- Describe the context surrounding the event, incident, or intervention.
- Describe the event, incident, or intervention itself.
- Explore the context of complex causal linkages.
- Confirm, challenge, or refute a theory or perspective through an in-depth analysis of a case.
- Present a unique, extreme, or rare case (Gray et al., 2016).

Case study analysis may generate both quantitative and qualitative data. Analysis requires rich, in-depth descriptions of the case. Some case study analysis techniques are pattern matching, explanation building, and time-series analysis. Pattern matching compares the expected patterns with the patterns in the case under investigation or patterns occurring among similar cases. Explanation building is an analysis that develops an explanation of weaving together or developing an explanation from the findings in the case. A time-series analysis reviews and provides an explanation of the variable's outcomes over a period of time, generally represented in a graphic display.

A case study of a simple individual's description of disease occurrence or health condition is sometimes referred to as a case report in the medical literature. The term *case report* is used interchangeably with case study; however, more precisely, a case report should refer to the written document, manuscript or presentation of a case study. A suggested format for writing a case report consists of:

- **Introduction:** Brief, one or two sentence description of the case, uniqueness, and epidemiology
- **Case report:** Case description (demographics, lifestyle, behaviors); brief history of case; details of case investigation; clinical features; physical examination findings; screening and diagnostic test and results; differential diagnoses considered (if appropriate); treatment plan and outcomes; expected outcome of treatment plan; and actual outcomes of treatment plan
- **Discussion:** Discuss the case within the context of existing literature; importance of the case and its results; patient experience; lessons learned; future recommendations for practice, policy, and research
- **Ethical:** Discuss consent and human protection of privacy and confidentiality
- **Reference citations:** Present references used in preparing the case report (Anwar et al., 2004; Guidelines to writing a clinical case report, 2017)

A case study has limited external validity (generalizability). Case studies are key to hypothesis generation (Celentano & Szkio, 2018). If there are multiple cases of a similar condition, situation, or event, a series of cases could present a more compelling study finding across the cases—a case series design.

Case Series Design

A case series design consists of multiple case studies synthesized. The case series design is an aggregation of multiple similar case studies into one unit of analysis (Aggarwal & Ranganathan, 2019). The case series design is a coherent presentation of a set of cases with a similar health condition or disease generally derived from practice. Generally the number of cases in a case series range from as few as 5 to more than 100, with an average range of 20 to 50 (Omair, 2015). A case series design does not have a comparison group but, due to the number of similar cases, hypotheses could be suggested for further investigation.

A case series design is epidemiologically valuable for studying predictive signs and symptoms, creating case definitions, exploring screening and diagnostic testing, and establishing prevention and control procedures. Some common points of analysis in a case series design are diagnostic criteria or case definition characteristics, cause of morbidity and mortality, date of onset or mortality, place characteristics inclusive of the physical and social environment, characteristics of the individual and the population from which the individual originates, and population size and at-risk characteristics of the individual and population. Precisely, a case series focuses on: What is the condition being studied? Who has the condition under investigation? Where does the condition originate from? Why did the disease develop? How did the disease develop or become transmitted?

Ecological Study Design

Ecological study design examines the association between an exposure and an outcome across populations, not individuals (Box 10.4;

BOX 10.4. Alcohol Outlet Density and Alcohol-Related Hospital Admissions in England: A National Small-Area Level Ecological Study

Summary: The aim of this ecological study was to examine the existing relation between the density of outlets (defined as within a 1 km radius of a residential postcode) selling alcohol and alcohol-associated hospital admission rates within certain local neighborhoods. This study employed the use of a national small-area level ecological study design and utilized 32,482 small geographic areas termed lower layer super output census areas (LSOAs) with approximately 1,500 people within each area. The sample analysis was based on a total of 42,227,108 individuals aged 15 years of age and older. The period of analysis was based on hospital admission data from 2002 to 2003 through 2013 to 2014. Four alcohol-related outcome categories were investigated—acute or chronic conditions and completely or partially attributed to alcohol. Emergency admissions were considered as acute conditions while nonemergency admissions were considered for chronic conditions. Overall, there were 1,007,137 admissions completely attributed to alcohol, and 2,153,874 admissions partially attributed to alcohol over the analysis period of 12 years within the sampled population. The obtained results demonstrated that higher hospital admission rates were observed in areas with higher density of outlets selling, especially for conditions wholly attributable to alcohol consumption.

Source: Maheswaran, R., Green, M. A., Strong, M., Brindley, P., Angus, C., & Holmes, J. (2018). Alcohol outlet density and alcohol related hospital admissions in England: A national small-area level ecological study. *Addiction (Abingdon, England), 113*(11), 2051–2059. https://doi.org/10.1111/add.14285

Aggarwal & Ranganathan, 2019). In an ecological study, the unit of observation is the population or community. Ecological study design examines the average exposure associated with a health condition in a population with the overall frequency of the disease within the population. For example, an ecological study design could be used to examine meat or fiber consumption association with colon cancer among several countries. Ecological variables are generally of three types: aggregate, environmental, or global. Aggregate measures are summaries of observations from individuals in each group, such as the proportion of cigarette smokers. Environmental measures are physical characteristics of the place or setting in which individuals live, work, or play, such as air pollution levels or water quality. Global measures are group level attributes that do not consider individual level characteristics such as population density in a location.

A limitation of ecological study design is the limited information present on the risk factor status or exposure. There is limited ability to link the exposure or risk factor to the disease or health condition. This can result in an ecological fallacy. An ecological fallacy is the ascribing to individuals within a group some characteristic that they in fact do not possess individually (Celentano & Szkio, 2018). In addition, ecological studies do not permit the accounting for or adjusting for other factors that may influence the outcome variable. Therefore, confounders may exist in ecological studies.

Cross-Sectional Study Design

A cross-sectional study design takes one "snapshot" in a defined period of time (Box 10.5). Cross-sectional study designs measure existing levels of an exposure and health condition at that single point of time. Some advantages of a cross-sectional study design are the ability to generate hypothesis, easy, inexpensive, examine multiple exposures or outcomes at one time, and ability to estimate prevalence of disease and exposure. Some disadvantages are the inability to infer causality, potential to miss latent disease, and presence of recall bias. An exemplar research question for a cross-sectional study is to determine the differences in the rate of cerebrovascular injury and myocardial infarction by age, race, and gender during January 1, 2018 to December 31, 2020.

BOX 10.5. Hypertension Awareness, Treatment and, Control in Ghana: A Cross-Sectional Study

Summary: The purpose of this cross-sectional study was to evaluate the rates of hypertension awareness, treatment, and control, and to examine the socioeconomic and demographic correlates of hypertension awareness and treatment in a nationally representative sample of Ghanaians. There were 5,526 respondents aged 18 years and older with information about their blood pressure (BP) who participated in this study. A stratified multistage cluster design based on the World Health Survey design was utilized. The sampling units were stratified by region and place of residence. There were 20 strata developed based on regional and residential information. Three BP measurements were collected from the participants, with the average of the measurements used as a measure of blood pressure. The prevalence of hypertension was defined as a former diagnosis of hypertension or systolic BP of ≥140 and/or diastolic BP of ≥90. Socioeconomic factors evaluated were education level and employment status, while the demographic factors were age, marital status, ethnicity, religion, and place of residence—all associated with hypertension awareness. The results obtained indicated that hypertension prevalence in the population was 58.9% with a larger population of women with hypertension when compared to men. Of these individuals with hypertension, 19% were aware of their hypertension; 68% aware of the hypertension were treating the condition. Of the hypertensives identified, only 12% were maintaining their BP within the parameters considered controlled. These cross-sectional findings suggest that hypertension is prevalent in Ghana, and along with it low levels of awareness, treatment, and control. Socioeconomic and demographic factors are vital correlates of hypertension awareness and treatment in Ghana.

Source: Sanuade, O. A., Awuah, R. B., & Kushitor, M. (2020). Hypertension awareness, treatment and control in Ghana: A cross-sectional study. *Ethnicity & Health*, 25(5), 702–716. https://doi.org/10.1080/1355 7858.2018.1439898

Cross-sectional studies do not have a comparison group. However, cross-sectional studies can produce estimates of the prevalence of a characteristic, exposure, or outcome in a population.

EXHIBIT 10.1. Prevalence Ratio

Exposure	Disease	Without Disease	Total
Exposed	A	B	A + B
Unexposed	C	D	C + D
Total	A + C	B + D	

$PR = A \div (A + B) \div C \div (C + D)$

A hypothetical example of calculating the PR for food-borne illness with *Escherichia coli* exposure to a fast-food restaurant is:

Exposure	Disease	Without Disease	Total
Exposed	20	1	21
Unexposed	5	74	79
Total	25	75	100

$PR = 20 \div (20 + 1) \div 5 \div (5 + 74) = 0.95/0.0632 = 15$; so PR is 15. This is interpreted to mean that the proportion of people with food-borne illness exposed to *E. coli* was 15-fold times greater than the persons not exposed to *E. coli*.

Data generated from a cross-sectional study can be used to calculate an odds ratio.

Prevalence ratio (PR) is generated from a cross-sectional study. It is similar to a risk ratio (RR) in a cohort study. The denominators for both populations are fixed populations. The PR is similar to the RR when the outcomes occur over a short period of time. If the period of risk extends over a longer period of time (months to years), it is preferred to calculate a prevalence odds ratio (see the following). The PR is basically the prevalence of disease in the exposed group divided by the prevalence of disease in the unexposed group. Exhibit 10.1 presents the formula for PR.

Prevalence odds ratio (POR) may also be calculated from a cross-sectional study. It is similar to an odds ratio in a case control study design. In cross-sectional studies, the odds ratio is also referred to as the POR when prevalent cases with long-lasting risk factors are included. The POR is the preferred measure of association in cross-sectional studies. If the prevalence of disease is low such as 10% or less in exposed and unexposed populations, then the POR is considered equal to the PR. Exhibit 10.2 presents the formula for a POR.

EXHIBIT 10.2. Prevalence Odds Ratio

Exposure	Disease	Without Disease	Total
Exposed	A	B	A + B
Unexposed	C	D	C + D
	A + C	B + D	

$$POR = \frac{A \times D}{C \times B}$$

A hypothetical example of calculating the POR below for food-borne illness with *E. coli* exposure to a fast-food restaurant is:

Exposure	Disease	Without Disease	Total
Exposed	20	1	21
Unexposed	5	74	79
Total	25	75	100

$$POR = \frac{20 \times 74}{5 \times 1} = \frac{1,480}{5} = 296$$

SYNTHESIS AND CRITICAL APPRAISAL

Epidemiologic research studies should be critically appraised to assess the scientific rigor of the study. Critical appraisal of an epidemiologic study provides confidence in the findings and a clear understanding of the limitations of translation into practice. To determine the state of epidemiologic science related to a topic, research articles should be synthesized into a body of knowledge that provides the current state of science on a topic. Refer to Appendix E for helpful documents to write a collective summary of findings table from which to generate the synthesis of the state of epidemiologic science.

The synthesized review of literature presents the current state of science, identifies gaps in the science, and provides a supportive rationale for the need to conduct the investigation along with justification for the proposed research design to improve and advance the "current" science. In nursing, this is what is frequently referred to as the "nursing state of science" paper.

END-OF-CHAPTER RESOURCES

SUMMARY POINTS

- Epidemiologic research studies are conducted to describe the burden of disease in a population, the presence of risk factors, health behaviors or other characteristics of a population that influence health alterations or disease processes.
- Primary data collection is when the epidemiologist collects the data.
- Secondary data collection is when the data have been collected by others.
- A research design is the "blueprint" from which to conduct a study.
- An independent variable is also known as predictor, exposure, intervention, or risk factor variable in epidemiology.
- A good research design attends to three types of validity: statistical conclusion, internal, and external.
- Statistical conclusion validity ensures that the statistical test supports the inferences between the empirical relationships of the independent and dependent research variables.
- Internal validity is the extent to which the researcher can make an inference that the independent variable is truly associated with or causally influencing the dependent variable.
- External validity is the extent to which the findings of a study are generalizable.
- "O" refers to an observation or measure.
- "X" refers to a treatment or intervention.
- "R" refers to random assignment.
- Descriptive or nonanalytical observational study designs describe the data of one or more characteristics of a group of individuals or sample.
- Descriptive analytical observational study designs attempt to establish relationships between variables or test hypotheses.
- Sampling is the process of selecting individuals for participation in a research study from the population.
- Random selection is the equal and independent chance of being selected from the population into the sample.
- Random assignment is the allocation of a subject from the sample into a subset or group of the sample such as an experimental or control group.

- **Type I Error:** The researcher decides there is a difference but in reality, there is no difference.
- **Type II Error:** The researcher decides there is no difference but in reality, there is a difference.
- A research proposal is a written plan that outlines the major elements of research study design.
- A research report is the formal method of communicating what occurred during the implementation of the research study and the study findings.
- A descriptive study design describes the characteristics of an attribute or the distribution of one or more variables, without determining relationships.
- A comparative descriptive design describes a phenomenon appearing in two groups or more and describes the differences in the variables in two or more groups in one setting.
- The case study design is an intensive exploration of a single unit of study, which could be an individual person, family, incident such as an outbreak, community, small population of individuals, or institution.
- The case series design is an aggregation of multiple similar case studies into one unit of analysis.
- In an ecological study, the unit of observation is the population or community.
- Cross-sectional study designs measure existing levels of an exposure and health condition at one point in time.

EPIDEMIOLOGY CRITICAL REASONING QUESTIONS

1. Compose a research question for a descriptive study design. Write a research proposal for a descriptive study design inclusive of the variable to be measured, sampling method, and data collection process.
2. Differentiate a descriptive study design and a comparative descriptive study design.
3. Identify a clinical case of interest for a case study design. Gather the data and compose a case study report.
4. Utilizing the clinical case of interest in #3, identify two or more similar cases. Conduct

a case series analysis. Compose a case series report.

5. Identify a phenomenon of interest and a population of interest. Describe the manner in which sampling would be different by contrasting at least two different sampling methods.

6. Explain the difference between Type I and Type II error.

ADDITIONAL RESOURCES

 A robust set of instructor resources designed to supplement this text is located at http://connect. springerpub.com/content/book/978-0-8261-8514-3. Qualifying instructors may request access by emailing textbook@springerpub.com.

REFERENCES

Aggarwal, R., & Ranganathan, P. (2019). Study designs: Part 2—Descriptive studies. *Perspectives in Clinical Research*, *10*(1), 34–36.

Anwar, R., Kabir, H., Botchu, R., Khan, S., & Gogi, N. (2004). How to write a case report. *Student British Medical Journal*, *12*, 60–66.

Celentano, D., & Szkio, M. (2018). *Gordis epidemiology* (6th ed.). Elsevier.

Chatburn, R. (2017). Basic study design: Practical considerations. *Cleveland Clinic Journal of Medicine*, *84*(Suppl 2), e10–e19.

Fain, J. (2017). *Reading, understanding, and applying nursing research* (5th ed.). F. A. Davis.

Gray, J., & Grove, S. (2020). *Burns and Grove's the practice of nursing research: Appraisal, synthesis, and generation of evidence* (9th ed.).Saunders.

Guidelines to writing a clinical case report. (2017). *Heart Views*, *18*(3), 104–105.

Maheswaran, R., Green, M. A., Strong, M., Brindley, P., Angus, C., & Holmes, J. (2018). Alcohol outlet density and alcohol related hospital admissions in England: A national small-area level ecological study. *Addiction (Abingdon, England)*, *113*(11), 2051–2059. https://doi.org/10.1111/add.14285

Omair, A. (2015). Selecting the appropriate study design for your research: Descriptive study designs. *Journal of Health Specialties*, *3*(3):153–156.

Pineda, P., Deluque, A., Peña, M., Diaz, O. L., Allepuz, A., & Casal, J. (2020). Descriptive epidemiology of classical swine fever outbreaks in the period 2013–2018 in Colombia. *PLoS One*, *15*(6). https://doi.org/10.1371/journal.pone.0234490

Ranganathan, P., & Aggarwal, R. (2018). Study designs: Part 1—An overview and classification. *Perspectives in Clinical Research*, *9*(4), 184–186.

Sanuade, O. A., Awuah, R. B., & Kushitor, M. (2020). Hypertension awareness, treatment and control in Ghana: A cross-sectional study. *Ethnicity & Health*, *25*(5), 702–716. https://doi.org/10.1080/13557858.2018.1439898

Tappen, R. (2015). *Advanced nursing research: From theory to practice* (2nd ed.). Jones & Bartlett Learning.

Chapter 11

COHORT STUDIES

Demetrius J. Porche

So never lose an opportunity of urging a practical beginning, however small, for it is wonderful how often in such matters the mustard-seed germinates and roots.

–Florence Nightingale

CHAPTER COMPETENCIES

At the conclusion of this chapter, the reader will be able to:

1. Describe an epidemiologic cohort study design
2. Differentiate a prospective and retrospective cohort study design
3. Calculate a risk ratio and rate ratio

ESSENTIAL TERMINOLOGY

The essential terminology for cohort study designs is:

- Cohort study design
- Prospective cohort design
- Rate ratio
- Retrospective cohort design
- Risk ratio

Cohort study designs are a population-based observational epidemiologic study. These population-based studies follow a larger sample of the target population over time (prospective or retrospective) to identify and predict etiologies and associated risk factors. Cohort studies evolve over time as diagnostic and medical science advances; for example, improved diagnostic screening and testing methods will be integrated into a cohort study design as they are developed or improved. Two historical cardiovascular cohort studies are the Framingham Study and Bogalusa Heart Study. In addition, there are Nurses' Health Studies that specifically use nurses as their cohort.

The Framingham Study was initiated in 1948 by the United States Public Health Service. The purpose of this cohort epidemiologic study was to investigate the epidemiology and risk factors for cardiovascular disease. This was a prospective longitudinal cohort study that collected data on biological and lifestyle factors related to cardiovascular disease for three generations. The original Framingham cohort was recruited from 1948 to 1950 consisting of 5,209 participants (2,873 women and 2,336 men) aged between 28 and 62 years old. This original cohort comprised two thirds of the adult Framingham, Massachusetts adult population. The sample is evaluated biennially. In 1971, children and spouses of the original cohort were enrolled as the offspring cohort. In 2002, a third generation of the original cohort was recruited into the Gen 3 cohort. This one cohort study has generated a dense and complex database of over 50 years.

The Bogalusa Heart Study was initiated in 1972. An interprofessional team of anthropologists, biochemists, cardiologists, epidemiologists, geneticists, nurses, nutritionists, psychologists, sociologists, and statisticians are exploring the hereditary and environmental factors associated with early coronary artery disease. From this longitudinal prospective study, there have been over 160 nested studies or studies generated exploring hypertension, lipidemia, genetic disorders, cardiac murmurs, diabetes, and other pathologies. This study has characterized the early natural history of cardiovascular disease risk factors, early coronary disease, type II diabetes, and essential hypertension.

COHORT STUDY DESIGN

Cohort study design selects research subjects that are representative of a larger population of interest based on some cohort characteristic. The cohort can be selected based on a key exposure of interest such as pregnancy, school age, or stage of life (Buka et al., 2018). In a cohort study design, the epidemiologist selects a target population and follows the target population over time to compare the incidence rate of the disease or death. The basic components of a cohort study design are presented in Figure 11.1.

Cohorts can also be selected based on risk status. A high-risk cohort study intentionally selects subjects with the key distinction of being a subject from a high-risk group that most likely had a known high-risk exposure (Buka et al., 2018). A basic requirement of a prospective cohort study design is that the outcome or endpoint under investigation should not have occurred in individuals in the cohort study (Bangdiwala, 2019).

The study population in a cohort study can be diverse and include a sample of the general population or specific geographical or political areas. A cohort can also be identified based on a common characteristic such as an occupational cohort to explore occupational hazards or a group with some identified behavioral or cultural commonality such as men who have sex with men. An essential element for a cohort design is the ascertainment of events that occur over time. Most cohort studies are known as prospective cohort studies since they follow the cohort forward in time examining the cohort characteristics and exposures to a specific outcome variable. A cohort study design can be constructed in a retrospective manner. In a retrospective cohort design, a cohort is identified and sampled in the past based on existing records and followed forward to the present time at which the study is being conducted. Prospective and retrospective cohort study designs are presented in Boxes 11.1 and 11.2.

Advantages of cohort study design are population-based incidence calculations, relative risk and risk ratio estimations, establishment of temporality, multiple exposures and outcomes measurements, and less likely to have selection and recall bias. Disadvantages of a cohort study design are its expense; study population issues such as attrition, migration, nonresponse, and loss to follow-up; and may be impractical for rate or diseases with long latency periods.

Risk Ratio

Risk ratio can be called relative risk (RR). The risk ratio or RR quantifies the proportion of a population's risk of disease due to a specific exposure. The formula for an RR or risk ratio is:

$$\text{Risk ratio} = \frac{\text{Risk in the exposure group}}{\text{Risk in the unexposed group}}$$

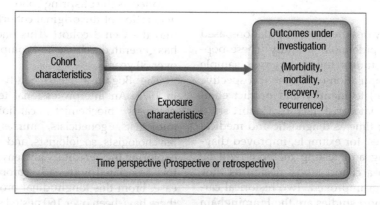

Figure 11.1 Basic cohort design component.

BOX 11.1. Cohort Study Example

Title: Weight History, All-Cause and Cause-Specific Mortality in Three Prospective Cohort Studies

Summary: There is ongoing debate regarding the optimal body mass index (BMI) in relation to all-cause mortality rates. This study used data from three prospective cohorts to examine all-cause and cause-specific mortality risks of overweight and obese health professionals in the United States. The study population consisted of the Nurses' Health Study (NHS) initiated in 1976 that enrolled 121,700 female nurses aged 30 to 55 years old, the Nurses' Health Study II (NHS II) initiated in 1989 with 116,686 female registered nurses aged 25 to 42 years old, and the Health Professionals Follow-up Study (NPFS) initiated in 1986 with 51,529 male health professionals aged 40 to 75 years old. Questionnaires were administered biennially on diet, lifestyle, and other health-related information. BMI was assessed every 2 years via self-report. A primary study outcome was death of a cause reported via next of kin or searches of the National Death Index. Cause of death was determined through an examination of the death certificate. Deaths were then classified using the International Classification of Diseases, 8th revision (ICD-8). Data was collected on maximum BMI ever reported on a health questionnaire regarding weight history. The findings from the analysis of these three prospective cohort studies indicate that the overweight, obese I, and obese II categories were associated with increased risk of all-cause mortality from cardiovascular disease and noncardiovascular disease such as cancer and respiratory diseases. Maximum overweight was associated with increased cause-specific mortality from cardiovascular disease and coronary heart disease. This study also reported methodological considerations. Compared to the use of BMI data from one baseline questionnaire, use of extended weight histories provided a stronger associative measure with mortality risk. In addition, stratified BMI analysis by maximum BMI and baseline BMI indicated that the highest risks of death occurred among subjects who experienced substantial decreases in weight most likely associated with unintentional weight loss caused by preclinical or clinical disease. In contrast, intentional weight loss was associated with decreased risk of early mortality.

Source: Yu, E., Stokes, A., Ley, S., Manson, J., Willett, W., Satija, A., & Hu, F. (2017). Weight history, all-cause and cause-specific mortality in three prospective cohort studies. Annals of Internal Medicine, 166(9), 613–620. https://doi.org/10.7326/M16-1390

BOX 11.2. Prospective Cohort Study Example

Title: Optimism and Cause-Specific Mortality: A Prospective Cohort Study

Summary: Positive psychological attributes such as optimism are associated with lower health risk such as cardiovascular health. Randomized controlled clinical trials have demonstrated evidence that optimism can be learned to improve health outcomes. The study population was the National Nurses' Health Study initiated in 1976 that enrolled 121,700 female registered nurses aged 30 to 55 years old. Subjects receive questionnaires about their health and health behaviors every 2 years. There is about a 90% follow-up rate. In 2004, the measure of optimism was included in the questionnaire. Optimism was measured using the Life Orientation Test-Revised in 2004 and in 2008. Mortality data were collected from systematic searches of state vital statistics records and the National Death Index with supplemental reports from family members. The cause of death was examined by a physician through a review of each death statistic. Death certificate causes were determined for 98% of this sample. The findings identified strong associations between higher optimism levels and lower risks of mortality ($p < .001$). A comparison of the more optimistic women to the least optimistic women, the hazard ratio (HR) was 0.71 (Confidence interval [CI] 95%: 0.66, 0.76) for all-cause mortality. Higher rates of optimism were associated with lower risk of mortality for major causes of death such as cancer, heart disease, and stroke. Optimism was also associated with reduced HR for mortality from respiratory disease (HR = 0.63, 95% CI: 0.48, 0.82) and infection (HR = 0.48, 95% CI: 0.29, 0.80). These findings were maintained after close control for potential confounding factors such as sociodemographic characteristics and depression. This is suggested to be one of the first studies in which there is a significant, broad-based association between optimism and health demonstrated in a general population.

Source: Kim, E., Hagain, K., Grodstein, F., DeMeo, D., De Vivo, I., & Kubzansky, L. (2016). Optimism and cause-specific mortality: A prospective cohort study. *American Journal of Epidemiology*, 185(1), 21–29. https://doi.org/10.1093/aje/kww182

Rate Ratio

The rate ratio compares the rate of disease in two groups that differ by a characteristic or exposure history. The formula to calculate a rate ratio is:

$$\text{Rate ratio} = \frac{\text{Rate for group of interest}}{\text{Rate for comparison group}}$$

As stated previously, a cohort study provides for a comparison of the incidence rate between the exposed and the unexposed group. If there is a positive association that exists between the exposure and the disease, it would be expected that the proportion of the exposed group in whom the disease develops (exposed group incidence) would be greater than the proportion of the unexposed group in whom the disease develops (unexposed group incidence). This can be calculated using the following data table and calculation. The cohort is first divided into the exposed and unexposed groups. Then the diseased and non-diseased cases are categorized into the exposed and unexposed groups. For example, in the exposed group (A + B), if the disease develops in the A but not the B group, then the incidence formula for the exposed group would be:

$$\frac{A}{A+B}$$

For example, in the unexposed group (C + D), if the disease develops, then the incidence formula for the unexposed group would be:

$$\frac{C}{C+D}$$

Therefore, a cohort study design of exposed and unexposed, diseased and nondiseased can provide associations with a health condition by comparing the incidence rates for each of the expected groups (Table 11.1).

A hypothetical example is of an exposed and unexposed cohort study that examines the association of atherosclerosis by selecting a study group exposed to a high saturated fat diet (2,000 exposed), and a group of 6,000 low saturated fat diet individuals, who are all without any evidence of atherosclerosis at baseline. The exposed and unexposed groups are followed over a period of 30 years for the development of atherosclerotic plaque in the carotid artery. The incidence rate of atherosclerotic plaque is calculated for each of these groups. The hypothetical incidence of atherosclerotic plaque formation is 600 per 1,000 with a high saturated fat diet and 133 per 1,000 with a low saturated fat diet (Table 11.2).

Table 11.1 Hypothetical Incidence of Atherosclerotic Plaque Formation With a High Saturated Fat Diet

	Disease Develops	Disease Does not Develop	Totals	Incidence Rate per 1,000
Exposed group	A	B	A + B	$\frac{A}{A+B}$
Unexposed group	C	D	C + D	$\frac{C}{C+D}$

Table 11.2 Hypothetical Incidence of Atherosclerotic Plaque Formation With a Low Saturated Fat Diet

	Atherosclerotic Plaque	No Atherosclerotic Plaque	Totals	Incidence Rate per 1,000
High saturated fat diet	1,200	800	2,000	$\dfrac{1,200}{1,200+800}=600$
Low saturated fat diet	800	5,200	6,000	$\dfrac{800}{800+5,200}=133$

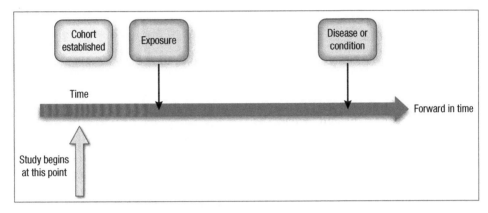

Figure 11.2 Prospective cohort study design.

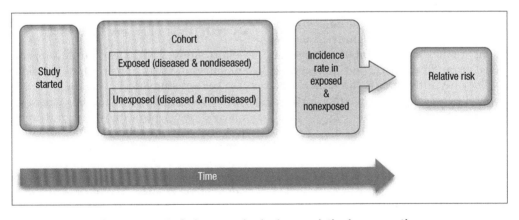

Figure 11.3 Cohort study design analytical perspective.

Prospective Cohort Study Design

Prospective cohort study design groups a cohort according to past or present exposure and follows them into the future to determine if an outcome occurs, as in the preceding example. Figure 11.2 presents the prospective cohort study design. Figure 11.3 presents a graphic representation of the analytical perspective of a cohort study. In a cohort study, the study population has to be followed for a long period of time to ascertain the development of a disease resulting from an exposure. A prospective cohort study is also sometimes referred to as a longitudinal or concurrent cohort study. Specifically, it is called a concurrent prospective study if the epidemiologist first identifies the cohort and follows the cohort forward in time until the point at which they develop the disease or do not develop the disease. A challenge with cohort studies is the length of time required to determine the association between an exposure and the development of a disease.

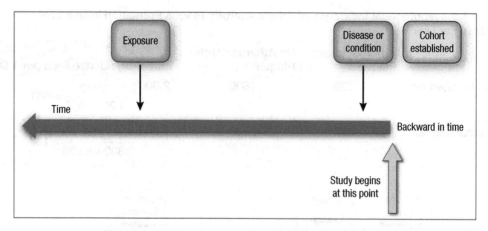

Figure 11.4 Retrospective cohort study design.

Retrospective Cohort Study Design

In a retrospective cohort design, when the study is initiated, the cohort has already experienced an outcome and exposure (Chapter 14). The epidemiologist conducts a retrospective review to identify characteristics and timing of the presence of the exposure and presentation of the outcome. A retrospective cohort study (Figure 11.4) is also known as an historical cohort study or a nonconcurrent prospective study. This design is identical to a prospective cohort study design as both compare the development of a disease as compared from an exposed and nonexposed group. The only difference is the time period or temporal perspective that is either forward or backward in time.

COHORT STUDY BIAS

Research study bias is discussed in Chapter 14. There are some potential biases associated with a cohort study design. These biases are selection and information bias. Selection bias in a cohort study can result from the subjects not responding or not participating in the study to generate the data needed. In addition, subjects can be lost to follow-up for numerous life-related reasons producing an attrition rate that impacts the study findings. Information bias is a concern in that subjects may not be honest or fail to provide sufficient quality and extent of data necessary.

COHORT STUDY VARIATIONS

Cohort study designs can be developed with an integration of other study designs. A case-control study design can be nested into a cohort study design. In addition, there can be a nested case-control study design within a cohort study design with matching of cases and controls to account for confounding variables. Other study designs can be combined with or integrated into a cohort study design as a strategy to increase internal and external validity of the research study design.

END-OF-CHAPTER RESOURCES

SUMMARY POINTS

- Cohort study designs are a population-based observational epidemiologic study.
- Cohort study design selects research subjects that are representative of a larger population of interest based on some cohort characteristic.
- Cohorts can be selected based on risk status.
- A high-risk cohort study intentionally selects subjects with the key distinction of being a subject from a high-risk group that most likely had a known high-risk exposure.
- A basic requirement of a prospective cohort study design is that the outcome or endpoint under investigation should not have occurred in individuals in the cohort study.
- Risk ratio can be abbreviated as RR.
- Risk ratio or RR quantifies the proportion of a population's risk of disease due to a specific exposure.
- Rate ratio compares the rate of disease in two groups that differ by a characteristic or exposure history.
- Prospective cohort study design groups a cohort according to past or present exposure and follows them into the future to determine if an outcomes occurs.
- In a retrospective cohort design, the cohort has already experienced an outcome and exposure when the study is initiated.

EPIDEMIOLOGY CRITICAL REASONING QUESTIONS

1. Design an epidemiologic prospective cohort study. Ensure that the prospective cohort study proposal includes the following:
   a. Research question or research purpose
   b. Rationale for study
   c. Study design description
   d. Target population description
   e. Sampling method/strategy
   f. Cohort characteristics
   g. Disease or health condition measurements
   h. Exposure measurements
   i. Data collection procedure and time intervals
   j. Proposed data analysis
2. Design an epidemiologic retrospective cohort study. Ensure that the retrospective cohort study proposal includes the following:
   a. Research question or research purpose
   b. Rationale for study
   c. Study design description
   d. Target population description
   e. Sampling method/strategy
   f. Cohort characteristics
   g. Disease or health condition measurements
   h. Exposure measurements
   i. Data collection procedure
   j. Retrospective time frame
   k. Proposed data analysis

ADDITIONAL RESOURCES

SPRINGER PUBLISHING **CONNECT™** | A robust set of instructor resources designed to supplement this text is located at http://connect. springerpub.com/content/book/978-0-8261-8514-3. Qualifying instructors may request access by emailing textbook@springerpub.com.

REFERENCES

Bangdiwala, S. (2019). Basic epidemiologic research designs III: Cohort prospective design. *International Journal of Injury Control and Safety Promotion, 26*(3), 322–325. https://doi.org/10.1080/17457300.2019.1625167

Buka, S., Rosenthal, S., & Lacy, M. (2018). Epidemiological study designs: Traditional and novel approaches to advance life course health development research. In N. Halfon, C. B. Forrest, R. M. Lerner, & E. M. Faustman (Eds.), *Handbook of life course health development* (pp. 541–560). Springer.

Chapter 12

CASE CONTROL, OTHER STUDY DESIGNS, AND RESEARCH APPRAISAL

Demetrius J. Porche

True wisdom comes to each of us when we realize how little we understand about life, ourselves, and the world around us.

–Socrates

CHAPTER COMPETENCIES

At the conclusion of this chapter, the reader will be able to:

1. Calculate an odds ratio from a case control study design
2. Differentiate prospective and retrospective research designs
3. Describe other research designs such as historical, exploratory, methodological, and correlational
4. Differentiate the types of triangulation

ESSENTIAL TERMINOLOGY

The essential terminology for case control and other study designs are:

- Analysis triangulation
- Case control
- Data triangulation
- Historical
- Investigator triangulation
- Longitudinal
- Methodological research
- Nested case control study
- Prospective
- Research appraisal
- Retrospective
- Secondary data analysis
- Theoretical triangulation
- Triangulation

Nursing as a practice discipline positions nurses to encounter unique events and situations that can serve as the foundation for future research exploration. Case control studies serve as a catalyst to differentiate the occurrence of disease among cases and controls to generate hypotheses. Nurses should remain astute and vigilant for unique situations encountered that could be the tipping point for exploration of unique cases.

CASE CONTROL STUDY DESIGN

A case control study design groups the research subjects into cases or controls. Cases are those individuals who are identified to have the condition or disorder under investigation. The controls are those individuals selected as a comparison group that does not have the condition or disorder under investigation. In a case control study design, the epidemiologist uses a case definition to select the cases. The case definition identifies the criteria used to select the cases into the sample. In a case control population-based study, the epidemiologist selects a sample of cases from the general population of those with the condition or disorder under investigation. In a hospital or healthcare facility-based study, the epidemiologist selects the cases from the patient list at the respective hospital or healthcare facility. A population-based study will provide greater generalizability than a hospital-based case control study. Controls are selected from the same population as those who had the health condition or disorder under investigation but are known not to have the criteria outlined in the case definition.

In a case control design (Box 12.1), the epidemiologist looks back in time, retrospectively, at the cases and controls to determine who was and was not exposed to the variable or risk factor under investigation. Figures 12.1 and 12.2 explain a case control study design. Case control study design is ideal for studying rare disease cases. Advantages of a case control study design are it is inexpensive, permits examination of multiple exposures, and estimates odds ratios. Disadvantages are the inability to study multiple outcomes at one time;

recall bias; sampling bias; and the inability to calculate prevalence, incidence, and population relative risks. Some other limitations of a case control study design are temporality (not knowing whether the exposure or outcome occurred first), case selection bias, potential confounding bias, and reliance on existing records or history taking (Ranganathan & Aggarwal, 2019).

An odds ratio can be calculated to determine level of risk using a case control study design. Exhibit 12.1 presents the table format and formula used to calculate an odds ratio for exposure to a factor or agent from a case control study design. Figure 12.3 presents the analytical perspective of a case control study design. Table 12.1 presents interpretative meaning of the odds ratio. A hypothetical case of odds ratio with lead poisoning is presented in Exhibit 12.2.

Nested Case Control Study Design

The nested case control study design is a variation on the case control and cohort study design. In a nested case control study design, cases (with the disease under investigation) that occur in a cohort study are identified and typically matched to controls (those in the cohort without the disease under investigation) that are also selected from the cohort study (Buka et al., 2018). In the nested case control study design, the case group consists of the individuals with the outcome under investigation (disease, health condition, or case) that occurs within the defined cohort being followed over time. The control group in the nested case control cohort design is selected from individuals who are either at risk at the time each case occurred or those individuals who are not affected in the cohort present for the baseline initiation of the cohort study.

BOX 12.1. Case Control Study Exemplar

Title: Racial/Ethnic Differences in the Epidemiology of Ovarian Cancer: A Pooled Analysis of 12 Case Control Studies

Summary: The aim of this study was to examine the relationship between 17 reproductive, hormonal and lifestyle factors and ovarian cancer risk by race/ethnicity using data from the African American Cancer Epidemiology Study (AACES) and the Ovarian Cancer Association Consortium (OCAC). Multivariable logistic regression was used to estimate the 17 factors and epithelial ovarian cancer (EOC) risk by race/ethnicity among 10,924 women with invasive EOC and 16,150 controls. The study found statistically significant racial/ethnic heterogeneity for hysterectomy and EOC risk, with the largest odds ratio (OR) observed in Black women compared with other racial/ethnic groups. Asian/Pacific Islander had the greatest magnitude of association for parity and Black women had the largest ORs for family history and endometriosis. The findings of this study support the validity of EOC risk factors across all racial/ethnic groups and suggest that all groups with a higher prevalence of a modifiable risk factor should be targeted to disseminate information about prevention.

Source: Peres, L. C., Risch, H., Terry, K. L., Webb, P. M., Goodman, M. T., Wu, A. H., Alberg, A. J., Bandera, E. V., Barnholtz-Sloan, J., Bondy, M. L., Cote, M. L., Funkhouser, E., Moorman, P. G., Peters, E. S., Schwartz, A. G., Terry, P. D., Manichaikul, A., Abbott, S. E., Camacho, F., ... African American Cancer Epidemiology Study and the Ovarian Cancer Association Consortium. (2018). Racial/ethnic differences in the epidemiology of ovarian cancer: A pooled analysis of 12 case control studies. *International Journal of Epidemiology, 47*(2), 460–472. https://doi.org/10.1093/ije/dyx252

EXHIBIT 12.1. Case Control Analysis Format

Exposure	Cases	Controls
Yes	A	B
No	C	D

Odds of being exposed among cases = A ÷ C

Odds of being exposed among controls = B ÷ D

Exposure odds ratio = (A ÷ C) ÷ (B ÷ D) = (A × D) ÷ (B × C)

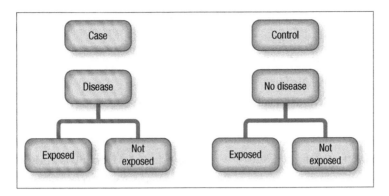

Figure 12.1 Case control research design.

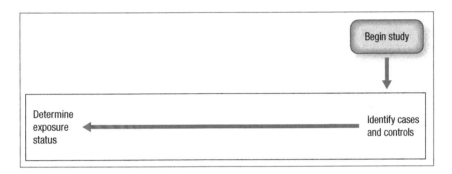

Figure 12.2 Case controls design: Time perspective.

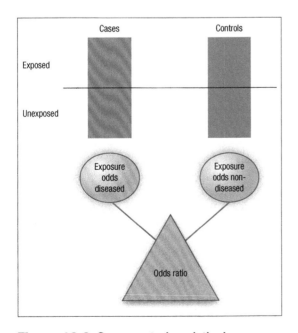

Figure 12.3 Case control analytical perspective.

Case Control Matching

Matching of subjects is implemented in a case control design when the epidemiologist is trying to reduce the impact of confounding factors. In case control matching, the epidemiologist attempts to ensure that the sample of cases and controls are as similar as possible. There are several types of matching that occur. Cases and controls can be matched on individual relevant characteristics from the target population. Some common characteristics that research subjects are matched on are gender, race/ethnicity, and age. Another matching option is frequency matching, which identifies the matching variable or factor for the cases and controls to be matched on first. With knowledge of the distribution of cases in the group with the matching variable, there can be an estimation of the number of controls needed to match the matching variable in the control group. Then the number of controls determined are selected with the matching variable so that it is proportional to the distribution of the matching variable in the case group.

Table 12.1 Odds Ratio Interpretation (or Relative Risk)

Odds Ratio	Interpretation
1.0	No association
>1.0	Positive association (may be causal)
<1.0	Negative association (may be protective effect)

EXHIBIT 12.2. Hypothetical Case of Lead Poisoning

Occupational Exposure	Cases	Controls
Yes	20	18
No	80	89

Exposure odds ratio = (A ÷ C) ÷ (B ÷ D) = (A × D) ÷ (B × C) = 20/80 ÷ 18/89 = 20 × 89 ÷ 18 × 80 = 1.23

TIME-BASED STUDY DESIGNS

Research study designs can simply be labeled or classified according to the temporal perspective of data collection. The time period can be prospective (forward in time) or retrospective (back in time). In addition, time-based studies can be classified in accordance with the number of times data are collected to monitor trends or patterns in data, such as with time-series designs (Pearce, 2012).

Prospective

A research design can be simply labeled as prospective. A prospective research design (Box 12.2) indicates that the epidemiologist begins the study and collects data moving forward in time. This research label does not provide specificity about the research methods and data collection procedures; it only defines the design in terms of temporal data collection forward in time.

Retrospective

The simple designation that a research design is retrospective indicates that the epidemiologist begins the study and looks back in time for data collection (Box 12.3). Like the prospective design label, a retrospective research design label alone does not provide specificity about the research methods or data collection procedures.

Time-Series Design

A time-series design involves the observation of a variable or outcome over a defined period

---

BOX 12.2. Prospective Study Exemplar

Title: Epidemiology of Invasive Pulmonary Aspergillosis Among Intubated Patients With COVID-19: A Prospective Study

Summary: The purpose of this study was to describe the incidence and outcome of corona virus-associated pulmonary aspergillosis (CAPA) in mechanically ventilated patients with COVID-19 and to evaluate the prognostic impact of different aspergillosis case definitions in this setting. There were 108 patients enrolled, and this was a prospective multicenter cohort study in patients hospitalized from February 22 through April 20, 2020 with laboratory confirmed SARS-CoV-2 virus infection in four ICUs from three hospitals in Bologna, Italy. The participants of this study went through a screening procedure for invasive pulmonary aspergillosis with broncheoalveolar lavage galactomannan and cultures that were taken on admission at 7 days and in cases of clinical status deterioration. The obtained results led to a conclusion that a high incidence of CAPA exists among critically ill COVID-19 patients, and changes the natural course of the disease.

Source: Bartoletti, M., Pascale, R., Cricca, M., Rinaldi, M., Maccaro, A., Bussini, L., Fornaro, G., Tonetti, T., Pizzilli, G., Francalanci, E., Giuntoli, L., Rubin, A., Moroni, A., Ambretti, A., Trapani, F., Vatamanu, O., Ranieri V. M., Castelli, A., Baiocchi, M., ... Viale, P. (2020). Epidemiology of invasive pulmonary aspergillosis among intubated patients with COVID-19: A prospective study. *Clinical Infectious Diseases: An Official Publication of the Infectious Diseases Society of America.* https://doi.org/10.1093/cid/ciaa1065

---

of time. Time-series designs can assist with the identification of subtle changes in patterns of morbidity occurrence over time. A time-series design (Box 12.4) is useful to measure the effect of an intervention or treatment at multiple points of time during a study. An interrupted time-series design is a type of time-series design that exposes the research subject to an intervention and withdraws the intervention, while measuring the impact of the intervention during periods of time before the intervention, while

BOX 12.3. Retrospective study exemplar

Title: Epidemiology and Predictors of NTM Pulmonary Infection in Taiwan—A Retrospective, 5-Year Multicenter Study

Summary: The purpose of this study was to provide a 5-year incidence rate of nontuberculosis mycobacteria (NTM) pulmonary infection (PI) in Taiwan and investigate nontuberculosis predictors. Six hospitals in Taiwan were recruited in the study that took place between 2008 and 2014. Medical records, laboratory data, and chest radiographs of patients were reviewed in these hospitals. The study identified a total of 1,674 new episodes of NTM-PI with 1,492 cases identified between 2010 and 2014. Among these, about 9.5% experienced multiple episodes of NTM-PI. The number of respiratory specimens was the lowest in 2010 and highest in 2012. New infection rate was stable in Northern Taiwan but peaked in 2014 in Southern Taiwan. Incidence rate of NTM-PI stabilized between 2010 and 2014.

Source: Huang, H. L., Cheng, M.-H., Lu, P.-L, Shu, C.-C., Wang, J.-Y, Wang, J.-T, Chong, I.-W., & Lee, L.-N. (2017). Epidemiology and predictors of NTM pulmonary infection in Taiwan—A retrospective, 5-year multicenter study. *Scientific Reports, 7*(1), 16300. https://doi.org/10.1038/s41598-017-16559-z

BOX 12.4. Times Series Study Exemplar

Title: The Role of Parental Self-Regulation and Household Chaos in Parent–Toddler Interactions: A Time-Series Study

Summary: This study aimed to study the effect of parental self-regulation on reactive negative parenting and how household chaos amplified or diminished these associations. The study also attempted to determine whether the associations between parental self-regulation, household chaos, and reactive negative parenting differed depending upon whether parental self-regulation was operationalized as self-reported, effortful control or as task-based executive functioning. The subjects included 62 Dutch toddlers and their parents aged 27 to 46 years. Examiners visited parents and their toddlers in their homes and assigned tasks to the children, while the parent–child interaction was videotaped. After the visit, the parents completed four computer-based tasks that assessed their level of executive functioning. At the end of the study it was found that lower parental self-regulation predicted more reactive negative parenting practices in chaotic households. Parents who are less regulated may benefit from home situations that provide a calm and tidy atmosphere with routine to remain neutral in situations where their toddler is noncompliant.

Source: Geeraerts, S. B., Endendijk, J., Deater-Deckard, K., Huijding, J., Deutz, M., van den Boomen, C., & Deković, M. (2020). The role of parental self-regulation and household chaos in parent–toddler interactions: A time-series study. *Journal of Family Psychology, 35*(2), 236–246. https://doi.org/10.1037/fam0000814

the intervention occurs, after the intervention is stopped, and again when the intervention is reinstated and interrupted again. Basically, an interrupted time-series design alternates between administering an intervention and withdrawing the intervention while continually measuring the outcome to determine effectiveness of the intervention over an extended period of time.

Longitudinal

A study design can be simply labeled longitudinal. A longitudinal research design indicates that the same sample has repeated measures or observations over a period of time. For example, a sample could be interviewed at regular intervals or complete a survey questionnaire at designated time intervals. A longitudinal research design's purpose is to identify changes over time and relate the temporal changes to a variable under investigation. Disease patterns over time can be studied using a longitudinal research design.

INCIDENCE STUDY DESIGN

An incidence study examines newly reported cases or diseases compared over time in relation to person, place, and time. Incidence studies provide the data necessary to calculate an incidence rate in a population during a specific time period (Pearce, 2012).

HISTORICAL STUDY DESIGN

Epidemiologists can use an historical research study design to examine the evolution of a disease process over time. Historical research involves a critical analysis of the events, documents, literature, and other sources of information to reconstruct past events as a means to understand what, how, and why a particular event occurred. Historical research can provide a foundation of knowledge from which to interpret and understand current epidemiologic events. Historical research uses an organizing framework to guide the search for authentic and verifiable data. Historical research is not a critical literature review or chronological presentation of a series of epidemiologic events over time. Historical research provides a contextual description of the past event with the incorporation of judgments, analyses, and inferences about the relationships of data discovered. These data are contextually organized and synthesized into a historical story from the past.

Historical research uses primary, original, and authentic data such as letters, photographs, eyewitness accounts, and direct recording of events. Historical research also uses secondary data from biographies, literature, and newspapers to support the understanding of the past event. One of the most critical elements of historical research is the establishment of the authenticity of the data which requires subjecting the data to external criticisms.

EXPLORATORY STUDY DESIGN

An exploratory research study is conducted when there is little to no earlier research on the phenomenon of interest. Exploratory studies are designed to gain insight and familiarity with the phenomenon. Exploratory research studies are somewhat unstructured and flexible, designed to increase familiarity with the setting, population, and situation under investigation. Exploratory study design may be combined with a descriptive study design called descriptive exploratory design.

TRIANGULATION

There are times when a single measurement approach to exploring a research concept is not sufficient to justify a valid interpretation of the findings. Triangulation is not considered so much of a research design but a method of combining measurements or analyses. Triangulation combines the use of two or more theories, methods, data sources, investigators, or analysis methods to examine the same phenomenon of interest. There are five general types of triangulation: data, investigator, theoretical, methodological, or analysis (Gray & Grove, 2020).

Data triangulation collects data from multiple sources for the same study. To be considered true data triangulation, the data collected should have the same foci. These multiple data sources provide the epidemiologist with the opportunity to examine how a phenomenon of interest is experienced by different individuals, groups, or populations at different times

or in different settings. Investigator triangulation involves two or more epidemiologic investigators with different research experience to examine the same phenomenon of interest. Theoretical triangulation uses two or more theoretical lenses to interpret the study findings. Methodological triangulation uses two or more research methods in a single study. The two types of methodological triangulation are within method and between method or across method. Within method triangulation uses two or more methods to study a phenomenon. For example, within method triangulation would use two different survey instruments to measure the same concepts or phenomena. Between method triangulation or across method triangulation combines two or more different research traditions in the same study. For example, a between method triangulation would use both quantitative and qualitative methods to examine the same phenomenon. Analysis triangulation uses two different analysis techniques to analyze the same data set (Gray & Grove, 2020).

METHODOLOGICAL RESEARCH

Methodological research is also sometimes referred to as psychometric research. Methodological research (Box 12.5) is the development and testing of measurement instruments, sometimes also referred to as instrument development. The instrument development could be for research and/or clinical practice purposes. These instruments could be screening and/or diagnostic instruments. Methodological research involves the establishment of an instrument's validity and reliability metrics.

SECONDARY DATA ANALYSIS

Secondary data analysis uses an existing database or data set to re-examine the variables. Generally, the epidemiologist poses a new or different research question for which the data have already been collected from a target population. Sometimes secondary data analysis is less expensive and time consuming since the data have already been collected. A limitation of secondary data analysis is the researchers' limited control over the data collection process.

CORRELATION STUDY DESIGN

Correlation study design measures the degree of association between two variables. A correlation

---

BOX 12.5 Methodological Research Exemplar

Title: The Healthcare Needs of Physically, Hearing, or Visually Impaired People: A Methodological Study

Summary: The purpose of this study was to evaluate the healthcare needs of individuals with disabilities, as well as those who have hearing or visual impairments through the development of an instrument to be validated by the Delphi technique. The study was conducted in two stages with three steps included in the second stage. Stage I identified the healthcare needs of the population studied by performing a thorough literature review. Stage II focused on the development and validation of the assessment tool for the healthcare needs of physically, hearing, or visually impaired people as it pertains to its content, reliability and applicability to people with disabilities. The content and reliability of the assessment tool were determined by the assessor's opinions, while applicability was determined by Cronbach alpha.

Source: Belmiro, S. S. D. D. R., Miranda, F. A. N. D., Moura, I. B. D. L., Carvalho, S. R. D., & Costa, I. K. F. (2016). The healthcare needs of physically, hearing or visually impaired people: A methodological study. *Online Brazilian Journal of Nursing, 15*(S1), 494–497. http://www.objnursing.uff.br/index.php/nursing/article/view/5565

---

study design is sometimes considered a type of descriptive or exploratory study design. Within the correlation design, correlation is considered a function of covariation in data. For example, correlation design provides data on the extent to which one variable changes or varies directly or indirectly with another variable. Trends and patterns in data are determined with correlation study designs. A correlation study design does not implement an intervention or attempt to control a variable under investigation. This design simply measures the extent to which one variable varies in relation or respect to another variable. Data from correlation study designs provide supportive data to establish the presence of causation between an independent and dependent research variable.

A predictive correlation study design uses statistical regression analysis to determine or predict a behavior or response of one variable based on observed relationships between the predictive behavior and other variables under investigation. Predictive correlation designs assist with developing clinical decision-making models to predict the success of an intervention. The ultimate aim of a predictive correlation study design is to determine the extent or level to which a dependent variable is predicted from an independent variable. In a predicative correlation design, the terms independent and dependent are used to describe the variables under investigation. In this design, a dependent variable is the variable or variables to be predicted. The independent variable is the term used to describe those variables that are considered predictors of the predictive variable.

MODEL TESTING

A model testing study design examines the relationships among all variables relevant to the model or framework under investigation. A model testing design is best used with a large, heterogeneous sample. In a model testing study design, the relationships or correlation paths are examined among all variables in the model. These relationships and the amount of correlation among the model variables are used to develop a conceptual map that confirms or challenges the proposed model.

Model testing uses three variable categories: exogenous, endogenous, and residual. Exogenous variables are those within the model being tested but caused by factors external to the model. Endogenous variables are those variables whose variation and correlations are explained within the model being tested. Residual variables are variables that impact the model but are not measured specifically in the model (Gray & Grove, 2020).

EPIDEMIOLOGIC RESEARCH STUDY APPRAISAL

Epidemiologic research study appraisal is the systematic evaluation of a research study's quality based on scientific merit and methodological rigor. The epidemiologic research study appraisal is dependent upon the research study design. Appendix E presents several sample questions for a research study appraisal based on the study design. Some general areas of evaluation for a research study appraisal are listed in the following:

- **Background:** Examine the merit and quality of the study rationale, significance, and background literature to support the study, problem statement or area, research question, purpose, objectives, or aims

- **Methods:** Identification of study design and evaluation of study design integrity, sampling method, validity, and reliability of measurement, sample size determination, power, and effect size, random selection and random assignment (as appropriate), data analysis and management, and human subjects' protection
- **Results/Findings:** Adequacy of findings; appropriate epidemiologic or statistical analysis; congruence between narrative, tables, and figures; results consistent with research question, purpose, objective or aims
- **Discussion:** Findings/results placed within context of existing science and knowledge base, limitations addressed, recommendations provided; generalizations are not presented beyond study capability and findings/results

END-OF-CHAPTER RESOURCES

SUMMARY POINTS

- A case control study design groups the research subjects into cases or controls.
- Cases are those individuals who are identified to have the condition or disorder under investigation.
- Controls are those individuals selected as a comparison group that does not have the condition or disorder under investigation.
- The case definition identifies the criteria used to select the cases for the sample.
- In a case control design, the epidemiologist looks back in time, retrospectively, at the cases and controls to determine who was and was not exposed to the variable or risk factor under investigation.
- An odds ratio can be calculated to determine level of risk using a case control study design.
- In a nested case control study design, cases that occur in a cohort study are identified and typically matched to controls that are also selected from the cohort study.
- In case control matching, the epidemiologist attempts to ensure that the sample of cases and controls are as similar as possible.
- Matching of subjects is implemented in a case control design when the epidemiologist is trying to reduce the impact of confounding factors.
- In a time-based study, the time period can be prospective (forward in time) or retrospective (back in time).
- A time-series design is useful to measure the effect of an intervention or treatment at multiple points of time during a study.
- Historical research can provide a foundation of knowledge from which to interpret and understand current epidemiologic events.
- Exploratory studies are designed to gain insight and familiarity with the phenomenon.
- Triangulation combines the use of two or more theories, methods, data sources, investigators, or analysis methods to examine the same phenomenon of interest.
- Data triangulation collects data from multiple sources for the same study.

- Investigator triangulation involves two or more epidemiologic investigators with different research experience to examine the same phenomenon of interest.
- Theoretical triangulation uses two or more theoretical lenses to interpret the study findings.
- Methodological triangulation uses two or more research methods.
- Analysis triangulation uses two different analysis techniques to analyze the same data set.
- Methodological research is the development and testing of measurement instruments, sometimes also referred to as instrument development.
- Secondary data analysis uses an existing database or data sets to re-examine the variables.
- Correlation study design examines why two or more variables vary together; measures association/correlation.
- A model testing study design examines the relationships between all variables relevant to the model or framework under investigation.
- Epidemiologic research study appraisal is the systematic evaluation of a research study's quality based on scientific merit and methodological rigor.

EPIDEMIOLOGY CRITICAL REASONING QUESTIONS

1. Identify a health condition or disease process of interest. Identify the definition for a case. Design a case control research study.
2. Select two types of triangulation. Describe how you would integrate these two types of triangulation into a research study.
3. Describe the design differences in a prospective and retrospective study design.
4. List at least four criteria to use in conducting an epidemiologic research study appraisal.
5. Design a case control study. In this case control study, integrate a nested study within the case control study design.
6. Describe the difference between primary data analysis and secondary data analysis.

ADDITIONAL RESOURCES

SPRINGER PUBLISHING CONNECT™	A robust set of instructor resources designed to supplement this text is located at http://connect.

springerpub.com/content/book/978-0-8261-8514-3.
Qualifying instructors may request access by emailing
textbook@springerpub.com.

REFERENCES

Buka, S., Rosenthal, S., & Lacy, M. (2018). Epidemiological study designs: Traditional and novel approaches to advance life course health development research. In N. Halfon, C. B. Forrest, R. M. Lerner, & E. M. Faustman (Eds.), *Handbook of life course health development* (pp. 541–560). Springer.

Gray, J., & Grove, S. (2020). *Burns and Grove's the practice of nursing research: Appraisal, synthesis, and generation of evidence* (9th ed.). Saunders.

Pearce, N. (2012). Classification of epidemiological study designs. *International Journal of Epidemiology, 41,* 393–397. https://doi.org/10.1093/ije/dys049

Ranganathan, P., & Aggarwal, R. (2019). Study designs: Part 3—Analytical observational studies. *Perspectives in Clinical Research, 10*(2), 91–94. https://doi.org/10.4103/picr.PICR_35_19

Chapter 13

EXPERIMENTAL STUDIES: QUASI-EXPERIMENTAL, EXPERIMENTAL, AND RANDOMIZED CLINICAL TRIALS

Demetrius J. Porche

You never fail until you stop trying.
–Albert Einstein

CHAPTER COMPETENCIES

At the conclusion of this chapter, the reader will be able to:

1. Describe the difference between a control and comparison group
2. Differentiate between an equivalent and nonequivalent research group
3. Demonstrate an understanding of quasi-experimental research designs
4. Demonstrate an understanding of the essential elements of an experimental research design
5. Differentiate the phases of a randomized controlled clinical trial
6. Discuss the design of a vaccine clinical trial

ESSENTIAL TERMINOLOGY

The essential terminology for experimental research designs are:

- Control group
- Comparison group
- Equivalent group
- Nonequivalent group
- Experimental design
- Quasi-experimental design
- Probabilistic equivalence
- Solomon four-group design
- Randomized block design
- Randomized controlled clinical trial
- Crossover study design
- Community interventional design

Experimental research designs provide the epidemiologist with the ability to make statements about relationships, associations, and supportive statements regarding causation. Hypotheses generated through observational research study designs can be tested with an experimental research design. Not all epidemiologic areas of inquiry are adaptable to an experimental research study design. Quasi-experimental research study designs provide an alternative research design to experimental research designs when all the essential elements required for a true experimental study cannot be established within the design.

CONTROL AND COMPARISON GROUPS

Control groups are used in experimental studies. Control groups are selected randomly from the same target population as the experimental group is selected. A control group, as explained in the experimental research design given in the following, does not receive any treatment or intervention. A control group assists the epidemiologist with the determination of differences between the treatment and control groups by reducing the risk of error.

A comparison group is used when the research study design does not randomly select the subjects. A comparison group, like a control group, does not receive any experimental treatment or intervention that is under investigation. There are four types of comparison groups:

1. Group receives no treatment or intervention
2. Group receives a placebo treatment
3. Group receives a usual or standard of care treatment
4. Group receives a different treatment that provides for a comparative effect analysis such as a different dosage (Chatburn, 2017; Gray & Grove, 2020)

QUASI-EXPERIMENTAL RESEARCH DESIGN

Quasi-experimental research designs provide an alternative research design when it is not possible to conduct a true experimental design. A quasi-experimental research design is a research design that lacks one of the three essential components of a true experiment. In a quasi-experimental design, one of the following three items are not present: randomization to group, comparison or control group, or the ability to manipulate the intervention or treatment (Box 13.1; Gray & Grove, 2020; Siedleck, 2020).

One-Group Posttest-Only Design

A one-group posttest-only design is also described as a pre-experimental design rather than a type of quasi-experimental design. This design limits the determination of causality. The one group under investigation is not protested and there is little control over the selection of subjects who receive the treatment or intervention. There is no comparison group with a one-group posttest-only design, which limits the ability to adequately determine the extent to which the posttest measure is a direct result of the treatment or intervention (Gray & Grove, 2020). The one-group posttest-only design is noted as follows, where X represents an intervention or treatment and O represents an observation or measurement:

X   O

BOX 13.1. Effectiveness of High-Fidelity Simulation in Nursing Education for End-of-Life Care: A Quasi-Experimental Design

Summary: The purpose of this study was to measure the effectiveness of high-fidelity simulation to teach end-of-life (EOL) care in a palliative care nursing course to nursing students in the undergraduate nursing education program at the School of Nursing and Midwifery at Aga Khan University in Karachi, Pakistan. A total of 42 nursing students participated in the study that used a pre- and postintervention quasi-experimental design without a control group. The study process was performed in three stages—the pre-brief about the scenario with role assignment of the participants, the actual simulation, and the debrief at the end of the simulation exercise. The study led to the conclusion that teaching EOL care via high-fidelity simulation improved the attitudes of students toward the care of dying patients and their family members, and simultaneously provided the students with an opportunity to deal with their own emotions.

Source: Rattani, S. A., Kurji, Z., Khowaja, A. A., Dias, J. M., & AliSher, A. N. (2020). Effectiveness of high-fidelity simulation in nursing education for end-of-life care: A quasi-experimental design. *Indian Journal of Palliative Care*, *26*(3), 312–318. https://doi.org/10.4103/IJPC.IJPC_157_19

Posttest-Only With Comparison Group Design

A posttest-only with comparison group design provides some improvement over the one-group posttest-only design. This is also considered a pre-experimental or quasi-experimental design type. This design combines the one-group posttest-only design with a comparison group. The comparison group is generally not randomly selected from the target population; therefore, it is considered a nonequivalent comparison group (Gray & Grove, 2020). The posttest-only with comparison group design is noted as follows, where X represents an intervention or treatment, and O represents an observation or measurement:

Experimental group   X   O
Nonequivalent group   O

One-Group Pretest–Posttest Design

A one-group pretest–posttest design is also considered a pre-experimental or quasi-experimental design type. This design is limited by the impact on the posttest scores by the pretest. In this design, it may not be clear what impact maturation, pretest administration, or instrumentation changes had on the posttest score, since there is no comparison group (Gray & Grove, 2020). This design is noted as follows, where X represents an intervention or treatment, and O represents an observation or measurement:

Experimental group   O   X   O

Pretest and Posttest With Comparison Group Design

The pretest and posttest with comparison group design improves the one-group pretest–posttest design by adding a comparison group. The major limitations or threats to internal validity are with the lack of randomization in this design (Gray & Grove, 2020). This design is noted as follows, where X represents an intervention or treatment, and O represents an observation or measurement:

Experimental group	O	X	O
Nonequivalent group	O		O

Pretest and Posttest Design With Two or More Comparison Groups

The pretest and posttest design (Box 13.2) can be improved with the addition of more comparison groups. A pretest and posttest design with two or more comparison groups can used when there is a known standard of care or identified effective treatment. This design is strengthened by adding one or more no treatment groups, a placebo treatment group, or a usual treatment group to the design. A pretest and posttest with two comparison treatment groups is noted as follows, where the X for treatment is replaced with a T to note the treatment and O represents the observation or measurement:

Experimental Group 1	O	T_1	O
Experimental Group 2	O	T_2	O

A pretest and posttest design with two comparison treatment groups and a standard of care or routine care group for comparison is noted as follows, where U represents the standard of care or usual treatment:

Experimental Group 1	O	T_1	O
Experimental Group 2	O	T_2	O
Comparison Group	O	U	O

BOX 13.2. A Clinical Teaching Blended Learning Program to Enhance Registered Nurse Preceptors' Teaching Competencies: Pretest and Posttest Study

Summary: The purpose of this study was to examine the effect of a geriatric day hospital (GDH) program on the functional independence of older adults and caregiver stress. A nonexperimental single group pre- and posttest design was utilized, with data collection via retrospective chart reviews and follow-up phone calls. The study measured outcomes such as fear of falling, balance, functional exercise capacity, and caregiver stress. The patient population consisted of 128 participants and included patients 65+ years old, referred by a physician and had two or more concerns related to mobility/falls, activities of daily living, cognitive issues, symptoms that affect function, medication concerns, and/or caregiver stress. Three-hour therapy sessions 2 days per week were given for a period of approximately 10 weeks. Therapy sessions consisted of large group and individual sessions with clinicians based on participants' needs. Although no statistically significant difference was found in the pre- and posttest scores in relation to caregiver stress, significant differences were found in the pre- and posttest mean scores for fear of falling, balance, and functional exercise capacity. This indicates that the GDH program positively impacted all outcomes except caregiver stress.

Source: Wu, X. V., Chi, Y., Panneer Selvam, U., Devi, M. K., Wang, W., Chan, Y. S., Wee, F. C., Zhao, S., Sehgal, V., & Ang, N. (2020). A clinical teaching blended learning program to enhance registered nurse preceptors' teaching competencies: Pretest and posttest study. *Journal of Medical Internet Research*, *22*(4), e18604. https://doi.org/10.2196/18604

Pretest and Posttest Reversed Treatment Design

The epidemiologist may desire to explore a known positive and negative treatment effect on a health condition or disease. If there is a known factor or agent that produces a positive impact on the health status and one that produces a negative impact on the same health status, these can be explored in a two-group design, known as a pretest and posttest reversed treatment design. One group is exposed to the positive effect and one group to the negative effect with the response monitored in both groups (Gray & Grove, 2020). This design is noted as +X represents the positive effect and −X represents the negative effect and O represents an observation or measurement:

Experimental Group 1   O   +X   O

Experimental Group 2   O   –X   O

EXPERIMENTAL RESEARCH DESIGN

Experimental research design provides the maximum amount of control in a research study design. An experimental study design provides data sufficient to support the examination of causation. An experimental design is considered the most "rigorous" research study design and the "gold standard" to which other study designs are compared in terms of internal and external validity. However, an experimental design should be structured with the intent to eliminate all factors that could influence the dependent variable under investigation to provide sufficient data for causation support (Gray & Grove, 2020). The three essential elements of an experimental research design are manipulation of an intervention or exposure under investigation, randomization, and existence of an experimental and control group. Figure 13.1 presents the basic elements of an experimental design.

In an experimental design, equivalent groups are created. With the establishment of equivalent groups, it is more likely that differences between the intervention or control group are due to the actual intervention. Group equivalence is best established through both random selection from the target population and random assignment to study groups. However, the minimum requirement to establish equivalent groups is random group assignment. The idea of "probabilistic equivalent" establishes that group equivalence is known.

Probabilistic equivalence does not mean that the two groups are equal to each other. Probabilistic group equivalence is based on the notion of probabilities. Probabilistic equivalence means that we know the odds that there will be a difference identified between the two groups. It does not mean that the two groups are equal or equivalent. Probabilistic equivalence calculates the chance that the two groups differ by chance alone even with random assignment. This provides some assurance that differences in findings are due to the known experimental intervention.

In summary, the basic hypothetical test in an experimental design is if X occurs, then Y happens. It can also further determine the opposite hypothetical test; if X occurs, then Y happens and if X does not occur, then Y does not happen. Satisfaction of both of these hypothetical statements provides more support to establish causation.

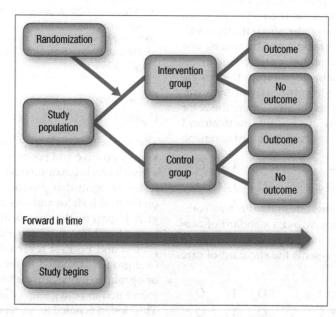

Figure 13.1 Basic experimental design elements.

Classic Experimental Design

The classic or original experimental design is a pretest–posttest control group design. Figure 13.2 provides the simple structure of a pretest and posttest control group design. In a classical experimental design, there are two groups randomized, one to a treatment or experimental group and one to a control group or comparison group. The dependent or outcome variable is measured before and after exposure to the intervention. The classic experimental design is noted as:

Experimental Group	R	O	X	O
Control Group	R	O		O

The classic experimental design provides the basic experimental research design from which other variations of the experimental design emerge.

Experimental Posttest-Only Control Group

If there is concern that the pretest will sensitize the subjects to the dependent or outcome variable, an experimental posttest-only control group design can be used. In this design, the posttest variable is not measured before the treatment. Figure 13.3 presents the posttest with control group design. The experimental posttest-only control group design is noted as:

Experimental Group	R	X	O
Control Group	R		O

RANDOMIZED BLOCK DESIGN

A randomized block design divides the sample into relatively homogenous groups or blocks, similar to strata in stratified sampling method. In a randomized block design, an intervention can be implemented within each homogenous sub-group. The thought with a randomized block design is that the variability within each sub-group or block will be less than the variability among the entire sample. An estimate of the treatment or intervention effect within a block may be more efficient than the efficient estimates across the entire sample. Figure 13.4 shows randomized block designs.

SOLOMON FOUR-GROUP DESIGN

The Solomon four-group design (Box 13.3) reduces the potential threat of testing or preintervention measurement. Basically, this design

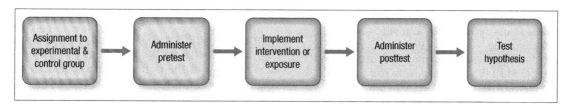

Figure 13.2 Pretest and posttest design.

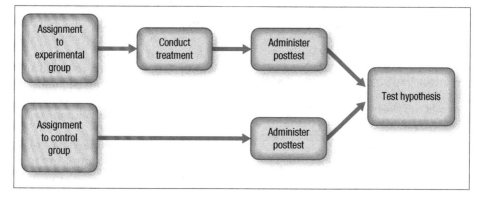

Figure 13.3 Posttest design.

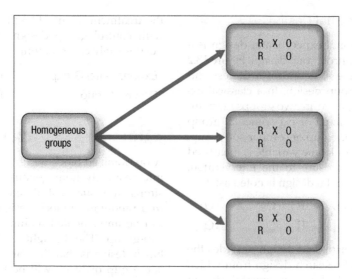

Figure 13.4 Randomized block design example (two-group posttest-only design).

BOX 13.3. Budget Over Health Unless Overweight: A Solomon Four-Group Study

Summary: The purpose of this study was to evaluate the influence of market prices targeting consumers' budget and health-related motivations for food purchase in a 2 (Price: recommended price, discount price) by 2 (Product: regular potato chips, potato chips with 75% less saturated fat) experiment using six Solomon four-group designs. Two groups measured the effect of price (S1, S6), two explored the effect of the products (S2, S5) and two examined the combined effect of price and product (S3, S4). There were two aspects to price—the recommended retail price (RRP) and the discount price (DP). The study involved 13 groups with 50 participants per group for a total of 650 randomly assigned participants. The sample was fairly distributed by gender with the majority 30-years-old or younger. According to BMIs, 9% were underweight, one third were overweight or obese, and the remaining were normal weight. Approximately 61% were married, and more than 27% had children. A 12-item questionnaire was used with five descriptive items collected—weight, height, gender, age and marital status. A 5-point scale was used to measure purchase intention regarding subjects' flavor choice for potato chips. Five remaining questions asked about consumption patterns and awareness of health messages on potato chips packets. The results of this study indicate that overweight consumers do not care much for discounts when compared to their normal weight counterparts. Price reductions on products essentially invalidate the influence of health messages on purchase intentions among normal weight buyers when the regular and healthier packaged foods are both on discount.

Source: Yin, Y., & Özdinç, Y. (2018). Budget over health unless overweight: A Solomon four-group study. *International Journal of Consumer Studies, 42*(2), 232–240. https://doi.org/10.1111/ijcs.12411

---

permits an assessment of whether there is an interaction between the treatment or intervention group and the pretest measurement. Testing threat occurs when the test or measurement affects the individual's response on the posttest. In the Solomon four-group design, two groups receive the treatment or intervention and two groups do not. The Solomon four-group structure consist of four groups:

- **Group 1:** Baseline data collected with subjects receiving the intervention (treatment/intervention group)
- **Group 2:** Baseline data collected and subjects are in the control group (standard treatment)
- **Group 3:** No baseline data collected and subjects receive the intervention (treatment/intervention group)
- **Group 4:** No baseline data collected and subjects are in the control group (standard treatment)

Two groups received a pretest and two do not receive the pretest. This design facilitates the examination of the extent to which a testing threat is operating in the findings. Exhibit 13.1 presents the Solomon four-group design notation.

Switching Replication Experimental Design

In a switching replication experimental design, there are two groups with three points of outcome measurement. The intervention or treatment is replicated in both groups. The two groups are considered to switch roles in which the control group becomes the treatment or intervention group in the second aspect of the study, and the original treatment or intervention group becomes the control group in the second aspect of the study. At the conclusion of the study, all subjects have served as a member of the control and treatment or intervention group. Exhibit 13.2 notes the switching replication experimental design.

RANDOMIZED CLINICAL TRIALS

As randomized controlled clinical trials (Box 13.4) are the gold standard for experimental research and the highest level of evidence in evidence-based practice, clinical trials are considered the gold standard for the development of new pharmaceutical agents and devices. Figure 13.5 outlines the phases and goals of clinical trials. Clinical trials are categorized as nonclinical and clinical trials. Nonclinical trials involve experimental testing in vitro (test tube) and in vivo (cell cultures or animal testing). Clinical trials involve experimental testing in humans, either healthy or with a specific disease condition. Clinical trial phases can be combined or eliminated depending on the level of scientific information available on the candidate pharmaceutical agent or device. Clinical trial phases ultimately desire to determine efficacy and effectiveness. Efficacy assesses the extent to which the pharmaceutical agent produces the desired outcome in a specific population. Effectiveness assesses the extent to which the pharmaceutical agent can produce the desired result in "real world" conditions. An Investigational New Drug (IND) application is filed prior to the initiation of clinical trials (Friedman et al., 2015).

EXHIBIT 13.1. Solomon Four-Group Design Structure

R	O	X	O
R	O		O
R		X	O
R			O

EXHIBIT 13.2. Switching Replication Experimental Design Notation

R	O	X	O		O (experiment then control group)
R	O		O	X	O (control then experimental group)

BOX 13.4. Effects of Early Integrated Palliative Care in Patients with Lung and GI Cancer: A Randomized Clinical Trial

Summary: The purpose of this study was to evaluate the effect of early integrated palliative care (PC) in patients with newly diagnosed, incurable cancers on quality of life (QOL). The 350 patients involved in this study were those from Massachusetts General Hospital (MGH) in a nonblinded, randomized trial of early PC with oncology care compared with usual oncology care. Participants were restricted to those within 8 weeks of a diagnosis of incurable lung or noncolorectal GI cancer. The patients were randomly assigned in a 1:1 manner to receive the early integrated PC intervention and oncology care versus the usual care. QOL was measured using a 27-item Functional Assessment of Cancer Therapy-General (FACT-G) scale that evaluates four areas of QOL (physical, functional, emotional, and social well-being). The Patient Health Questionnaire-9 (PHQ-9) and the Hospital Anxiety and Depression Scale (HADS) were both used to evaluate mood and anxiety. At the end of the study it was concluded that patients with newly diagnosed incurable cancers benefited from early integrated PC by improving QOL and other outcomes. It was also determined that early integrated PC may be most effective when aimed toward patients' specific needs.

Source: Temel, J. S., Greer, J. A., El-Jawahri, A., Pirl, W. F., Park, E. R., Jackson, V. A., Back, A. L., Kamdar, M., Jacobsen, J., Chittenden, E. H., Rinaldi, S. P., Gallagher, E. R., Eusebio, J. R., Li, Z., Muzikansky, A., & Ryan, D. P. (2017). Effects of early integrated palliative care in patients with lung and GI cancer: A randomized clinical trial. *Journal of Clinical Oncology: Official Journal of the American Society of Clinical Oncology, 35*(8), 834–841. https://doi.org/10.1200/JCO.2016.70.5046

To protect from bias, many clinical trials use double blinding. In double blinding, neither the research subject nor the investigator is aware of the group (control or experimental) to which the research subject is assigned (Gray & Grove, 2020).

Sometimes a clinical trial intervention cannot be easily administered to individuals but can be applied to groups. In this case, the groups are "clustered" to receive or not receive the intervention under investigation. These are best known as cluster randomized clinical trials. For example, a cluster controlled clinical trial could randomly allocate an intervention into different schools within the same or similar geographical area (Aggarwal & Ranganathan, 2019).

In addition to pharmaceutical clinical trials, there are other types of clinical trials. The following are the other types of clinical trials that follow a similar structure and goals as identified in Figure 13.5.

- Diagnostic trials examine diagnostic tests for safety, sensitivity, specificity, positive predictive value, and negative predictive value
- Treatment nonpharmacologic trials examine a therapeutic intervention compared to a standard of care
- Vaccine clinical trials

VACCINE CLINICAL TRIALS

Vaccine development involves an extensive vaccine clinical trial prior to utilization in humans. Vaccine clinical trials typically follow the four phases of clinical trials described in Figure 13.5. In the exploratory phase, basic laboratory research lasts about 2 to 4 years to identify natural or synthetic antigens that could enable a host response to prevent the disease in humans. Viral antigens identified can be either virus-like particles, weakened virus or bacteria, weakened viral or bacterial toxins, or other substances derived from the pathogen. The pre-clinical phase, which can last for 1 to

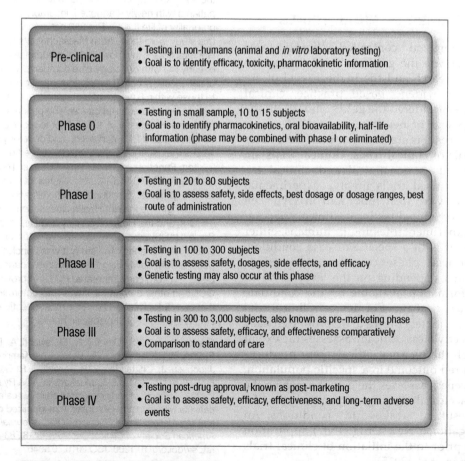

Figure 13.5 Clinical trial phases.

2 years, uses tissue or cell culture along with animal testing to assess the safety of the candidate vaccine. Immunogenicity is also studied during the pre-clinical phase to gain an understanding of immunologic cellular response to the candidate vaccine. The pre-clinical phase can also begin to identify a safe starting dose of the vaccine. After the exploratory and pre-clinical phase in the laboratory, an Investigational New Drug application is filed and once approved, human clinical trials are initiated (Plotkin et al., 2017; Singh & Mehta, 2016).

Phase I vaccine clinical trials involve about 20 to 80 subjects with the first trials involving adults. The goal of phase I vaccine clinical trials is to assess the safety of the candidate vaccine and determine the type and extent of immune response in humans. During phase I vaccine clinical trials, adults may be challenged with the pathogen after vaccination with the candidate vaccine. Phase II vaccine clinical trials involve several hundred subjects with a randomized placebo control group. The goal of phase II vaccine clinical trials is to assess the safety, immunogenicity, dosage, method or route of delivery, and schedule of immunizations of the candidate vaccine. Phase III vaccine clinical trials generally involve thousands of subjects randomized into a double-blinded experiment with a placebo group. The goal of phase III is to continue to assess the safety of the candidate vaccine along with the efficacy of the vaccine. After phase III trials are completed, the vaccine manufacturer can submit a biologics license application to the Food and Drug Administration (FDA). Phase IV vaccine clinical trials continue to assess the vaccine for safety, efficacy, other potential uses, and long-term adverse events (Plotkin et al., 2017; Singh & Mehta, 2016).

Vaccine Adverse Event Reporting System

The Centers for Disease Control and Prevention (CDC) and FDA established the Vaccine Adverse Event Reporting System (VAERS). The goal of VAERS is to detect possible indicators of adverse events associated with the administration of vaccines. VAERS is a voluntary reporting system. Patients, providers, or others can voluntarily report potential vaccine adverse events through the VAERS (Plotkin et al., 2017).

Crossover Study Design

A crossover study design is a type of experimental or interventional study design in which the research subjects serve as their own control. In this design, the subjects intentionally "crossover" to both intervention groups. In this study design, research subjects exposed to the first intervention, will then "crossover" to the other intervention group after the first intervention and postintervention measurements are complete. Typically, the period between the research subjects' exposures to the two interventions are separated by a "washout" period. A washout period is a period of time provided for the effect of the first intervention to dissipate and the research subject to return to their baseline or normal state before moving into the second intervention group (Aggarwal & Ranganathan, 2019).

Community Interventional Study Designs

Interventional study designs are prospective in nature. The controlled clinical trials already described are an interventional study design. An additional type of intervention study design is the community trials or field trials. A community or field trial involves an entire village, neighborhood, or geopolitical district being assigned to intervention groups (Agartala & Ranganathan, 2019).

END-OF-CHAPTER RESOURCES

SUMMARY POINTS

- Not all epidemiologic areas of inquiry are adaptable to an experimental research study design.
- A control group does not receive any treatment or intervention.
- A comparison group is used when the research study design does not randomly select the subjects.
- Quasi-experimental research designs provide an alternative research design when it is not possible to conduct a true experimental design.
- A quasi-experimental research design is a research design that lacks one of the three essential components of a true experiment.
- The pretest and posttest with comparison group design improves the one-group, pretest–posttest design by adding a comparison group.
- Experimental research designs provide the maximum amount of control in a research study design.
- The three essential elements of an experimental research design are manipulation of an intervention or exposure under investigation, randomization, and existence of an experimental and control group.
- In an experimental design, equivalent groups are created to each other.
- Probabilistic equivalence does not mean that the two groups are equal to each other.
- Probabilistic equivalence means that the odds are known that there will be a difference identified between the two groups.
- The classic or original experimental design is a pretest–posttest control group design.
- A randomized block design divides the sample into relatively homogeneous groups or blocks.
- In the Solomon four-group design, two groups receive the treatment or intervention and two groups do not.
- Randomized controlled clinical trials are the gold standard for experimental research and the highest level of evidence in evidence-based practice.
- Randomized clinical trials are considered the gold standard for the development of new pharmaceutical agents and devices.
- In double blinding, neither the research subject nor the investigator is aware of the group (control or experimental) to which the research subject is assigned.
- There are four phases for randomized controlled clinical trials.
- Vaccine development involves an extensive vaccine clinical trial prior to utilization in humans.
- Goal of the Vaccine Adverse Event Reporting System (VAERS) is to detect possible indicators of adverse events associated with the administration of vaccines.
- A crossover study design is a type of experimental or intervention study design in which the research subjects serve as their own control.

EPIDEMIOLOGY CRITICAL REASONING QUESTIONS

1. VARIVAX (Varicella Virus Vaccine Live) is a vaccine administered to prevent varicella infection in individuals 12 months of age and older. Each dose of VARIVAX is administered 0.5 mL subcutaneously via injection. Adults require the administration of two doses with a minimum of 4 weeks between doses. A pharmaceutical company is interested in producing a varicella vaccine that can be administered subcutaneously or intramuscularly once to children aged 12 months and older and adults. Design and describe each phase of the clinical trial for a new vaccine.
2. Compare and contrast the phases of a randomized controlled clinical trial and a vaccine clinical trial.
3. What are the essential required elements of a true experimental design?
4. Describe the differences in a quasi-experimental research design and an experimental research design.
5. What events would be reported to the Vaccine Adverse Event Reporting System (VAERS)?

ADDITIONAL RESOURCES

SPRINGER PUBLISHING CONNECT™ | A robust set of instructor resources designed to supplement this text is located at http://connect. springerpub.com/content/book/978-0-8261-8514-3. Qualifying instructors may request access by emailing textbook@springerpub.com.

REFERENCES

Aggarwal, A., & Ranganathan, P. (2019). Intervention studies. *Perspectives in Clinical Research, 10*(3), 137–139. https://doi.org/10.4103/picr.PICR_91_19

Chatburn, R. (2017). Basics of study design: Practical considerations. *Cleveland Clinic Journal of Medicine, 84*(Suppl 2), e10–e19. https://doi.org/10.3949/ccjm.84.s2.03

Friedman, L., Furberg, C., DeMets, D., Reboussin, D., & Granger, C. (2015). *Fundamentals of clinical trials* (5th ed.). Springer.

Gray, J., & Grove, S. (2020). *Burns and Grove's the practice of nursing research: Appraisal, synthesis, and generation of evidence* (9th ed.). Saunders.

Plotkin, S., Orenstein, W., Offit, P., & Edwards, K. (2017). *Vaccines* (7th ed.). Saunders.

Siedlecki, S. (2020). Quasi-experimental research designs. *Clinical Nurse Specialist, 34*(5), 198–202. https://doi.org/10.1097/NUR.0000000000000540

Singh, K., & Mehta, S. (2016). The clinical development process of a novel preventive vaccine: An overview. *Journal of Postgraduate Medicine, 62*(1), 4–11. https://doi.org/10.4103/0022-3859.173187

EPIDEMIOLOGIC DESIGN BIAS, CONFOUNDERS, AND INTERACTION

Demetrius J. Porche

I was afraid that by observing objects with my eyes and trying to comprehend them with each of my other senses I might blind my soul altogether.

—Socrates

CHAPTER COMPETENCIES

At the conclusion of this chapter, the reader will be able to:

1. Demonstrate an understanding of the different types of research bias
2. Describe strategies to impact research bias
3. Demonstrate an understanding of confounding and interaction

ESSENTIAL TERMINOLOGY

The essential terminology for research bias, confounding, and interaction are:

- Confounding
- Interaction
- Research bias
- Effect modification

Epidemiologic investigations and research studies attempt to explore the occurrence of a health event or disease within a population. Epidemiologic studies that examine the relationship between an exposure and a health event or disease attempt to extrapolate those findings to a broader population. Factors that impact a study's internal validity will directly impact the external validity of a study. Bias can be introduced at multiple points in an epidemiologic investigation or research study and can have a direct impact on both the internal and external validity of the epidemiologic findings (refer to Chapter 10). The ability to determine the extent of association and causal inference is impacted by research bias, confounding variables, and interaction of variables. Randomization can reduce the chance of both bias and confounding.

Bias reduction or elimination is the responsibility of the nurse researcher, nurse epidemiologist, or public health epidemiologist. Nurses themselves should also explore the extent to which their behavior or method of data collection introduces bias into the epidemiologic research study.

RESEARCH BIAS

Research bias is defined as any actual or potential action that prevents the unprejudiced consideration of the study findings (Delgado-Rodriguez & Llorca, 2004). Research bias can occur at any phase of the research process. Research bias can be considered present or absent; however, most interpretation of research bias is considered in the degree of bias present. Researchers and individuals who utilize research findings must consider the extent to which the bias impacts the internal and external validity of the study and ultimately influences the interpretation of the study's conclusions. Care in designing of research studies can reduce the interjection of potential bias (Pannuci & Wilkins, 2010). The designing of research studies requires the compromise between balancing factors that impact the internal and external validity of the study. Table 14.1 provides several types of bias that should be considered

Table 14.1 Research Bias Types and Definitions

Bias Term	Definition
Allocation of intervention	When the intervention is assigned to groups differently
Berkson (admission rate)	Occurs with the recruitment of cases or controls from hospitalized patients, hospitalization of cases and controls differ in impacting case control studies
Citation	Articles that are frequently cited are more easily found and included in research such as systematic reviews and meta-analysis
Compliance	There is a difference in the adherence requirements between groups
Confirmation	Researcher intentionally focuses on information or data patterns to confirm their ideas or opinions they hold
Contamination	Other factors are found in the study unintentionally that influence the results
Design	Bias is a result of improper study design, a broad term
Dissemination	Bias resulting from the manner in which information is retrieved, including language bias in publications
Ecological fallacy	The association observed on an aggregate level does not necessarily represent the association that exists at the individual level
Exclusion	Controls with the condition related to exposure are excluded but the cases that have the same comorbidities are included in the study
Healthcare access	Subjects receiving healthcare services do not represent the cases that originate in the community
Inclusive	A type of sampling bias in which samples are selected for convenience
Information	Introduce bias during the collection of data from the information provided
Interviewer	The interviewer interjects intentional or subconscious subtle clues via language, voice tone, or body language to answers or expected responses that skew the interviewee's opinions, answers, or values
Length-bias sampling	Cases with long duration of illness are more likely to be included in research
Loss/withdrawals to follow-up	Loss/withdrawals to follow-up are uneven in the exposure and outcome categories
Missing information	Records with complete data are selected over those without complete data
Neyman (incidence-prevalence bias, selective survival bias)	Sample of cases is distorted by the survival, incidence, or prevalence rates
Nonresponse	Failure to secure responses from subjects in the selected sample
Nonresponse	Subjects who participated differ from those who did not participate
Observational (Hawthorne effect)	Subjects who are observed either consciously or unconsciously alter the manner in which they act or answer a question because they are being observed

(continued)

Table 14.1 Research Bias Types and Definitions *(continued)*

Bias Term	Definition
Observer	Observer's prior knowledge influences the manner in which data are collected, measured, or interpreted
Omission	A type of sampling bias in which certain groups of the population are not recruited
Procedural	The application of unfair pressure on subjects to complete their responses quickly
Publication	Bias that may result from decision regarding which manuscripts to publish; publication bias is influenced by statistical significance, sample size, funding source, design type, study quality, and researcher prestige
Recall	Subjects respond to questions about historical events or events that must be recalled from memory which may not be completely recalled due to memory failure
Reporting	There is an intentional or error made in the manner in which results are disseminated
Researcher	Also known as experimenter bias, the investigator influences the results to demonstrate a certain outcome
Response	Subject consciously or subconsciously responds in a manner in which they think the interviewer wants or expects
Sampling	Sample selection introduces bias
Selection	Error in the identification of the study population; sampling method leads to systematic error introduced through the screening and selection of research subjects
Spectrum	Case definition does not represent the entire spectrum of the illness
Survivor treatment selection	Subjects who live longer have a greater probability of receiving treatment
Temporal ambiguity	It cannot be established that exposure precedes effect
Work up (verification)	When the gold standard diagnostic test is administered and influences the results of the assessed test validity

in the design of a research study and balancing the compromise between internal and external validity. Table 14.1 also provides the definitions of the multiple types of research bias (Delgado-Rodriguez & Llorca, 2004).

CONFOUNDING

A confounder is a factor or variable that correlates with both the exposure and outcome (Vetter & Mascha, 2017). The confounding correlation can be either a positive or negative correlation. Positive confounding occurs when the observed association is biased away from the null hypothesis. Negative confounding occurs

when the observed association is biased toward the null hypothesis. In confounding, there is another factor impacting the associations observed. Simply, there is a distortion of the association or relationship between an exposure and outcome due to the presence of another variable. Confounding occurs when the effect of two associated exposures have not been separated, which results in the interpretation that the effect is a result of one variable rather than multiple or a silent variable. Confounding impacts the estimated association between an exposure and an outcome because the result is not a measure of a true effect due to the confounding variable's interaction. Stated in statistical

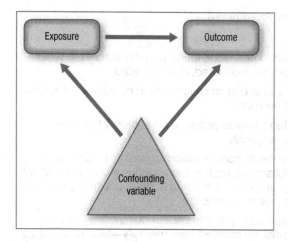

Figure 14.1 Confounding variable interaction.

terms, a confounder variable (Figure 14.1) correlates both with the regressor variable and the dependent variable. Confounding can mask the true effect of a risk factor on an outcome or disease. A variable is considered a confounder if the following exist:

1. The confounder variable is independently associated with the outcome.
2. The confounder variable is associated with the exposure under investigation in the population.
3. The confounder variable does not necessarily lie on the causal pathway between the exposure and the disease.

The temporal relationship between the purported confounding variable and the exposure variables should be discerned to determine the extent to which confounding is occurring. A confounder that occurs after the exposure and the outcome may only be a contributing factor and not a true confounder.

For example, a nurse epidemiologist is exploring the incidence and prevalence of colorectal cancer. Correlated with the incidence and prevalence of colorectal cancer is the amount of fat and fiber consumption. A possible confounding variable may be socioeconomic status or other nondietary lifestyle factors.

Failure to control a confounding variable results in an inaccurate interpretation of the effect of the exposure on the outcome. Confounding can result in the following erroneous interpretations:

1. There is an observed difference in study population when in fact there is no real difference.
2. There is no observed difference in the study population when in fact there is a real difference.
3. There is an underestimation of the exposure's effect.
4. There is an overestimation of the exposure's effect.

Confounding can be reduced with the integration of several research strategies. Some research strategies to reduce confounding are:

1. *Randomization:* Random assignment of subjects to different groups, such as experimental, comparison, or control groups
2. *Restriction:* Restrict subject's inclusion criteria to potential confounding variables
3. *Matching:* Subjects in exposed and nonexposed or cases and noncases are matched for one or more potential confounding variables or factors (individual and group matching)
4. *Multivariate analysis:* Conduct multivariate analysis with examination for covariance among variables
5. *Standardization:* Adjust or standardize mortality rates for the purpose of homogenizing the confounding variable in different groups
6. *Stratification:* Stratify the groups under investigation during data analysis in relation to the confounding variable and factor (Rivas-Ruiz et al., 2012)

Epidemiologists should be astute to the possibility of confounding. If an association is observed, the epidemiologist should question whether there is an association that suggests a causal relationship or whether there could be the possibility of a third or silent factor that is associated with the disease and the exposure in question.

Epidemiologists can attempt to control for the confounding variables through measurement of the variable in the study design. However, residual confounding may remain present if the variable being controlled is not a perfect surrogate of the true confounding variable. Positive confounding occurs when the confounding effects result in an overestimation of the effect present in the outcome variable. A negative confounding occurs when the confounding effects result in an underestimation of the effect present in the outcome variable.

It is important to remember that confounding variables can be a source of bias introduced into the study design.

INTERACTION (EFFECT MODIFICATION)

Interaction is also known as effect modification. Interaction among variables exists when the effect of one explanatory variable on the outcome depends on another explanatory variable. The joint effect of two explanatory variables can be larger or smaller than the individual effects, suggesting interaction is occurring. Interaction can be considered positive or negative. In relation to exploring risk factors, if there is interaction between risk factors or exposures present, the factors are not independent as a causative etiology of an outcome. In statistical terms, interaction means that two separate regressors are correlating together to create a variable that coalesces in an effect on the dependent variable (Vetter & Mascha, 2017). Interaction differs from confounding, in that the interacting variable is known to contribute to the correlation of the variable under investigation to the outcome.

END-OF-CHAPTER RESOURCES

SUMMARY POINTS

- Factors that impact a study's internal validity will directly impact the external validity of a study.
- Research bias is defined as any actual or potential action that prevents the unprejudiced consideration of the study findings.
- Researchers and individuals who utilize research findings must consider the extent to which the bias impacts the internal and external validity of the study.
- A confounder is a factor or variable that correlates with both the exposure and outcome.
- Confounding impacts the estimated association between an exposure and an outcome because the result is not a measure of a true effect due to the confounding variable's interaction.
- Failure to recognize a confounder can result in an incorrect estimate of the association or treatment effect.
- The temporal relationship between the purported confounding variable and the exposure variables should be discerned to determine the extent to which confounding is occurring.
- Confounding can be reduced with the integration of several research strategies: randomization, restriction, matching, multivariate analysis, standardization, and stratification.
- Interaction among variables exists when the effect of one explanatory variable on the outcome depends on another explanatory variable.

EPIDEMIOLOGY CRITICAL REASONING QUESTIONS

1. Differentiate between internal and external validity.
2. Identify and describe at least four types of bias that impact both internal and external validity.
3. Identify at least five bias types and research design strategies to reduce each bias type.
4. Compare and contrast confounding and interaction.

ADDITIONAL RESOURCES

 A robust set of instructor resources designed to supplement this text is located at http://connect. springerpub.com/content/book/978-0-8261-8514-3. Qualifying instructors may request access by emailing textbook@springerpub.com.

REFERENCES

Delgado-Rodriguez, M., & Llorca, J. (2004). Bias. *Journal of Epidemiological Community Health, 58*, 635–641. https://doi.org/10.1136/jech.2003.008466

Pannucci, C., & Wilkins, E. (2010). Identifying and avoiding bias in research. *Plastic Reconstructive Surgery, 126*(2), 619–625. https://doi.org/10.1097/PRS.0b013e3181de24bc

Rivas-Ruiz, F., Perez-Vicente, S., & Gonzalez-Ramirez, A. (2012). Bias in clinical epidemiological study designs. *Allergologia et Immunopathologia, 41*(1), 54–59. https://doi.org/10.1016/j.aller.2012.04.005

Vetter, T., & Mascha, E. (2017). Bias, confounding, and interaction: Lions and tigers, and bears, oh my! *Anesthesia & Analgesia, 125*(3), 1042–1048. https://doi.org/10.1213/ANE.0000000000002332

Chapter 15

BIOSTATISTICS PRIMER

Donald E. Mercante

Statistics is the grammar of science.
–Karl Pearson
(1857–1936, influential English mathematician)

CHAPTER COMPETENCIES

At the conclusion of this chapter, the reader will be able to:

1. Differentiate scales of measurement
2. Apply descriptive statistics to population level data
3. Apply probability statistics to population level data
4. Calculate sensitivity and specificity rates
5. Differentiate relative risk and odds ratio

ESSENTIAL TERMINOLOGY

Essential statistics primer terms are:

- Arithmetic mean
- Continuous random variable
- Continuous variable
- Descriptive statistics
- Discrete random variable
- Discrete variable
- Frequency distribution
- Geometric mean
- Interval scale
- Measures of central tendency
- Median
- Mode
- Nominal scale
- Odds ratio
- Ordinal scale
- Percentiles
- Random variable
- Range
- Ratio scale
- Relative risk
- ROC curves
- Sample variance
- Scale of measurement
- Sensitivity
- Specificity
- Variables

BASIC CONCEPTS

Statistics is all about recognizing and addressing sources of variability, either through study design or statistical analysis. Variability is both essential for understanding associations and a nuisance that encumbers our efforts at measuring them. We begin with a description of the properties of variables. Variables are measurable characteristics or traits that vary from object to object. It is useful to classify variables by their scale of measurement (Figure 15.1). Beginning with the least informative scale, nominal variables describe objects that differ in name or type. Blood type, gender, and ethnicity are examples of nominal variables.

Variables measured at the next higher scale, the ordinal scale, comprise a more diverse collection of variables that not only allow identification of object type, but also allow arrangement by natural ordering, ranking, or hierarchy of levels. Examples include Likert-type responses to survey opinion questions,

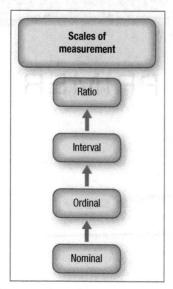

Figure 15.1 Scales of measurement.

- strongly disagree
- disagree
- no opinion
- agree
- strongly agree

and, an ordered listing of levels of administrative responsibilities for hospital-employed nursing positions:

1. Licensed Practical Nurse
2. Staff/Bedside Nurse
3. Advanced Practice Registered Nurse
4. Nurse Practitioner
5. Nurse Manager/Supervisor
6. Director of Nursing
7. Chief Nursing Officer

Categories may be numerically coded (as in the preceding example) for convenience or as an aid in analysis by statistical software. The numerical code is arbitrary, other than to impart order, as the distance between adjacent categories is not measurable. Variables on the nominal and ordinal scales are also described as being qualitative.

Variables on the two highest levels of measurement, interval and ratio, allow measurement of the distance between objects. The primary difference between the two scales is that ratio scale variables contain a true zero. Temperature in Fahrenheit (or Celsius) is an example of an interval level variable. Other examples include:

- pH scale for measuring the acidity or basicity of a solution

- Graduate Record Examination (GRE) Quantitative Scores
- Medical College Admissions Test Scores (MCAT)

Ratio scale variables contain the greatest amount of information, allowing measurement of distances between values and interpretation of ratios of values. For example, a dose of 10 mg is twice that of a 5 mg dose. Variables on the interval and ratio scales are also described as being quantitative.

Quantitative variables measure the numbers or amounts of objects. Examples of quantitative variables include:

- Number of ICU admissions per month to a level-1 trauma center
- Volume of IV fluids given to burn victims
- Wait times for a walk-in clinic
- Body mass index (BMI) of cardiac patients

Notice that the first variable is discrete and the last variable, BMI, is not directly measurable, but rather determined by an arithmetic expression,

$$BMI = \frac{\text{Height in meters}}{\text{Weight in kg}^2}.$$

Each of these variables conveys a sense of amount or quantity.

Qualitative variables identify differences in kind between objects, such as in the following examples:

- Gender designation
- Blood type, e.g., O, A, B, AB
- Treatment outcome: Cured/not cured

The frequency or count of the number of objects in each qualitative category is the quantity usually of interest.

When the observed value of a variable is subject to chance and cannot be determined with certainty *a priori*, the variable is referred to as a **random variable**. The observed values of a random variable (such as resting systolic blood pressure) may fluctuate randomly from subject to subject in a population or sample, or from observation to observation within the same subject over repeated measurements. The understanding of the sources of random and systematic variability plays a key role in statistics.

Another useful dichotomy is to classify variables as **discrete** or **continuous**.

A **discrete random variable** is a variable that has values that represent unique, noncontinuous attributes or characteristics of an object. Discrete variables typically describe objects that are inherently different, such as eye color or biological sex, or measure the number of objects, such as the number of children in a household or the number of decayed, missing, and filled teeth in a patient.

Continuous random variable is a random variable whose possible values cannot be put into one-to-one correspondence with the set of natural integers and do not possess discrete gaps in values. A continuous random variable can assume any value within a range of possible values, although it is quite common to record values of a continuous variable as discrete values for convenience or limitations in measurement.

SAMPLING AND STATISTICAL INFERENCE

Populations

Two goals of research are to characterize attributes or features of a population and assess associations of interest. These activities necessitate the need for observing characteristics of members of a population. However, populations tend to be large, possibly infinite, or intractable and obtaining direct measurements on every member is impractical or impossible. The role of statistics is to use measurements on variables of interest from a representative sample from a population to achieve the aforementioned goals. If the purpose is to simply characterize a particular attribute of a population, then the role of statistics is descriptive. The real strength in the use of statistical methods is to extrapolate findings of associations of interest to the population of interest, referred to as the target population. This area of statistics is called inferential statistics (see Chapter 10).

- **Population:** We define a population as the entire collection of objects of interest. Populations may be finite or infinite, but they are LARGE. Examples include:
  - First generation of individuals from immigrant families who earn college diplomas (finite)
  - Enrollees in a large national private healthcare plan (finite)
  - Bacterial cells on Earth, now and in the future (practically infinite)
- **Sample:** A sample is a fraction or subset of a population. Samples are much SMALLER and more manageable than populations (see Figure 15.2).

Samples and Sampling

Samples should reflect the essential characteristics of the parent population. Care must be exercised in obtaining samples to ensure that the sample members are reflective of the makeup of the population (Figure 15.3). Samples drawn haphazardly or arbitrarily cannot guarantee representative samples. To ensure representative

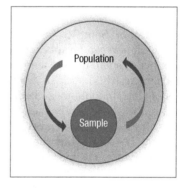

Figure 15.2 Populations and samples.

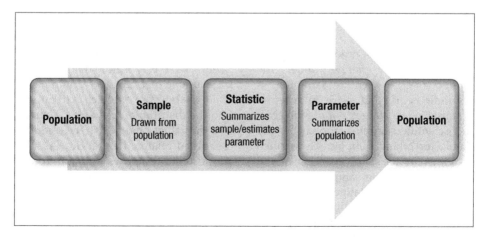

Figure 15.3 Populations, samples, statistics, and parameters.

samples and accuracy of our inferences, a sound scientific approach to obtaining samples is required. There are many types of scientific sampling approaches. The three most common are listed in the following:

- **Simple Random Sample (SRS):** This sample process is akin to drawing lottery numbers. Every object in the population has an equal chance of being selected into the sample.
- **Stratified Random Sample:** A population is divided into groups, or strata, by some characteristic (variable) so that members within each strata are more similar than to those in other strata. After the population is stratified, take SRSs independently from each stratum. Common strata variables include age groupings, gender, and ethnicity.
- **Systematic Random Sample:** To reduce selection bias, some form of randomness is generally introduced at the start of the sampling process, then members are included systematically according to a predefined sequence. For example, after a random start, every fourth eligible patient presenting at an emergency department may be included in a sample.
- **Cluster Random Sample:** In some situations, a population can be subdivided into a large number of small units, each possessing similar characteristics, such as members of a household or students in a classroom. In these cases, the cluster is the sampling unit rather than the individual member. This sampling scheme is useful when the population is large and diverse. The more similar the responses of individual members to each other, the more the cluster behaves like a single unit. Cluster random sampling may provide a less precise, cost-effective alternative to simple random or stratified random sampling.

There are many other random sampling approaches, collectively falling under the general framework of scientific sampling. A scientific sample is one that results in a representative subset of the target population. Numerous nonscientific sampling approaches are also available for taking samples. These often provide savings in terms of cost, time, and simplicity. However, these sampling methods do not guarantee representative samples and should be avoided when possible. Examples of nonscientific sampling methods include convenience sampling, quota sampling, and snowball sampling. A convenience sample selects members that are easily accessible, such as individuals exiting a polling station. A quota sample may specify that a sample consists of a predetermined proportion of individuals selected conveniently from distinct subpopulations. An example would be a sample of individuals with blood types in the following proportions: 40% Type O, 35% Type A, 15% Type B, and 10% Type AB. Snowball sampling uses peer-to-peer, person-to-person, social networking, or similar tactics to recruit individuals and is particularly useful for hard-to-reach populations such as illicit drug users.

Descriptive Statistics

Once a sample of individuals has been drawn, information is obtained from study subjects in the form of direct measurements, interviews, self- or investigator elicited questionnaires, observations, abstractions, or any several other means. Although these data may be stored as paper records, it has become increasingly more common to store data as electronic records. Spreadsheet programs such as Microsoft Excel are widely used as both data collection tools and for data storage. Spreadsheet programs work well for small studies with straightforward data collection. Larger and more complicated research studies may benefit greatly from software specifically designed for data collection, such as RedCap. These software platforms incorporate many additional features such as creating audit trails and incorporating conditional logic and quality control checks.

Whether the amount of data collected is modest or massive requires effective and appropriate summarization. Descriptive statistical summaries provide insight into key characteristics of a sample of individuals. The choice of summary measures depends heavily on the type and scale of the particular variable of interest. The frequency table is a useful summary of a categorical variable measured on a nominal or ordinal scale, the purpose of which is to provide insight into the distribution of values. That is to say, it lists the values observed in the sample and their associated relative frequencies. As an example, suppose the responses to a question asking recently employed nurses about their work environment, 287 reported working at a hospital, 153 at a multi-specialty clinic, and 60 at a single specialty facility. A more formal presentation of a frequency table is presented in the next section.

Frequency Distribution

A **frequency distribution** can be a tabular or graphical display of each value in the distribution of values and the relative frequency (estimated probability) of occurrence. Consider the following data set on ages of participants in a study of the effect of obesity on risk and severity of periodontitis (Exhibit 15.1; Auerkari, 2021).

Examples of a frequency table and histogram for the age data set can be seen in Table 15.1 and Figure 15.4.

The next step in summarizing data is to compute relevant descriptive statistics. There are a number of measures and graphical displays that can effectively be used to summarize a set of data to provide insight into the characteristics of the sample, and if the sample is representative of the population, the characteristics of the population as well. Descriptive statistics are often grouped into three categories as follows:

- Measures of location
- Measures of dispersion or variability
- Graphical methods

Measures of Central Tendency or Location

These are some of the most widely used and recognized measures of central tendency or location.

- Arithmetic mean
- Median
- Mode
- Geometric mean

Table 15.1 Frequency Table of Ages

Age Category	Freq.	Percent	Cum.
10–19	4	1.53	1.53
20–29	61	23.28	24.81
30–39	29	11.07	35.88
40–49	67	25.57	61.45
50–59	84	32.06	93.51
60–69	17	6.49	100.00
Total	262	100.00	

EXHIBIT 15.1. Example of Frequency Table

44	46	57	43	49	43	49	46	57	48	51	48	44	44	23	21
22	26	32	24	21	35	22	26	24	32	25	30	30	36	40	23
26	21	20	38	20	20	28	24	34	21	23	24	25	21	19	28
29	25	22	36	21	38	38	36	29	35	18	22	34	32	23	37
19	25	31	22	29	34	21	21	24	39	36	35	27	22	24	22
31	22	22	22	22	21	38	39	22	21	20	22	23	24	23	22
21	25	31	21	28	33	38	25	20	55	45	54	48	58	52	45
45	59	57	47	58	58	49	54	54	55	47	66	50	60	57	55
63	61	62	57	65	53	57	53	60	61	63	55	59	53	58	49
47	45	48	51	47	47	53	49	47	53	55	52	64	64	54	62
52	50	56	61	57	58	53	41	57	50	52	44	52	51	46	46
44	48	63	60	53	46	42	57	58	50	51	58	48	45	47	53
51	52	47	43	54	43	50	44	54	60	55	48	49	49	48	51
53	50	45	50	49	53	47	47	53	52	53	50	54	55	49	55
50	50	47	47	47	47	60	55	45	46	46	45	49	50	48	55
45	53	52	50	51	57	49	52	53	55	47	49	56	52	50	53
45	47	36	39	23	18										

Source: From Auerkari, E. (2021). *Raw data of effect of obesity on risk and severity of periodontitis*. Harvard Dataverse. https://doi.org/10.7910/DVN/MBVN3O

Note: Unsorted dataset.

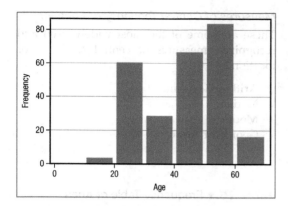

Figure 15.4 Histogram of ages.

Arithmetic Mean

- Uses all of the data in the sample
- Preferred for continuous data
- Susceptible to extreme values (outliers)

If we let x = variable of interest (e.g., age), then the mean, $\bar{x}$, is calculated as:

$$\bar{x} = \frac{1}{n}\sum_{i=1}^{n} x_i = \frac{x_1 + x_2 + \ \ + x_n}{n} = 42.63.$$

The mean can be quite affected by the presence of outliers or extreme data values. The following data set, 55, 45, 54, 48, 58, 52, 45, 45, 59, 57 has a mean of 51.8. Suppose the last observation, 59, is replaced with 295, giving 55, 45, 54, 48, 58, 52, 45, 45, 59, 295. The new mean is 75.6, which is now 23.8 units larger.

Median

- Easy to compute
- Uses at most two observations and order of the data
- Represents the middle value in ordered array of observations
- Resistant to extreme values (outliers)
- Preferred when distribution is skewed

Let X = variable of interest (e.g., age), then the median is determined as:

- Middle value if N is odd
- Average of two middle values if N even

The value of the median can be determined from an ordered array as:

- $\frac{n+1}{2}$ largest observation if n is odd;
- Average of the $\frac{n}{2}$ and the $\frac{n}{2}+1$ largest observation if n is even.

Continuing with the obesity dataset, the median age is the average of the two middle values since the sample size is even. The average of the 131st and 132nd observations with values of 47 and 47, respectively, is = 47.

Most software can easily produce a set of useful summary statistics, as illustrated here using the summary function in R, Min.: 18.00, 1st Qu.: 30.00, Median: 47.00, Mean: 42.63, 3rd Qu.: 53.00, Max.: 66.00.

To illustrate how the median is less affected by an outlier than the mean, consider the same example as before.

Again, consider the following dataset, 55, 45, 54, 48, 58, 52, 45, 45, 59, 295, that has a median of 53. Suppose the last observation, 295, is replaced with 1475, giving 55, 45, 54, 48, 58, 52, 45, 45, 59, 1475. The new median is 53, which did not change.

Mode

- Most frequently occurring value(s)
- Easily determined
- Not unique
- Uses very few of the data
- Preferred when distribution is skewed
- Let X = variable of interest (e.g., age), then the mode is given as:

The mode of age is 47, which occurs 16 times.

Geometric Mean

Particularly useful for right-skewed data where numbers represent population counts that are highly variable (e.g., growth in number of bacteria on a petri dish over time or HIV viral counts). Calculation:

Let $\bar{x}$ = age

1. Compute logs of each value, $\log(x_i)$
2. Sum all log-transformed values,

$$\sum_{i=1}^{n} \log(x_i)$$

3. Compute mean of log-transformed values,

$$\frac{1}{n}\sum_{i=1}^{n} \log(x_i)$$

4. Take anti-log,

$$\exp(\frac{1}{n}\sum_{i=1}^{n} \log(x_i))$$

The geometric mean of all 262 subjects (geometric mean) = 40.17, which for right-skewed data will always fall between the arithmetic mean and the median.

Measures of Measures of Spread
- Range
- Quantiles/percentiles
- Interquartile range
- Variance/standard deviation
- Coefficient of variation

Range
Properties of the sample range include the following:

- Easy to compute
- Very susceptible to outliers or extreme values
- Uses at most two observations and order of the data
- Computed as the max − min = 66 − 18 = 48.

Percentiles
Values determined from an ordered sample measuring the proportion of smaller values in the sample.

Example
50th percentile, or median, is the value such that 50% of all values in the sample fall below it and 50% are above it.

- Common percentiles of interest are the 25th, 50th, and 75th percentiles.
- These values are also known as quartiles since they divide the sample into four groups with equal numbers of observations.
- The difference between the 25th and 75th percentiles is called the interquartile range (IQR). It is a measure of spread.

For the obesity study data set containing participant's ages, we have the following percentiles:

- 25th percentile (1st quartile, i.e., Q1) = 30
- 50th percentile (median, or 2nd quartile, i.e., Q2) = 47
- 75th percentile (3rd quartile, i.e., Q3) = 53
- IQR = 23

Sample Variance/Standard Deviation
The sample variance and its square root, the standard deviation, are the most widely used measures of variability. When the distribution of a variable is normally distributed, the sample variance (or S.D.) are the best measures of variability. **Characteristics of the sample variance include:**

- Uses all of the data, which can be a disadvantage in that it is very susceptible to outliers.
- Uses the mean as a reference point.

- Only non-negative values are possible.
- Computed as the average of the sums of squared deviations from the mean. Thus, the sample variance uses the sample mean as a reference point to measure variability or deviations.

Definitional form:

$$S^2 = \frac{1}{n-1} \sum_{i=1}^{n} (x_i - \bar{x})^2$$

The sample standard deviation is simply the square root of the variance,

$$S = \sqrt{\frac{1}{n-1} \sum_{i=1}^{n} (x_i - \bar{x})^2}$$

which has the advantage of being expressed in the original units of the variable rather than in the square of the units as in the variance. Using our example dataset, the sample variance of ages, $S^2 = 177.54$ years^2, with a standard deviation of $S = 13.32$ years. The interpretation of the standard deviation is that ages of individuals in our sample vary, on average, from individual to individual approximately 13.32 years from the sample average of 42.63 years. It is common in research publications when reporting the mean of a variable to also present the standard deviation in the form mean ± S.D., or mean (SD). For example, as either 42.63 ± 13.32, or 42.63 (13.32).

Coefficient of Variation
The coefficient of variation has the following properties:

- Is a unitless measure of variability
- Useful for comparing variability of data measured in different units
- Can only be applied to data measured on a ratio scale

The coefficient of variation (CV) is the ratio of the standard deviation to the sample mean,

$$CV = \frac{s}{x} = \frac{13.32}{42.63} = 0.3125.$$

It is often reported as a percentage by multiplying by 100%:

$$\% CV = 100\% \times \frac{13.32}{42.63} = 31.25\%.$$

Guidance on Reporting Measures of Location and Variability (Dispersion)
When reporting descriptive statistics, it is customary to pair a measure of location with a measure of spread or variability.

- When the distribution is symmetric and no outliers are present, the mean is the preferred measure of center, and the standard deviation is the preferred measure of spread or dispersion.
- For nonsymmetric distributions and/or those with outliers, the median is the preferred measure of center, and the IQR is the preferred measure of spread.

INTRODUCTION TO PROBABILITY

Basic Probability Concepts

We begin with a few definitions of terms and basic notions of probability that form the basis for studying inferential statistics.

The **sample space** is the set of all possible outcomes of an experiment. Let this set be denoted by $\{\mathbb{S}\}$. An **event** is the set of all outcomes of interest. The **probability** (of an event) is defined as the relative frequency of a set of outcomes (event) over an infinitely large number of trials.

Since we can't perform an experiment an infinite number of times, we estimate probabilities by:

- Empirical probabilities calculated from large samples
- Theoretical probability models such as the binomial or normal

The axioms for probabilities dictate that (a) all probabilities are bounded by 0 and 1, that is, for any event E, $0 \le P(E) \le 1$, and, (b) the sum of the probabilities across a set of mutually disjoint and exhaustive events is 1.

The **complement** of an event A, denoted by $\bar{A}$, is the set of all objects in the sample space that are not in set A. Thus, $\bar{A}$ is the event that event A does not occur. As a consequence,

$$P(A) = 1 - P(\bar{A})$$

$$P(A) + P(\bar{A}) = 1$$

EXAMPLE:

Let A = Diastolic BP ≤ 90. Then, $\bar{A}$ = Diastolic BP > 90. If $P(A)$ = 0.75, then p($\bar{A}$) = 1 − 0.75 = 0.25.

The **union** of events A and B, $A \cup B$, is the event that either event A or B occurs, or both. That is, it is the set of objects in either set A or set B or in both sets A and B.

EXAMPLE:

Let A = {DBP ≥ 90}; B={75 ≤ DBP ≤ 100}. Then, A∪B = {DBP ≥ 75}.

In Figure 15.5, $\mathbb{S}$ is the sample space or universe of all outcomes. The probability of the union of the two sets A and B correspond to the area of the shaded region proportional to the total area of the sample space, which is scaled to 1. Computationally, the probability of the union of events A and B is defined as, $P(A \cup B) = P(A) + P(B) - P(A \cap B)$.

The **intersection** of events A and B, A∩B, is the event that both events A and B occurs. That is, it is the set of objects common to both sets A and B.

EXAMPLE:

Let A = {DBP ≥ 90}; B = {75 ≤ DBP ≤ 100}. Then, A∩B = {90 ≤ DBP ≤ 100}.

In Figure 15.6, $\mathbb{S}$ the sample space or universe of all outcomes. The probability of the intersection of the two sets A and B correspond to the area of the shaded region proportional to the total area of the sample space, which is scaled to 1. Computationally, the probability of the union of events A and B is defined as, P(A∩B) = P(A) + P(B) − P(A∪B).

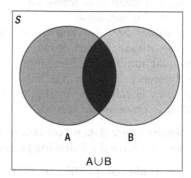

Figure 15.5 Illustrating the principle of the union of two sets using a Venn diagram.

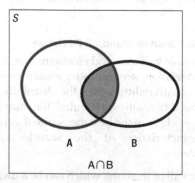

Figure 15.6 Illustrating the principle of the intersection of two sets using a Venn diagram.

Two events A and B are **mutually exclusive** if they have no elements in common. The intersection of mutually exclusive sets is the empty set, $A \cap B = \emptyset$. Empty sets have probability zero, $P(\emptyset) = 0$.

EXAMPLE:

Let A = {DBP ≥ 110}; B = {75 ≤ DBP ≤ 100}. Then, A∩B, and $P(A \cap B) = 0$. Hence, the probability of the union of two disjoint sets is given as, $P(A \cup B) = P(A) + P(B)$, since $P(A \cap B) = \emptyset = 0$.

Given two events A and B, these are said to be **independent** if knowing whether one event occurs tells us nothing about whether the other event occurs. Stated in a slightly different way, if the occurrence/nonoccurrence of an event A does not affect the probability of occurrence of event B, then the two events, A and B, are said to be independent events. Independence is an extremely important concept in statistics.

THEOREM

Multiplication Law of Probabilities for Independent Events

If A and B are independent events, then $P(A \cap B) = P(A)P(B)$.

EXAMPLE:

Let A = {Father has hypertension} and B = {Father has hypertension}

Suppose, $P(A) = 0.2; P(B) = 0.1; P(A \cap B) = 0.02$

To check for the independence of events A and B, we have that $0.02 = P(A \cap B) - (0.2)(0.1) = P(A)P(B) = 0.02$, Thus, events A and B are independent.

The **conditional probability** of an event A given an event B has occurred is defined as,

$$P(A \mid B) = \frac{P(A \cap B)}{P(B)}.$$

The independence of two events can be stated in terms of conditional probability. If two events, A and B, are independent, then $P(A \mid B) = P(A)$, and $P(A \cap B) = P(A)P(B)$.

EXAMPLE:

Suppose in a certain adult population of women who have received a mammogram screening for breast cancer, it is desired to compute the conditional probability that a randomly chosen woman from this population who has a positive mammogram actually has cancer.

Let the event, A = {mammogram is positive}
Let the event, B = {positive for breast cancer}

In addition, suppose it is known that 5% of women in this population have positive mammograms, 2% have breast cancer, and 1% have positive mammograms and have breast cancer. Thus,

- $P(A) = 0.05$,
- $P(B) = 0.02$, and
- $P(A \cap B) = 0.01$

The probability that a randomly chosen member of this population has breast cancer given she has a positive mammogram

$$= P(B \mid A) = \frac{P(A \cap B)}{P(A)} = \frac{0.01}{0.05} = 0.2.$$

Note: If events A and B were independent, then $P(B \mid A) = P(A)P(B)$, which it clearly not the case here. Hence, events A and B are not independent.

As an application of conditional probability, consider the "gold standard" risk estimator, relative risk (RR) or risk ratio. RR is the ratio of the risks of a particular outcome given the presence or absence of a risk factor. In this context, risk is defined as the conditional probability of an event occurring given another event (presence of a risk factor) has or has not occurred. More formally, the relative risk of event occurring relative to the occurrence (nonoccurrrence) of event A can be expressed as,

$$RR(B \mid A) = \frac{P(B \mid A)}{P(B \mid \bar{A})},$$

which clearly illustrates risks as conditional probabilities and relative risk as a ratio of conditional probabilities. To further illustrate, consider the following example.

EXAMPLE:

Define event = {person is a smoker}, and event = {person develops lung cancer}, with associated probabilities:

- $P(A) = 0.3$,
- $P(B) = 0.02$,
- $P(A \cap B) = 0.015$,

The relative risk of developing lung cancer given a person is a smoker can be determined as:

$$RR(B \mid A) = \frac{P(B \mid A)}{P(B \mid \bar{A})} = \frac{\dfrac{P(A \cap B)}{P(A)}}{\dfrac{P(\bar{A} \cap B)}{P(\bar{A})}} = \frac{\dfrac{0.015}{0.3}}{\dfrac{0.005}{0.7}} = 7.$$

The trick to solving this is to find: $P(\bar{A} \cap B)$ Note that B can be expressed as the union of two disjoint events, $B = (A \cap B) \cup (\bar{A} \cap B)$. Since

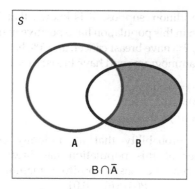

Figure 15.7 Determining probability.

these two events are mutually exclusive, the probability of their union is the sum of their probabilities, $P(B) = P(A \cap B) + P(\bar{A} \cap B)$, or solving for $P(\bar{A} \cap B)$ we obtain $P(\cap B) = P(B) - P(A \cap B) = 0.02 - 0.015 = 0.005$. It is easier to solve this by visualizing the shaded area in the related Venn diagram (Figure 15.7).

Diagnostic/Screening Tests

Although diagnostic testing measures are discussed elsewhere in this publication, it is instructive to note that another important application of conditional probability is in constructing measures of diagnostic test accuracy (see Chapter 8). In random samples, **sensitivity** can be expressed as the conditional probability that a diagnostic test produces a positive test result given an individual has the disease. Similarly, **specificity** is the conditional probability that a diagnostic test produces a negative test result given an individual is disease free. The complementary misclassification rates to sensitivity and specificity, the **false negative** and **false positive** rates, can also be defined as conditional probabilities.

Another set of useful measures are the predictive values. In studies where subjects are selected completely at random, the positive predictive value (PPV) and negative predictive value (NPV) can be expressed as the conditional probabilities. A summary of measures of diagnostic test performance is provided below. Let $D+$ and $D-$ denote the events an individual has and does not have disease, respectively. Also, let $T+$ and $T-$ denote the events that a test produces a positive or negative result. Then, measures of diagnostic test accuracy can be defined using conditional probability notation as,

- Sensitivity $= P(T+ \mid D+) = \dfrac{P(T+ \cap D+)}{P(D+)}$

- Specificity $= P(T- \mid D-) = \dfrac{P(T- \cap D-)}{P(D-)}$

- False negative rate $= P(T- \mid D+) = \dfrac{P(T- \cap D+)}{P(D+)}$

- False positive rate $= P(T+ \mid D-) = \dfrac{P(T+ \cap D-)}{P(D-)}$

- PPV $= P(D+ \mid T+) = \dfrac{P(T+ \cap D+)}{P(T+)}$

- PPN $= P(T- \mid D-) = \dfrac{P(T- \cap D-)}{P(D-)}$

In designs where the subjects are selected based on a nonrandom sample as case-control designs, sensitivity and specificity are not conditional probabilities, but are determined as relative frequencies or proportions. Also, predictive values cannot be directly computed. If an external estimate of prevalence is available Bayes' Theorem can be used to estimate predictive values.

$$PVP = P(D+ \mid T+) = \frac{(\text{Sensitivity})(\text{Prevalence})}{\substack{(\text{Sensitivity})(\text{Prevalence}) \\ + (\text{Specificity})(1 - \text{Prevalence})}}$$

$$PVN = P(D- \mid T-) = \frac{(\text{Specificity})(1 - \text{Prevalence})}{\substack{(\text{Specificity})(1 - \text{Prevalence}) \\ + (1 - \text{Sensitivity})(\text{Prevalence})}}$$

Receiver Operating Characteristic Curves

- In some diagnostic tests there may be multiple categories of test response, rather than $+/-$, and in other instances the test response may be continuous.
- In either case, the choice of cut-off (or categories) representing positive and negative test response is arbitrary.
- The cut-off can be varied over the range of test response values and a plot constructed of sensitivity versus (100% – specificity) to help determine and compare the operating characteristics of the diagnostic test.
- This plot is known as the Receiver Operating Characteristic curve or ROC curve. Generally, the areas under such curves are useful for comparing competing diagnostic tests.

In the following example taken from Hanley and McNeil (1982), CT scans on 109 individuals with neurological problems were rated by a single reader using a 5-point scale. To compute sensitivity and specificity the minimum rating for positive finding of neurological problem is progressively increased from 1 to >5, each time recalculating sensitivity and specificity as demonstrated in the Tables 15.2 through 15.8 that follow.

Table 15.2 Diagnostic Test for Neurological Problems

True Disease Status	Rating					
	Definitely Normal (1)	Probably Normal (2)	Questionable (3)	Probably Abnormal (4)	Definitely Abnormal (5)	Total
Normal	33	6	6	11	2	58
Abnormal	3	2	2	11	33	51
Total	36	8	8	22	35	109

We wish to assess the behavior of the rating scale by determining how sensitivity and specificity change in response to varying the definition of a positive finding for abnormality from ≥ 1 to > 5.

Table 15.3 Rule: Any Rating ≥ 1 Interpreted as Positive for Abnormality

(≥1)	Rating		
True Disease Status	+	−	Total
Normal	58	0	58
Abnormal	51	0	51
Total	109	0	109

Cut-off criterion (≥ 1): Rating is interpreted as a positive finding of abnormality if rating is 1 or higher.

$$\text{Sensitivity} = \frac{51}{51} = 1.00 \text{ or } 100\%$$

$$\text{Specificity} = \frac{0}{58} = 0 \text{ or } 0\%$$

Table 15.4 Rule: Any Rating ≥ 2 Interpreted as Positive for Abnormality

(≥2)	Rating		
True Disease Status	+	−	Total
Normal	25	33	58
Abnormal	48	3	51
Total	73	36	109

Cut-off criterion (≥ 2): Rating is interpreted as a positive finding of abnormality if rating is 2 or higher.

$$\text{Sensitivity} = \frac{48}{51} = 0.941 \text{ or } 94.1\%$$

$$\text{Specificity} = \frac{33}{58} = 0.569 \text{ or } 56.9\%$$

Table 15.5 Rule: Any Rating ≥ 3 Interpreted as Positive for Abnormality

(≥3)	Rating		
True Disease Status	+	−	Total
Normal	19	39	58
Abnormal	46	5	51
Total	65	44	109

Cut-off criterion (≥ 3): Rating is interpreted as a positive finding of abnormality if rating is 3 or higher.

$$\text{Sensitivity} = \frac{46}{51} = 0.902 \text{ or } 90.2\%$$

$$\text{Specificity} = \frac{39}{58} = 0.672 \text{ or } 67.2\%$$

Table 15.6 Rule: Any Rating ≥ 4 Interpreted as Positive for Abnormality

(≥4)	Rating		
True Disease Status	+	−	Total
Normal	13	45	58
Abnormal	44	7	51
Total	57	52	109

Cut-off criterion (≥ 4): Rating is interpreted as a positive finding of abnormality if rating is 4 or higher.

$$\text{Sensitivity} = \frac{44}{51} = 0.863 \text{ or } 86.3\%$$

$$\text{Specificity} = \frac{45}{58} = 0.776 \text{ or } 77.6\%$$

Table 15.7 Rule: Any Rating ≥ 5 Interpreted as Positive for Abnormality

(≥5)	Rating		
True Disease Status	+	−	Total
Normal	2	56	58
Abnormal	33	18	51
Total	35	74	109

Cut-off criterion (≥5): Rating is interpreted as a positive finding of abnormality if rating is 5 or higher.

$$\text{Sensitivity} = \frac{33}{51} = 0.647 \text{ or } 64.7\%$$

$$\text{Specificity} = \frac{56}{58} = 0.966 \text{ or } 96.6\%$$

Table 15.8 Rule: Any Rating >5 Interpreted as Positive for Abnormality

(>5)	Rating		
True Disease Status	+	–	Total
Normal	0	58	58
Abnormal	0	51	51
Total	36	35	109

Cut-off criterion (≥5): Rating is interpreted as a positive finding of abnormality if rating is greater than 5.

$$\text{Sensitivity} = \frac{0}{51} = 0 \text{ or } 0\%$$

$$\text{Specificity} = \frac{58}{58} = 1.00 \text{ or } 100\%$$

Sensitivity and 100% – Specificity values calculated as the criterion or rule for interpreting a positive finding of abnormality is varied and are presented in Table 15.9.

Table 15.9 Sensitivity and 100% – Specificity Values Used in Constructing the Receiver Operating Characteristic **Curve**

+Test Criterion	% Sensitivity	100% – % Specificity
≥1	100	100
≥2	94.1	43.1
≥3	90.2	32.8
≥4	86.3	22.4
≥5	64.7	3.4
≥5	0	0

The calculated area under the ROC curve (AUC) is an overall summary of the accuracy of a diagnostic test (rating system). In Figure 15.8, the AUC = 0.893. Interpretation: A clinician can distinguish between normal and abnormal cases with probability of 0.893 based on this rating. Another way of saying the same thing: A clinician has an 89.3% chance of distinguishing between normal and abnormal cases based on these gradings.

RELATIVE RISK AND ODDS RATIO

It was previously shown that relative risk (RR) can be expressed as a ratio of two conditional probabilities. We now further expand on relative risk and introduce the concept of odds as

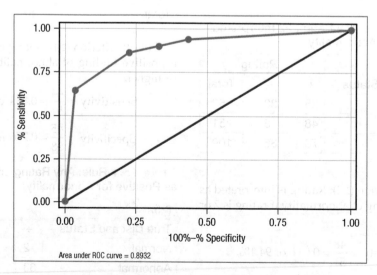

Figure 15.8 Receiver operating characteristic graph.

Table 15.10 Association of Low Bone Mineral Density (BMD) with Development of Osteoporosis by Age 75

Low BMD at Age 40?	Hip Fracture by Age 75?		
	Yes	No	Total
Yes	a	b	a+b
No	c	d	c+d
Total	a+c	b+d	a+b+c+d

Table 15.11 Association of Low Bone Mineral Density (BMD) with Development of Osteoporitis by Age 75

Low BMD at Age 40?	Hip Fracture by Age 75?		
	Yes	No	Total
Yes	35	205	240
No	60	900	960
Total	95	1,105	1,200

an alternate measure to probability of chance, leading to an important alternative relative measure of association, the odds ratio. Consider the following example involving assessment of the association of a potential risk factor, low bone mineral density (BMD) at 40 years of age, and the development of hip fractures in women by age 75. In this first scenario, assume that the sample was taken completely at random from a population of women 75 years or older, all of whom had BMD measured at age 40. To illustrate the calculation of risks, odds, and their ratios, frequency counts for a 2×2 contingency table appear as the variables a, b, c, and d (Table 15.10).

The (estimate of) risk of a randomly chosen individual who had low BMD at age 40 of developing a hip fracture by age 75 is calculated as

$$\frac{a}{a+b}.$$

Similarly, the risk of a randomly chosen individual who did not have low BMD at age 40 of developing hip fracture by age 75 is calculated as

$$\frac{c}{c+d}.$$

Then, RR, defined as the ratio of risks in the group of individuals with and without the risk factor (low BMD at age 40), is calculated as,

$$RR = \frac{\frac{a}{a+b}}{\frac{c}{c+d}} = \frac{a(c+d)}{c(a+b)}.$$

The odds ratio is an alternate measure of association often computed when the study design does not permit computation of RR, such as when using a case-control design. Odds provide an alternative to probability for computing the chance of an event. In the generic 2×2 table (Table 15.10), the odds in favor of developing hip fracture as opposed to not developing hip fracture in the group of individuals with low BMD at age 40 is computed as,

$$\frac{a}{b}.$$

Similarly, the odds in favor of developing hip fracture in the group of individuals with normal BMD at age 40 is computed as,

$$\frac{c}{d}.$$

Then, the odds ratio (OR), defined as the ratio of odds in favor of developing hip fracture in the group of individuals with low versus normal BMD at age 40, is calculated as,

$$OR = \frac{\frac{a}{b}}{\frac{c}{d}} = \frac{a \cdot d}{c \cdot b}.$$

The OR provides an accurate estimate of RR when the disease (event) of interest is relative rare.

Now, as a concrete example of computing the various measures of risk and association, consider the data appearing in Table 15.11, with the accompanying calculation of RR and odds ratio that follow.

$$RR = \frac{\frac{35}{240}}{\frac{60}{960}} = \frac{35(960)}{60(240)} = 2.33.$$

$$OR = \frac{\frac{35}{205}}{\frac{60}{900}} = \frac{35(900)}{60(205)} = 2.56.$$

The RR estimate of 2.33 indicates that individuals who have low BMD at age 40 experience 2.33 times the risk of developing osteoporosis by age 75. A similar interpretation would hold for the OR of 2.56.

The interpretations of the RRs and ORs are similar across their range of values. For example, RR (OR) = 1 implies equal risks (odds) in the groups of individuals with and without the presumed risk factor. RR (OR) >1 implies an increased risk (odds) of outcome (e.g., development of disease) in the group possessing the presume risk factor, while RR (OR) <1 implies a decreased risk (odds) in the risk factor group.

In practice, statistical models, such as Cox or logistic regression, are often used to calculate RRs or ORs and allow for adjusting these estimates for potential confounding effects from other variables, such as demographic characteristics. The adjusted estimates are the preferred measures of association and should be the primary measures for interpretation and reporting of results.

END-OF-CHAPTER RESOURCES

SUMMARY POINTS

- Variables are measurable characteristics or traits that vary from object to object.
- The primary difference between the two scales is that ratio scale variables contain a true zero.
- Ratio scale variables contain the greatest amount of information, allowing measurement of distances between values and interpretation of ratios of values.
- Quantitative variables measure the numbers or amounts of objects.
- The observed values of a random variable may fluctuate randomly from subject to subject in a population or sample, or from observation to observation within the same subject over repeated measurements.
- Discrete Random Variable is a variable that has values that represent unique, noncontinuous attributes, or characteristics of an object.
- Continuous Random Variable is a random variable whose possible values cannot be put into one-to-one correspondence with the set of natural integers.
- The role of statistics is to use measurements on variables of interest from a representative sample from a population to achieve the aforementioned goals.
- A sample is a fraction or subset of a population.
- A frequency distribution can be a tabular or graphical display of each value in the distribution of values and the relative frequency (estimated probability) of occurrence.
- Relative risk (RR) or risk ratio is the ratio of the risks of a particular outcome given the presence or absence of a risk factor.
- Sensitivity can be expressed as the conditional probability that a diagnostic test produces a positive test result given an individual has the disease.
- Specificity is the conditional probability that a diagnostic test produces a negative test result given an individual is disease free.

CRITICAL REASONING QUESTIONS

1. Identify clinical data for the following scales of measurement: nominal, ordinal, interval, and ratio.
2. Provide an example of quantitative and qualitative data from your area of nursing practice.
3. Identify an example of a continuous random variable.
4. Identify a population of interest. Describe what would be considered a sample from your population of interest.
5. Explain the difference among a mean, median, mode, and range.
6. Explain the concept of a false negative and false positive result.

ADDITIONAL RESOURCES

 A robust set of instructor resources designed to supplement this text is located at http://connect. springerpub.com/content/book/978-0-8261-8514-3. Qualifying instructors may request access by emailing textbook@springerpub.com.

REFERENCES

Auerkari, E. (2021). *Raw data of effect of obesity on risk and severity of periodontitis*. V1. Harvard Dataverse. https://doi.org/10.7910/DVN/MBVN3O

Hanley, J., & McNeil, B. (1982). The meaning and use of the area under a receiver operating characteristic (ROC) curve. *Radiology, 143*(1), 29–36. https://doi.org/10.1148/radiology.143.1.7063747

Chapter 16

FIELD, FORENSIC, AND LEGAL EPIDEMIOLOGY

Demetrius J. Porche

The best way to do field work is never to come up for air until it is all over.
–Margaret Mead, American anthropologist

A just law is a man-made code that squares with the moral law, or the law of God. An unjust law is a code that is out of harmony with the moral law.
–Martin Luther King Jr.

CHAPTER COMPETENCIES

At the conclusion of this chapter, the reader will be able to:

1. Differentiate field epidemiology, forensic epidemiology, and legal epidemiology
2. Describe the steps of a field investigation
3. Discuss the legal implications of a field investigation
4. Discuss the competencies needed for legal epidemiology practice

ESSENTIAL TERMINOLOGY

Essential terminology is:

- Field epidemiology
- Forensic epidemiology
- Legal epidemiology

Field epidemiology is the practical application of epidemiology knowledge, skills, and methods to resolve population-based public health problems. The core functions of field epidemiology are outbreak investigation, conduct of public health surveillance, collection and analysis of epidemiologic data, engaging in epidemiologic judgment, and dissemination and communication of epidemiologic findings (Dicker, 2017). Even though epidemiologists frequently work in the field, the specialty of field epidemiology characteristically refers to field investigations initiated in response to an urgent public health problem. Nursing and epidemiology are both practice disciplines. In the field is where the intersectionality of nursing practice, public health practice, and epidemiology intersect.

A primary goal of field epidemiology is to determine the characteristics of the epidemiologic event along with the appropriate public health interventions to decrease or prevent the negative health impact within a population (Goodman et al., 2019). The Centers for Disease Control and Prevention (CDC) specifically defines field epidemiology as that application of epidemiology under the following conditions:

- Timing of the problem is unexpected
- A timely response is necessary
- Epidemiologists must work in the field to solve the public health event
- The extent of the investigation is likely to be limited in scope with the need for timely intervention (Goodman et al., 2019).

In a field epidemiologic investigation, the epidemiologist does not start with a specific hypothesis about the public health event's cause or source of illness. Through descriptive epidemiologic investigations, the epidemiologist is able to generate hypotheses before conducting analytic studies to examine hypotheses generated later during the investigation in the field. In field epidemiology, the epidemiologist is focused on determining the appropriate public health interventions needed to take sufficient action to protect the health and welfare of the public as the epidemiologist is conducting the investigation in the field. Nurses, specifically public/community health and primary care nurses, engage in program planning activities based on the health interventions identified as appropriate through field epidemiology. Field epidemiology initiates preventive and control measures concurrently with the field investigation. Therefore, intervention determination is occurring as the field investigation unfolds. Generally, the field epidemiologist begins with immediate recommendations for interventions based on initial assessments (Goodman et al., 2019).

Field epidemiologists are dependent on data from multiple sources. Data sources for field epidemiology consist of hospital, outpatient, and school health records; clinical laboratory data; and environmental or other biological specimen information. In addition to collecting data, during a "real time" public health event, field epidemiologists must communicate with the public. Field epidemiologists assist with informing the public by developing information, identifying cases, and recommending interventions to reduce or eliminate the event. Field epidemiologists are obligated to communicate what is known, what is unknown, and the recommended public health interventions directly or through the media (Goodman et al., 2019).

A statement that every nurse should be familiar with is "If it is not documented, it is not done." This statement can also be used to support the critical contribution of nursing documentation to field epidemiology, especially to the conduct of outbreak or epidemic investigations. Nursing documentation of events that the patient experienced are critical to a field epidemiologic investigation. Critical aspects of nursing documentation include signs and symptoms, physical findings, date and timing of all events, historical events, and lifestyle practices associated with the event.

The inherent nature of field epidemiology requires a rapid response with quick and appropriate decisive actions. They ensure the scientific quality of field investigations and that the standards for field epidemiology investigations that have been established are followed. The field epidemiology investigation standards are:

- Timely response is given.
- Important public health problem in the community based on epidemiological data such as morbidity and mortality information are addressed.
- Resources are assessed and deployed early in the investigation.
- Appropriate descriptive and analytical epidemiological methods for the investigation are used.
- The expertise of multiple disciplines as necessary such as microbiology, toxicology, psychology, anthropology, informatics, economics, laboratory and environmental sciences is engaged.
- Causality to determine etiology, source of the event, and modes of transmission is investigated.
- Evidence-based interventions are identified.
- Interprofessional collaboration to ensure optimal and effective use of investigative information is enforced (Goodman et al., 2019).

FIELD OUTBREAK INVESTIGATION METHOD

The method for conducting a field outbreak investigation involves several steps that are nonlinear and many times iterative. The order of field outbreak investigation methods and processes will depend on the presentation of the outbreak and the existing information available regarding the outbreak and the causative or etiologic agent. Field outbreak investigation methods are as follows:

1. Determine that an outbreak exists based on number of cases, and eventually determine incidence and prevalence rates when the health condition or case definition is known.
2. Characterize the outbreak in terms of the epidemiologic triad: agent, host, and environment; determine reservoir or carrier status.
3. Hypothesize about modes of transmission and etiologic agent.
4. Characterize the outbreak in terms of person, place, and time—who is affected, geographic location of exposure and presentation of symptoms, and information regarding timing of exposure to presentation of symptoms (incubation period).
5. Determine if this is a known health condition. Use established case definitions. If this is an unknown or emerging condition/infection, develop and continually refine the case definition.
6. Graph epidemic curves.
7. Describe clinical presentation: signs and symptoms.

8. Conduct screening and diagnostic testing or develop screening and diagnostic testing. Determine sensitivity, specificity, positive predictive value, negative predictive value.
9. Conduct traceback investigation. A traceback investigation identifies the source of contamination to implement prevention and control measures. A traceback investigation may need to include the entire aspect of the source of exposure; for example, in foodborne outbreaks, this could include food harvesting, food production, food distribution, and food preparation and cooking
10. Investigate each case for risk or associative factors.
11. Develop a surveillance system to monitor and evaluate ongoing outbreaks.
12. Conduct contact tracing and develop further understanding of the outbreak. Develop surveys to explore the outbreaks within the community.
13. Implement control and prevention strategies early in the outbreak investigation when the condition is known.
14. Conduct case–control studies to further understand the outbreak etiology, natural history of the disease, risk factors, associated factors, and prevention and treatment strategies.
15. Conduct other studies or investigations to confirm the hypotheses generated about the outbreak and future prevention and control strategies.

FIELD EPIDEMIOLOGY: INTERVENTIONS

Field epidemiologists are challenged with determining the best evidence-based interventions to implement as a public health event is occurring. In addition, field epidemiologists are integral to facilitating the implementation of the interventions and evaluation of the intervention effectiveness. Some guiding principles for developing interventions are:

- Intervene early to minimize preventable morbidity and mortality.
- Base interventions on current and established facts and data along with knowledge from previous field investigations.
- Manage salient sociopolitical forces from negatively impacting the investigation.
- Tailor the intervention or interventions to the scope of the problem.

- Maintain open communication regarding the interventions (Hadler et al., 2019).

Each intervention deployed should have a sound scientific rationale. The urgency and necessity for the intervention should be determined by the severity of the problem. Several factors impact the determination about the aggressiveness, extent, and need for an intervention. These primary factors are the etiology, source of the problem, and mode of transmission. In addition to these primary factors, other factors to be considered are:

- Reservoir of the agent
- R_0 or R-naught
- Host risk factors
- Environmental and other mediating factors
- Known effectiveness of interventions
- Operational and logistic feasibility
- Legal authority and issues (Hadler et al., 2019)

Box 16.1 presents field epidemiology categories. Registered nurses and advanced practice nurses are essential frontline providers in the implementation of field interventions.

FIELD OUTBREAK LEGAL CONSIDERATIONS

As stated, field epidemiologists are investigating a public health event in "real time." Therefore, field epidemiologists must be aware of the legal and ethical parameters that impact their epidemiologic investigation. Field epidemiologists are expected to be cognizant of federal and state regulations that impact their investigative actions.

The U.S. Constitution provides the federal authority to protect the health and safety of the public. States gain their "police power" from their respective state constitution statutes. It is important for field epidemiologists to understand the different types and levels of legal authority. A statute is a congressional or state legislative act signed into effect by the U.S. president or state governor. A regulation or rule is promulgated under administrative law codes by an executive agency of the federal or state government. A regulation has legal enforcement powers by the respective executive agency. An executive order, such as a disaster declaration, is a directive provided by the U.S. president or state governor that can have legal force. A state has police power to protect the health, safety,

---

BOX 16.1. Field Epidemiology Intervention Categories

■ Source directed interventions
  □ Treat infected or affected individuals and/or animals
  □ Isolate infected individuals
  □ Use barrier precautions and personal protective equipment for healthcare workers
  □ Monitor exposed individuals for illness
  □ Quarantine contaminated sites or sources
  □ Implement cordon sanitaire—closing public spaces, reducing size or eliminating public gatherings, limit movement and mixing of groups
  □ Conduct contact tracing and partner notification
  □ Seize or destroy contaminated sources
  □ Eliminate environmental vectors
  □ Behavior modification to reduce risks
  □ Deter civil suits or criminal prosecution
  □ Restricted or control dangerous drugs or contaminants
■ Susceptible host- or animal-directed interventions
  □ Administer postexposure prophylaxis
  □ Administer vaccinations to immunize population
  □ Use barrier methods and person protective equipment
  □ Implement cordon sanitaire
  □ Behavior modification to reduce risk
  □ Shelter in place to reduce exposure
  □ Communicate with public via health alerts, press releases, and news reports about status of field investigation and necessary precautions with supporting rationales

Source: From Hadler, J., Varma, J., Vugia, D., & Goodman, R. (2019). Developing interventions. In S. Rasmussen & R. Goodman (Eds.), *The CDC field epidemiology manual*. Oxford University Press.

---

and welfare of its citizens. Police power is the authority of the state to enact laws and promulgate regulations that protect, preserve, and promote the health, safety, morals, and general welfare of the people. This police power does include the ability to place sanctions and restrictions on individuals within the state (Holt et al., 2019).

There are limitations to the state's police power. These limitations are provided by the Fourth, Fifth, and Fourteenth Amendments of the U.S. Constitution. These amendments protect citizens from unreasonable search and seizures (Fourth Amendment) and provide a requirement of due process of law before an individual can be deprived of life, liberty, or property (Fifth Amendment). The Fourteenth Amendment requires that actions should not be unreasonable, arbitrary, or capricious (Holt et al., 2019). Therefore, during a field investigation, epidemiologists should ensure that the interventions enacted are the least restrictive alternative to achieve the best possible public health outcomes.

The state police powers do provide state and local public health officials with the authority to conduct field epidemiology investigations. Generally, this authority includes the ability to:

- Obtain microbiological and laboratory specimens from hospitals and private laboratories.
- Review patient medical records in all types of clinical settings.
- Administer questionnaires and collect specimens from individuals affected in the outbreak.
- Administer questionnaires to unaffected persons who are necessary for field epidemiology investigations and analytical studies.
- Retain health-related information with confidentiality protections in place.
- Implement interventions for the immediate problem, prevent recurrences, and evaluate the effectiveness of interventions.
- Recall goods or products implicated in the public health event.
- Close businesses or restrict activities related to an outbreak source.
- Use isolation and quarantine measures.
- Administer vaccinations and other therapeutics to exposed individuals and groups (Holt et al., 2019).

Some other federal laws that should be considered during a field investigation are:

- **Part 46 of Title 45 of the Code of Federal Regulations (CFR):** Requires data collection that is deemed to be research to be reviewed and approved by an institutional review board with the insurance of research subject consent.
- **Privacy Act of 1974:** Protects the confidentiality of an individual's identifiable information when the records are maintained by a federal agency.
- **Freedom of Information Act (FOIA):** Provides that any person has a right to obtain access to federal agency records, except to the extent those records are protected from public disclosure by the FOIA exclusions.

- **Health Insurance Portability and Accountability Act of 1996 (HIPAA):** Provides privacy protection for an individual's identifiable health information, known as protected health information (PHI).
- **Genetic Information Nondiscrimination Act of 2008:** Protects an individual against health coverage discrimination based on their genetic information (Holt et al., 2019).

FORENSIC EPIDEMIOLOGY

Forensic epidemiology is an area of field epidemiology developing as an area of specialization. Forensic epidemiology uses epidemiologic field methods to support criminal investigations. Field-based forensic epidemiology is described as the application of public health methods in a field-based setting to investigate health-related criminal events, an integration of public health, epidemiology, and law (Mountcastle, n.d.).

Forensic epidemiologists' primary role has been in providing legal depositions, courtroom testimony, and expert witness testimony for other disciplines such as law enforcement and toxicology. Epidemiologic information is critical to forensic investigations. Forensic investigations require an associated or causal linkage between some exposure and a criminal act or health alteration. Epidemiologists are experts with the capability of providing this associated or causal forensic linkage by serving as an investigative expert, conducting case interviews, explaining scientific principles, explaining epidemiologic data related to the health problem, and presenting data collected on the exposure and criminal outcome under scrutiny (Mountcastle, n.d.).

The International Association of Forensic Nurses define Sexual Assault Nurse Examiners (SANE) as registered nurses who have completed specialized education and clinical preparation in the medical forensic care of the patient who has experienced sexual assault or abuse. These SANE are considered practitioners of forensic epidemiology. SANE nurses collect and testify about critical forensic evidence used in criminal cases of both adults and children who experienced some type of sexual assault.

LEGAL EPIDEMIOLOGY

Black's Law Dictionary defines law as a rule or method; a system; or principles or rules of human conduct that are either prescribed or recognized by a governing or authoritative power within an organized society (Garner, 2019). From this definition, it is evident that law creates the authority from which policies are developed and enforced. These laws that are intended for the general public's health and welfare are known as public health laws (Benjamin, 2020). Public health law is a recognized specialty within the professions of law and public health. Public health law practice is defined as the application of professional legal skills in the formulation of health policy and the practice of public health (Burris et al., 2016, 2020; Gable, 2020).

Public health laws have the potential to impact the health, safety, and general welfare of a population, both positively and negatively. The enactment of public health laws can be a key determinant of the public's health (Thompson et al., 2020). Laws could be enacted that serve as a primary driver to influence an individual's behaviors or encourage healthy decision-making (Ramanathan et al., 2017). Laws regarding living conditions, education, employment, and housing are a few exemplars that have the potential to affect the social determinants of health that have an impact on the public's health.

Legal epidemiology is an advancing area of epidemiology practice. The legal epidemiology field is an area of scientific study and the deployment of law as a factor in the cause, distribution, determinants, and prevention of health and disease in a population (Ramanathan et al., 2017). In legal epidemiology, the law text is researched into empirical data as a measure of the impact on public health outcomes (Ramanathan et al., 2017).

Legal Epidemiology Competencies

The minimum competencies required for legal epidemiology focus on research and knowledge translation and the required skills for public health practitioners, attorneys, and policy experts to practice in the specialized area of legal epidemiology. Legal epidemiology is an evolved specialty in multiple disciplines. This competency model suggests that attorneys and non-attorneys practicing legal epidemiology should have basic competence in public health law, policy making, and basic principles of administrative and constitutional law.

The legal epidemiology competency model is organized into three domains: general legal epidemiology, legal mapping, and legal evaluation. In the general legal epidemiology domain, the focus is on transdisciplinary knowledge that includes basic research and epidemiology skills. The legal mapping domain addresses the skills needed for legal mapping studies and the designing of policy surveillance projects. The legal evaluation domain focuses on evaluating the impact and outcomes of laws on health (CDC and Office for State, Tribal, Local, and Territorial Support, 2018). The competencies for each domain are further classified according to three practitioner tiers: entry level, mid-level, and senior manager/ principal investigator level. The reader is referred to the specific CDC website (https://www.cdc.gov/phlp/publications/topic/resources/legalepimodel/index.html) for a more in-depth review of the legal competency by domain and tiers. The three domain competencies are:

1. Domain 1—General Legal Epidemiology
   a. **Competency statement 1:** Articulate the importance of legal epidemiology concepts to inform health, fiscal, administrative, legal, social, and political research and discourse.
   b. **Competency statement 2:** Apply legal epidemiology principles to research studies, funding opportunities, and policy agendas.
   c. **Competency statement 3:** Communicate legal epidemiology findings, methodologies, and recommendations to lay and professional audiences.
   d. **Competency statement 4:** Analyze the use of legal epidemiology findings to inform health, fiscal, administrative, legal, social and political activities.
2. Domain 2—Legal Mapping Studies
   a. **Competency statement 1:** Identify opportunities for legal mapping to inform the process, nature, and impact of policies and laws on public health.
   b. **Competency statement 2:** Develop policy surveillance or legal assessment studies to address specific research questions.

   c. **Competency statement 3:** Analyze laws, policies, and political and programmatic priorities using evidence-based or empirical guidelines (including health-related principles or trends, stakeholder or special interests, and other key developments or concerns).
   d. **Competency statement 4:** Validate and synthesize results that compare and contrast meaningful variations in law and policy related to health.
3. Domain 3—Legal Evaluation Studies
   a. **Competency statement 1:** Identify opportunities for legal evaluation study to address existing legal, health, or other issues.
   b. **Competency statement 2:** Design a legal evaluation to study potential associations between law and health.
   c. **Competency statement 3:** Collect and analyze quantitative and qualitative study data using generally accepted research methodologies.
   d. **Competency statement 4:** Interpret results, draw conclusions, and formulate key findings toward the improvement of public health.

A competency of legal epidemiology is the ability to conduct a legal mapping study. A legal mapping study examines the key provisions of a law on a particular public health issue; identifies the patterns in the nature, content, and distribution of the law; and analyzes the legal components of the law to public health measures. The legal mapping process consists of defining the scope of the research project by identifying the law to be examined; conducting an explicit, reproducible research strategy to identify all applicable laws; creating and executing a valid and reliable coding schematic to code the text of each law; analyzing the legal code schematic from the text to the public health outcomes; and disseminating the legal mapping findings and conclusions.

END-OF-CHAPTER RESOURCES

SUMMARY POINTS

- Field epidemiology is the practical application of epidemiology knowledge, skills, and methods to resolve population-based public health problems.
- The core functions of field epidemiology are outbreak investigation, conduct of public health surveillance, collection and analysis of epidemiologic data, engagement of epidemiologic judgment, and dissemination and communication of epidemiologic findings.
- A primary goal of field epidemiology is to determine the characteristics of the epidemiologic event along with the appropriate public health interventions to initiate to decrease or prevent the negative health impact within a population.
- In a field epidemiologic investigation, the epidemiologist does not start with a specific hypothesis.
- Data sources for field epidemiology consist of hospital, outpatient, and school health records, clinical laboratory data, environmental or other biological specimens information.
- Standards for field epidemiology investigations have been established.
- Field outbreak investigation methods and processes will depend on the presentation of the outbreak and the existing information available regarding the outbreak and the causative or etiologic agent.
- Field epidemiologists are integral to facilitating the implementation of the interventions and evaluation of the intervention effectiveness.
- Each intervention deployed should have a sound scientific rationale.
- The U.S. Constitution provides the federal authority to protect the health and safety of the public.
- A statute is a congressional or state legislative act signed into effect by the U.S. president or state governor.
- A regulation or rule is promulgated under administrative law codes by an executive agency of the federal or state government.
- An executive order, such as a disaster declaration, is a directive provided by the U.S. president or state governor that can have legal force.
- Police power is the authority of the state to enact laws and promulgate regulations that protect, preserve, and promote the health, safety, morals, and general welfare of the people.
- There are limitations to the state's police power.
- The enactment of public health laws can be a key determinant of the public's health.
- Laws could be enacted that serve as a primary driver to influence an individual's behaviors or encourage healthy decision-making.
- Legal epidemiology field is an area of scientific study and the deployment of law as a factor in the cause, distribution, determinants, and prevention of health and disease in a population.
- Forensic epidemiology uses epidemiologic field methods to support criminal investigations.

EPIDEMIOLOGY CRITICAL REASONING QUESTIONS

1. A rural critical access hospital emergency department had 15 patients present within the last 72 hours with the presentation of blood diarrhea. The emergency department records indicate that all individuals report eating a hamburger at a local family-owned restaurant about 20 miles from the local hospital. Patients implicated the presentation of their symptoms being related to eating the hamburger. Notification to the local health department indicated that there were also additional reported cases of bloody diarrhea associated with eating at the local family-owned restaurant. Using field outbreak investigation methods, respond to the following:
   a. What are possible causes for an increase in these reported cases?
   b. What information is necessary to determine if this is an outbreak?
   c. What is (are) your initial hypothesis(es)?
   d. What information is necessary to confirm your hypothesis(es)?
   e. What laboratory testing would you recommend on the presenting patients?
   f. What traceback measures would you suggest?

g. What environmental and employee testing would you recommend at the family-owned restaurant?
h. Propose a working case definition.
i. Describe the data that would be collected and analyzed to characterize this outbreak in terms of person, place, and time.
j. During the surveillance and contact tracing interviews, what questions would you propose to be asked of the symptomatic patients and of individuals potentially exposed?
k. Given your knowledge of *Escherichia coli*, salmonella, and other food-borne organisms, provide explanations, descriptions, or hypothesis(es) about the initial cases, source of the outbreak, modes of transmission, and control and prevention measures.

2. Compare and contrast the practice of field epidemiology, legal epidemiology, and forensic epidemiology.

3. As a forensic epidemiologist subpoenaed to provide expert testimony in a legal case resulting from an outbreak of foodborne illness at a local restaurant, list the sources of epidemiologic evidence you would plan to review and provide during your deposition.

ADDITIONAL RESOURCES

 A robust set of instructor resources designed to supplement this text is located at http://connect. springerpub.com/content/book/978-0-8261-8514-3. Qualifying instructors may request access by emailing textbook@springerpub.com.

REFERENCES

Benjamin, G. (2020). Perspectives from the field: Using legal epidemiology to advance public health practice. *Journal of Public Health Management and Practice, 26*(2), S93–S95. https://doi.org/10.1097/PHH.0000000000001108

Burris, S., Ashe, M., Levin, D., Penn, M., & Larkin, M. (2016). A transdisciplinary approach to public health law: The emerging practice of legal epidemiology. *Annual Review of Public Health, 37*(1), 135–148. https://doi.org/10.1146/annurev-publhealth-032315-021841

Burris, S., Cloud, L., & Penn, M. (2020). The growing field of legal epidemiology. *Journal of Public Health Management and Practice, 26*(S4–S9); doi: 10.1097/PHH.0000000000001133

Centers for Disease Control and Prevention and Office for State, Tribal, Local, and Territorial Support. (2018). *The legal epidemiology competency model version 1.0.* https://www.cdc.gov/phlp/publications/topic/resources/legalepimodel/index.html

Dicker, R. (2017). Case studies in applied epidemiology. *The Pan African Medical Journal, 27*(Suppl. 1), 1–2. https://doi.org/10.11604/pamj.supp.2017.27.1.12886

Gable, L. (2020). Teaching the future: Legal epidemiology as a model for transdisciplinary education. *Journal of Public Health Management and Practice, 26*(2), S96–S99. https://doi.org/10.1097/PHH.0000000000001135

Garner, B. (2019). What is law? In *Black's law dictionary* (11th ed.). Thomson Reuters.

Goodman, R., Buehler, J., & Mott, J. (2019). Defining field epidemiology. In S. Rasmussen & R. Goodman (Eds.), *The CDC field epidemiology manual.* Oxford University Press.

Hadler, J., Varma, J., Vugia, D., & Goodman, R. (2019). Developing interventions. In S. Rasmussen & R. Goodman (Eds.), *The CDC field epidemiology manual.* Oxford University Press.

Holt, J., Ghosh, S., & Black, J. (2019). Legal considerations. In S. Rasmussen & R. Goodman (Eds.), *The CDC field epidemiology manual.* Oxford University Press.

Mountcastle, S. (n.d.). Introduction to forensic epidemiology. *FOCUS on Field epidemiology, 2*(5), 1–5.

Ramanathan, T., Hulkower, R., Holbrook, J., & Penn, M. (2017). Legal epidemiology: The science of law. *Journal of Law and Medical Ethics, 45*(1_Suppl), 69–72. https://doi.org/10.1177/1073110517703329

Rasmussen, S., & Goodman, R. (2019). *The CDC field epidemiology manual.* Oxford University Press.

Thompson, B., Cloud, L., & Gable, L. (2020). Advancing legal epidemiology: An introduction. *Journal of Public Health Management and Practice, 28*(2), S1–S2. https://doi.org/10.1097/PHH.0000000000001119

Section IV:
Fields of Epidemiology in Practice

Chapter 17

PANDEMIC EPIDEMIOLOGY

Demetrius J. Porche

The worst pandemic in modern history was the Spanish flu of 1918, which killed tens of millions of people. Today with how interconnected the world is, it would spread faster.

–Bill Gates

If we can provide even a few months of early warning for just one pandemic, the benefits outweigh all the time and energy we are devoting. Imagine preventing health crises, not just responding to them.

–Nathan Wolfe (American virologist)

CHAPTER COMPETENCIES

At the conclusion of this chapter, the reader will be able to:

1. Characterize the aspects of a whole-of-society multisector approach to pandemic risk assessment
2. Compare and contrast the World Health Organization pandemic phases and Centers for Disease Control and Prevention pandemic intervals
3. Compose a list of epidemiologic data used to characterize a pandemic risk assessment
4. Plan appropriate pandemic prevention measures to include medical countermeasures and community mitigation
5. Discuss the legal authority for declaration of an emergency and liability immunity

ESSENTIAL TERMINOLOGY

- Acceleration interval
- Alert phase
- All-hazards approach
- Community mitigation
- Community resilience
- Comprehensive risk management
- Deceleration interval
- Efficient transmission
- Exposure assessment
- Genetic mutation
- Genetic reassortment
- Initial assessment
- Initiation interval
- Interpandemic phase
- Investigation interval
- Medical countermeasures
- Multidisciplinary approach
- Multisectoral approach
- Pandemic
- Pandemic influenza preparedness framework
- Pandemic interval
- Pandemic phase
- Pandemic risk assessment
- Prepandemic interval
- Preparation interval
- Recognition interval
- Refined assessment
- Sustainable development
- Sustained transmission
- Transition phase

A pandemic impacts the entire health of the community and multiple countries at the same time. During a pandemic, it is imperative to engage the entire community, healthcare system, and create international exchanges of information and science, what is considered a multisector approach. To effectively respond to and control a pandemic, it is necessary to have integration of all aspects of the healthcare system inclusive of but not limited to public health, primary care, episodic care, acute care, convalescent or long-term care, and care provided by nontraditional care settings such as community-based or non-profit organizations. One of the concerns during a pandemic is overstressing the healthcare system to the point of collapse or inability to appropriately and effectively respond to the crisis.

In a pandemic situation, clinical disease can range from mild to severe even to the point of causing significant mortality within the population. Historically, pandemics have occurred as a result of genetic reassortment, genetic mutation, or a combination of both. Genetic reassortment involves the genes from different viruses combining to create a new strain with a new genetic complement. In genetic mutation, a gene in an animal virus changes permitting the virus to infect humans and continue transmission from human to human (World Health Organization [WHO], 2017). Since about the 16th century, influenza pandemics have occurred in intervals ranging from 10 and 50 years with different levels of severity and impact. Table 17.1 presents some characteristics of the past four influenza pandemics.

WORLD HEALTH ORGANIZATION PANDEMIC GUIDANCE

The World Health Organization (WHO) purports that influenza pandemics are unpredictable but recurring events that have a significant consequence to human health and economic well-being of the world (2017). The mitigation of a pandemic needs advance planning and preparedness. WHO provides an emergency risk management health guide that strives to strengthen capacities to manage health risk from all hazards, embed comprehensive emergency risk management activities into healthcare systems, and enable and promote the linkage and integration of societal sectors across the government and society for a coordinated response (WHO, 2017). Figure 17.1 characterizes the whole-of-society multisector approach. The whole-of-society multisector approach involves all governmental levels and industry sectors of society. The whole-of-society multisector approach integrates pandemic activities of prevention, control, and restoration from each of the sectors listed in Figure 17.1.

World Health Organization Risk Management Guidance

The Pandemic Influenza Preparedness (PIP) Framework provides a global approach to pandemic preparedness and response. PIP goals are to improve and strengthen sharing of information about influenza viruses with human pandemic potential and achieve efficient and equitable access for all countries in need of life-saving vaccines and medicines during a pandemic. The Emergency Risk Management for Health (ERMH) principles recognize that risks are managed with a specific hazards approach, but hazard-specific risk management requires similar preparedness and response systems common to all hazards. Foundational principles of ERMH are comprehensive risk management, all-hazards approach, multisectoral approach, multidisciplinary approach, community resilience, sustainable development, and ethical basis of all decision-making. Table 17.2 summarizes the ERMH principles (WHO, 2017). ERMH objectives are to:

Table 17.1 Past Four Influenza Pandemics: Characteristics

Pandemic	Origin	Influenza A Viral Subtype	R_0	Case-Fatality Rate	Population Affected
1918 Spanish Flu	Not sure	H1N1	1.2–3.0	2%–3%	All ages
1957–1969 Asian Flu	Southern China	H2N2 (avian)	1.5	<0.2%	All ages
1968–1969 Hong Kong Flu	Southern China	H3N2 (avian)	1.3–1.6	<0.2%	All ages
2009–2010	North America	H1N1 (swine)	1.1–1.8	0.02%	All ages
2019–2020	Wuhan China	SARS-CoV-2	2–3	0 to >10%	All ages

Source: Adapted from World Health Organization. (2017). *Pandemic influenza risk management: A WHO guide to inform and harmonize national and international pandemic preparedness and response.* Author.

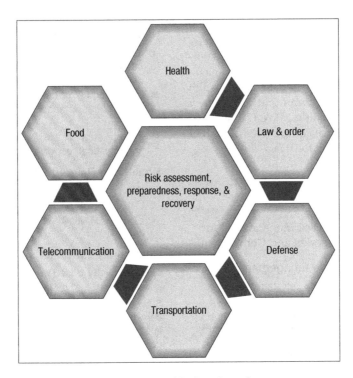

Figure 17.1 Multisector: Whole-of-society approach.

Table 17.2 Emergency Risk Management for Health (ERMH) Principles

Principle	Descriptor
Comprehensive Risk Management	Focus on assessment and management of emergency risk rather than actual emergency events
All-Hazards Approach	Use, develop, and strengthen the capabilities of all systems that are common to all risks and emergencies
Multisectoral Approach	Recognize the need to integrate all societal sector capabilities—government, businesses, and civil society
Multidisciplinary Approach	Recognize and utilize many disciplines in health to manage health risks through risk assessment, mitigation, prevention, preparedness, response, recovery, and capacity building
Community Resilience	Utilize capabilities at the community level for risk assessment, reporting, provision of basic services, risk communication for disease prevention and long-term care and rehabilitation
Sustainable Development	Recognize the need for long-term development approach to promote health and build resilience
Ethical Basis	Ethical principles integrated throughout ERMH activities

- Strengthen country and community capacity to manage health crises arising from all types of hazards
- Ensure essential components are required in a comprehensive risk management program
- Link and integrate the healthcare system, multisectoral disaster management systems, and other entities across society as a whole for relevant risk management with nonhealth-related sectors
- Enable the health sector to advocate for and strengthen national and international policies and frameworks to respond to emergencies and disasters to reduce the risk and health impacts from all hazards (WHO, 2017).

There are six essential component categories of ERMH. These essential components are policies and resource management, planning and coordination, information and knowledge management, health infrastructure and logistics, health and related services, and community emergency risk management capabilities. Box 17.1 summarizes the ERMH essential components of each of these six categories (WHO, 2017).

BOX 17.1. Emergency Risk Management for Health Essential Categories and Components

Policies and Resource Management

■ Appropriate policies, plans, strategies and legislation that supports effective governance of ERMH
■ Policies, plans, strategies, and legislation uses an all hazards approach
■ Management of human and material resources
■ Specify role, responsibilities, and authority of responders
■ Healthcare workforce capacity development

Planning and Coordination

■ All levels of government represented
■ Stakeholder involvement in planning and coordination
■ Prevention and mitigation actions planned after detailed risk assessment
■ Implementation of prevention, mitigation, and preparedness measures with all governmental levels, businesses, and civil society
■ Effective coordination of all aspects of the response
■ Recovery should be an essential component of response planning
■ Business continuity management

Information and Knowledge Management

■ Technical guidance provided for risk management, communications, and early warning and surveillance systems
■ Effective risk communication to build capacity
■ Communication strategy provides information in a timely manner with attention to how people react to and act on advice
■ Implement early warning and surveillance systems that capture data on assessment of severity
■ Early warning and surveillance system should include minimum data sets of information

Health Infrastructure and Logistics

■ Infrastructure and logistics about transportation, telecommunications, stockpiling, and distribution of medications and supplies
■ Establishment of temporary health services
■ Logistical assistance during health emergencies
■ Identify, support, train, and deploy operational and logistical response teams as needed

Health and Related Services

■ Provision of healthcare services
■ Provision of public health measures
■ Provide specialized services for the specific hazard

Community Risk Management Capabilities

■ Community-based healthcare workforce development and capacity building

Source: From World Health Organization. (2017). *Pandemic influenza risk management: A WHO guide to inform and harmonize national and international pandemic preparedness and response.* Author.

Naming of New Human Infectious Diseases: World Health Organization

WHO established identified best practices for naming of new human infectious diseases. The International Classification of Diseases (ICD), managed by WHO, provides the final standard name for each human disease. WHO best practices naming principles considers that disease names can include generic description (such as clinical symptoms, physiologic processes, and anatomical or pathological references to affected systems—respiratory, neurological, syndrome, disease), specific descriptive terms representative of age, time of origin, severity, seasonality, or environment (such as juvenile, pediatric, acute, chronic, severe, summer, desert, ocean), causal pathogen and associated descriptors (such as coronavirus, novel, variant, subtype), year of first detection or reporting (such as 2019), and an arbitrary identification (such as alpha, beta, or a letter or number). WHO does not recommend that names include geographic locations (cities, countries, regions, or continents); people's names; species or class of animal or food; cultural, population, industry or occupational references; or terms that incite anxiety or fear (WHO, 2015). Other naming recommendations are for the name to be short with easy pronunciation.

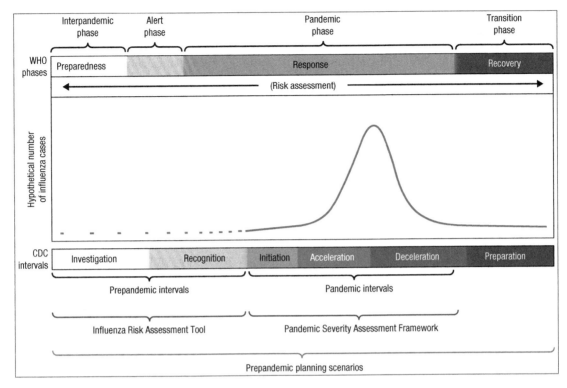

Figure 17.2 Pandemic continuum intervals: Response framework—Preparedness and response framework for novel influenza A virus pandemics, with Centers for Disease Control and Prevention intervals and World Health Organization phases.

Source: Adapted from Holloway, R., Rasmussen, S. A., Zaza, S., Cox, N. J., Jernigan, D. B., & Influenza Pandemic Framework Workgroup. (2014). Updated preparedness and response framework for influenza pandemics. *MMWR Recommendations and Reports, 63*(RR-6); Qualls, N., Levitt, A., Kanade, N., Wright-Jegede, N., Dopson, S., Biggerstaff, M., Reed, C., & Uzicanin, A. (2017). Community mitigation guidelines to prevent pandemic influenza — United States, 2017. *MMWR Recommendations and Reports, 66*(RR-1), 1–34. https://doi.org/10.15585/mmwr.rr6601a1.

World Health Organization Pandemic Phases

WHO considers that there are four phases of a pandemic. Figure 17.2 presents WHO pandemic phases. The four pandemic phases are interpandemic, alert, pandemic, and transition. Interpandemic is the period between influenza pandemics. The alert phase is the period in which a new influenza subtype has been identified in humans. In the alert phase, there is increased vigilance and careful risk assessment at all levels—local, state, federal, and international. In the pandemic phase, there is global spread of human influenza caused by a new subtype. Movement into the pandemic phase is dependent upon epidemiologic surveillance data, virologic information, and clinical data. The transition phase emerges as the global risk is reduced, global actions are de-escalated, and

response activities are reduced. It is the WHO Director who has the authority to declare the determination of a public health emergency of international concern (PHEIC) or declaration of a pandemic (WHO, 2017). WHO embraces the all-hazards approach to emergency risk management. The all-hazards phases of preparedness, response, and recovery are outlined in Figure 17.2 as they correspond to pandemic phases.

CENTERS FOR DISEASE CONTROL AND PREVENTION PREPAREDNESS AND RESPONSE FRAMEWORK

The CDC (2014) provides a framework of preparedness and response for a novel influenza virus infection that causes a pandemic. This framework presents the evolutionary phases for an influenza pandemic but is considered by some authorities to be applicable for other pandemics. These intervals provide for an understanding of the unfolding dynamics during a pandemic. These pandemic intervals are not exclusively linear. They are divided into prepandemic and pandemic intervals. Within the prepandemic interval, there are two intervals. Within the pandemic interval, there are four intervals (CDC, 2014). Figure 17.2 presents the intervals.

The prepandemic intervals are investigation and recognition. In the investigation interval, there is the identification of a novel influenza virus. During the investigation interval, public health actions are targeted toward epidemiologic surveillance and investigations to identify infected humans and assess the potential of the virus to cause several human diseases. The investigation interval also investigates the presence of the influenza virus outbreaks within the animal population. This interval assesses modes of transmission. The recognition interval begins with the increasing number of reported human cases or reporting of infection clusters of a novel infection. This increase in cases indicates human-to-human transmission with the need for activation of outbreak control measures (CDC, 2014).

In the pandemic interval of initiation, there is confirmation of human cases of the viral infection throughout the world with demonstrated efficient and sustained human-to-human transmission. Efficient transmission is considered household or an institutional attack rate of greater than 20% in more than two communities. Sustained is defined as transmission of the virus for three or more generations in more than one cluster. During the initiation interval, case-based control measures and routine personal protective measures such as hand hygiene are critical to reducing transmission. In the acceleration interval, there is a consistent increase in the incidence rate of viral cases. The acceleration interval requires the implementation of community mitigation measures to include isolation, quarantine, and treatment. The deceleration interval is the consistent decreasing rate of viral cases. During the deceleration interval, community mitigation measures may begin to be suspended with recovery efforts implemented. In the final interval, the preparation interval, there is low pandemic activity with the occasional occurrence of outbreaks in some areas. The preparation interval is characterized

by actions such as suspending community mitigation measures, promoting the recovery phase of healthcare and other industry infrastructures, resuming surveillance protocols to detect subsequent waves of the viral activity, evaluating the pandemic response, and preparing for potential additional and future pandemic infections. A pandemic is declared as ended when surveillance evidence indicates worldwide that the viral infection is transitioning to a seasonal pattern of transmission (CDC, 2014).

NATIONAL RISK ASSESSMENTS

Risk assessment is the systematic process to collect, analyze, and document information for the purpose of assigning a risk level. A pandemic risk assessment aims to determine the likelihood that an infection will impact the health of individuals and the extent to which the impact will occur throughout multiple countries simultaneously. The information from a risk assessment informs the pandemic response to prevent, mitigate, or eliminate the pandemic. In an all-hazards approach, the risk assessment specifically informs the pandemic preparedness, response, and recovery efforts inclusive of all types of potential hazards. The risk assessment suggests what to be prepared for in relation to preparedness, informs actions for the response, and prioritizes areas of greatest need for system and service recovery (WHO, 2017). The pandemic risk assessment should consist of an interprofessional team with multisector representation from multiple industry sectors. The pandemic risk assessment should consider the hazard, exposure, and context along with risk characterization. For a viral pandemic, the hazard assessment should include the virus of concern, virologist and clinical information, and rank the pandemic potential of the virus.

The exposure assessment defines the individuals who have been, are likely to be, and were exposed to the virus of concern. The exposure assessment incorporates epidemiologic and susceptibility information to include mode/route of transmission and incubation period.

The context assessment evaluates the environment in which the event occurs. The context assessment evaluates those factors that affect risk such as social, technical and scientific, economic, ethical, and policy and political.

Assessment Tools: Influenza Risk Assessment Tool and Pandemic Severity Assessment Framework

There are two tools used to facilitate the assessment of an influenza pandemic, the Influenza Risk Assessment Tool (IRAT) and the Pandemic Severity Assessment Framework (PSAF).

Influenza Risk Assessment Tool

The IRAT assesses the pandemic risk of a novel virus based on the likelihood of emergence and the public health impact should the novel virus pandemic emerge. For the IRAT, emergence refers to the risk of a novel virus acquiring the ability to easily and efficiently spread to and among humans. In the IRAT, public health impact is considered the potential severity of human disease caused by the viral infection along with the societal impact (CDC, 2014). The purposes of the IRAT are to:

- Prioritize and maximize investments in pandemic preparedness.
- Identify key information and knowledge gaps.
- Document transparently the data and scientific processes that inform management decisions.
- Provide a flexible means to easily and regularly revise and update the risk assessment.
- Communicate effectively for policy makers and the community.
- Provide a means to weigh the 10 evaluation criteria differently depending on whether the intent of the risk assessment is to measure the ability of a virus to "emerge" into a pandemic capable of human-to-human transmission or to measure the human population impact if the virus emerged as a pandemic (CDC, 2014, 2019).

The IRAT has 10 evaluation criteria divided into three sections—virus properties, population attributes, and ecology and epidemiology. Box 17.2 presents the 10 IRAT evaluation criteria (CDC, 2019).

Pandemic Severity Assessment Framework

Historically, influenza pandemic effects have been assessed by using an estimate of the overall case-fatality ratio (CFR). Using the CFR ratio alone presents several challenges: reporting bias due to mortality, the overall CFR does not account for the seasonal epidemic or pandemic affecting vulnerable populations, and the CFR does not take into account societal effects such

---

BOX 17.2. Influenza Risk Assessment Tool Criteria

Viral Properties

1. **Genomic analysis:** Measures the extent of genetic diversity or presence of unknown molecular signatures for human infection and disease
2. **Receptor binding:** Host preferences, types of tissues and cells infected by the virus
3. **Lab animal transmission:** Ability of the virus to be transmitted efficiently in an animal laboratory environment
4. **Antiviral treatment options:** Predicted effectiveness of antiviral medications

Population Attributes

1. **Existing population immunity:** The extent to which the human population has existing immune protection against the virus
2. **Disease severity and pathogenesis:** Measures the severity of illness caused by the virus in humans
3. **Antigenic relatedness:** Measures the antigenic similarity of the virus to seasonal influenza vaccines, prepandemic candidate vaccines, and stockpiled prepandemic vaccines

Ecology and Epidemiology

1. **Global distribution:** Measures the amount of widespread infection in animals, rate of spread over time, and management factors that may impact the distributions
2. **Infection in animal species:** The types of animals impacted by the virus and likelihood of human contact with these animals
3. **Human infections:** Evidence and frequency of human infections with the virus not currently capable of sustained human-to-human transmission

Source: From Centers for Disease Control and Prevention. (2019). *Influenza risk assessment tool.* https://www.cdc.gov/flu/pandemic-resources/national-strategy/risk-assessment.htm

---

as absenteeism or healthcare service demands. The PSAF was developed in consideration of these challenges. It is used to determine the actual or potential impact of the pandemic. The PSAF is primarily determined by the clinical severity of the infection and the transmissibility of the infection from human to human. These two combined factors guide decisions and actions during a pandemic.

The PSAF is divided into two parts, initial assessment and refined assessment. The initial assessment is conducted early during the pandemic. During the initial assessment, there is minimal epidemiologic data and the early indicators of the pandemic may be very variable. The initial assessment collects epidemiologic data in two areas, transmissibility and clinical severity. Based on the data, each of the transmissibility and clinical severity parameters are categorized into one of two scales as low-moderate or moderate-high. Box 17.3 presents the initial assessment parameters for transmissibility and clinical severity (Reed et al., 2013). The on-line article in *Prevent Epidemics*, located at https://preventepidemics.org/covid19/science/insights/covid-19-pandemic-severity-assessment-framework-by-age/, presents an example of the PSAF for COVID-19.

In the second refined assessment, the pandemic is progressing with an increase in known epidemiologic data. The refined assessment provides a more refined and accurate perspective of the pandemic's impact. Box 17.4 presents the transmissibility and clinical severity parameters

---

BOX 17.3. Initial Assessment Parameters Measured: Transmissibility and Clinical Severity

Transmissibility

- Secondary attack rate, household, %
- Attack rate, school or university, %
- Attack rate, workplace or community, %
- R_0
- Underlying population immunity
- Emergency or other outpatient influenza-like illnesses, %
- Virologic characterization (genetic markers of transmissibility present)
- Animal models of transmission (efficiency compared to seasonal influenza)

Clinical Severity

- Upper boundary of case-fatality ratio, %
- Upper boundary of case-hospitalization ratio, %
- Death ratio, hospitalizations, %
- Virologic characterization (genetic markers for virulence—absent or present)
- Animal models of transmission (less or more virulent than seasonal influenza)

Source: From Reed, C., Biggerstaff, M., Finelli, L., Koonin, L. M., Beauvais, D., Uzicanin, A., Plummer, A., Bresee, J., Redd, S. C., & Jernigan, D. B. (2013). Novel framework for assessing epidemiologic effects of influenza epidemics and pandemics. *Emerging Infectious Diseases*, 19(1), 85–91. https://doi.org/10.3201/eid1901.120124.

BOX 17.4. Refined Assessment Parameters Measured: Transmissibility and Clinical Severity

Transmissibility

- Symptomatic attack rate, community, %
- Symptomatic attack rate, school, %
- Symptomatic attack rate, workplace, %
- Household secondary attack rate, symptomatic, %
- R_0
- Peak % outpatient visits for influenza-like symptoms

Clinical Severity

- Case-fatality ratio, %
- Case-hospitalization ratio, %
- Death ratio, hospitalization, %

---

used in the refined assessment. The refined assessment assigns a rating to each parameter on a scale of 1 to 7 (with 7 being the higher end of the scale; Reed et al., 2013).

Both the initial and refined assessments are compared to the existing knowledge base regarding past influenza pandemics. This comparison provides the pandemic assessment team with information from which to advise the public on the pandemic's potential impact. This information provides a measure of the pandemic's severity and potential for transmission. From these assessments on severity, pandemic intervention strategies can be implemented to decrease the viral spread (Reed et al., 2013).

U.S. FEDERAL PLAN FOR EMERGING INFECTIOUS DISEASE THREATS AND BIOLOGICAL INCIDENTS

The Pandemic Prediction and Forecasting Science and Technology Working Group of the National Science and Technology Council identified challenges and proposed recommendations for responding to infectious disease outbreaks that threaten global health, economic viability, and the United States' national security interest (2016). This group's report identified critical uncertainties to be aware of when modeling epidemic outbreaks. These uncertainties are:

- **Outbreak growth rate and future course of the epidemic:** Determine R_0, number of cases, incidence and prevalence rates, and mortality rates

- **Geographical spread:** Identify geographical areas of high risk
- **Possible interventions and clinical trials:** Assessment, comparison, and implementation of possible control measures
- **Pathogen evolution and functional genetic determinants:** Determine relationship of outbreak strain to known pathogen characteristics
- **Pathogen origin and drivers of emergence:** Predict the time and place of the outbreak before it occurs

The Executive Office of the United States developed an Early Response to High-Consequence Emerging Infectious Disease Threats and Biological Incidents, commonly referred to as the "epidemic/pandemic playbook." This "playbook" identified Executive Branch Offices and Agencies critical to the development of an early response while embracing the recommendations of WHO for assessing the risk of an infectious disease threat that may become a public health emergency of international concern (PHEIC). This "playbook" provides assessment dashboards to serve as a guidance for planning best strategies to assess the risk of evolving infectious disease threats using four critical dimensions—epidemiology; humanitarian, development, and public health impacts; security and political stability; and transmission, outbreak potential, and potential for public concern in the United States.

Each of these four critical dimensions are rated on the following scale for international assessment—1a. Normal operations (no unusual infectious disease outbreak); 1b. Elevated threat (infectious disease outbreak with high mortality or high morbidity, clinical severity, or public health consequences, high transmission or outbreak potential, case reports or clusters of high consequence with limited countermeasures, case reports, and clusters of novel pathogen); 1c. Credible threat (infectious outbreak with high mortality, clinical severity, high transmission, infectious disease outbreak with limited countermeasures, novel pathogen, community transmission, rate of transmission higher than average rate or number of cases prior to outbreak threshold, and cases imported to the United States); 2a. Public health emergency of international concern (official WHO declaration of PHEIC); 2b. Worsening public health emergency indicators/PHEIC; and 2c. Improving public health emergency/PHEIC.

Each of these four critical dimensions are rated on the following scale for a domestic assessment: 1a. Normal operations (no specific pandemic threat); 1b. Elevated threat (identification of a human case of a pathogen of pandemic potential [PPP] anywhere); 1c. Credible threat (confirmation of multiple human cases of PPP anywhere or the determination of a significant potential for a public health emergency [PHE]); 2a. Initial response-activation, situation assessment, and movement (documented efficient and sustained human-to-human transmission of a novel or re-emerging PPP anywhere or declaration of PHE); 2b. Employment of resources and stabilization (increasing number of cases in the United States or healthcare system burden that exceeds local, state, tribal/territorial [LSTT] resources of request for assistance); 2c. Intermediate operations (case count continues to increase with long-term service disruption and critical infrastructure impact or Presidential Stafford Act Declaration or LSTT request for assistance; and 3a. Sustained operations (long-term recovery operations with or without continuous incidence of new cases).

Key pathogen questions that must be considered according to this "playbook" are mode of transmission of the pathogen (tier 1—respiratory pathogens, tier 2—transmission via fluid contact, tier 3—vector transmission); what is the actual and potential impact of the pathogen in the future; what is the potential for successful transmission; and what are the known tools to mitigate the spread of the pathogen. Other key considerations identified in the "playbook" are medical countermeasures; deployment of medical personnel; biological sample sharing (nationally and internationally); financial and staffing resources; risk rating adaptations (trigger criteria to evaluate an emerging infectious threat—epidemiology, geographic location, host nation's response, disruption of healthcare system); triggers for activating the United Nations' public health emergency response; coordination of simultaneous domestic response and international governmental response; and standardization of clinical care. This "playbook" provides substantive guidance on actions to respond to potential or actual pandemic threats.

PANDEMIC INTERVENTION STRATEGIES

Medical Countermeasures

During a pandemic, especially of an infectious nature, medical countermeasures (MCMs) are central to the response and mitigation process. MCMs include vaccines, pharmacologic therapeutic agents (such as antiviral and antibiotics), diagnostics, ventilators, and respiratory protective devices (CDC, 2020).

Community Mitigation

The goal of community mitigation is to control the spread of an infectious pandemic agent in the community. Community mitigation efforts include medication administration and/or nonpharmacologic interventions (NPIs). Nonpharmacologic interventions include travel restrictions even to the extent of country border closures; everyday preventive strategies such as face coverings, hand hygiene, social distancing; and routine and frequent cleaning of frequently touched surfaces. Community mitigation may also include closure of businesses and restriction of service delivery to reduce person-to-person contact. Community level NPI can also include restriction or closure of schools and universities (Qualls et al., 2017). Box 17.5 summarizes community mitigation NPI.

BOX 17.5. Community Mitigation Measures: Nonpharmacologic Interventions (NPIs)

Personal NPIs

- Everyday personal protective measures
  - □ Voluntary home isolation of ill individuals for at least 24 hours after a fever or signs of a fever
  - □ Respiratory etiquette (covering nose for sneeze and cough), dispose of tissue, and practice hand hygiene
  - □ Hand hygiene is understood as cleaning hands with soap and water or alcohol-based hand sanitizers with at least 60% ethanol or isopropanol
- Pandemic personal protective measures
  - □ Home quarantine of exposed household members for up to 3 days
  - □ Face masks in community settings when ill
- Community NPIs
  - □ School closure and dismissal
  - □ Social distancing
  - □ Avoidance of mass gatherings
- Environmental Surface Cleaning Measures
  - □ Cleaning surfaces in all settings (home, schools, workplaces) with detergent based cleaners or disinfectants registered with the Environmental Protection Agency (EPA)

- Mobilizing Public Engagement
  - □ Provide a clear purpose and goal
  - □ Establish relationships with community members, build trust, work with formal and informal leaders, seek commitment from community organizations
  - □ Ensure attention to community's culture, economic conditions, social networks, political and power structures, norms and values, history, and previous experiences
  - □ Accept collective self-determination is the responsibility and right of all people
  - □ Recognize the community's diversity
  - □ Mobilize community assets
  - □ Be prepared to release control of action and interventions to the community
  - □ Prepare for a long-term commitment with the community

As evidenced with the recent COVID-19 pandemic, there is reporting of the epidemic curve and the need to "flatten the curve." Community mitigation goals from a pandemic, as described in Box 17.5, are essential in "flattening the curve." In the midst of each pandemic, these epidemic curves are used to demonstrate the number of cases over time and what is the desired goal to decrease the number of cases—reducing the morbidity and mortality as graphic epidemic curves. Figure 17.3 presents typical epidemic curves used to present data during an epidemic or pandemic displaying projected cases in an epidemic curve with no interventions, means to slow the acceleration, or flatten the curve with interventions over time.

LEGAL BASIS FOR PANDEMIC CONTROL

Mitigation and control strategies during a pandemic involve the request and sometimes requirement of behavior change. The Public Health Service (PHS) Act forms the legal foundation of authority for the Department of Health and Human Services (DHHS) to respond to public health emergencies such as a pandemic. PHS empowers the Secretary of the DHHS to lead the public health and medical response, declare public health emergencies, assist states with meeting their state-level needs, maintain and mobilize the Strategic National

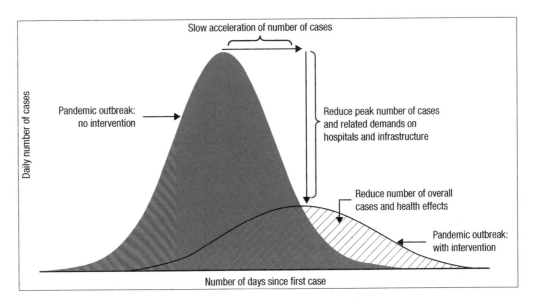

Figure 17.3 Community mitigation goals for influenza pandemic.

Source: Adapted from the Centers for Disease Control and Prevention. (2007). *Interim pre-pandemic planning guidance: community strategy for pandemic influenza mitigation in the United States— early, targeted, layered use of nonpharmaceutical interventions.* U.S. Department of Health and Human Services, CDC. https://stacks.cdc.gov/view/cdc/11425; Qualls, N., Levitt, A., Kanade, N., Wright-Jegede, N., Dopson, S., Biggerstaff, M., Reed, C., & Uzicanin, A. (2017). Community mitigation guidelines to prevent pandemic influenza — United States, 2017. *MMWR Recommendations and Reports, 66*(RR-1), 1–34. https://doi .org/10.15585/mmwr.rr6601a1.

Stockpile, and implement measures to control communicable diseases (CDC, 2016).

An emergency response to a pandemic begins with the state governor or chief executive of the Indian tribe requesting the president of the United States to declare a national emergency. The president of the United States can declare a national emergency without the governor's request if the primary responsibility for the emergency response rests with the federal government. Section 319 of the PHS authorizes the Secretary of the DHHS to take actions during a pandemic that include but are not limited to providing grants; entering into contractual agreements; conducting and/or supporting investigations into the pandemic cause, treatment, prevention, or control measures; and waiving some requirements of social programs such as Medicare, Medicaid, Children's Health Insurance Program (CHIP), and Health Insurance Portability and Accountability Act (HIPAA).

The PHS Public Readiness and Emergency Preparedness (PREP) Act authorized the DHHS Secretary to issue declarations that provides immunity from liability for the use of MCMs, except if there is intentional willful misconduct. The authority of the DHHS Secretary to use MCM during a declared national emergency is provided for in the Federal Food, Drug and Cosmetic (FD&C) Act, Section 564. Also, this provision permits the FDA Commissioner to use unapproved medical products such as vaccines or diagnostic tests or medical products to diagnose, treat, or prevent a serious or life-threatening disease or condition caused by a chemical, biological, radiological, or nuclear agent. Community mitigation measures are authorized under Section 361 of the PHS Act. These measures include the prevention of entry and spread of communicable diseases from foreign countries into the United States and between states (CDC, 2016).

PANDEMIC INSIGHTS FROM THE PAST

Boxes 17.6 through 17.11 give specific historical details about polio, influenza A-H1N1, Zika, the Spanish flu of 1918, HIV, and Ebola.

BOX 17.6. Pandemic Insights from the Past: Poliomyelitis (p)

Epidemiology: About 90% of the infected population remains asymptomatic, with 10% developing flu-like symptoms within 3 to 5 days (incubation period). There has not been a polio outbreak in the United States since the early 1900s. The first major epidemic of polio in the United States occurred in 1916. There was a seasonal presentation with higher rates during the summer months. The number of cases sharply decreased after 1952 when a vaccine was developed. Since there has been viral eradication in several countries, surveillance testing remains only in Africa and Eastern Mediterranean regions.

Etiologic Agent: Viral agent—poliovirus. There are three forms, P1, P2 and P3, each producing similar signs and symptoms. Reservoir of poliovirus is humans, residing in the gastrointestinal tract. A host is considered infectious 3 days prior to the onset of prodromal symptoms and remains infectious for as long as 2 months after the initial onset of symptoms.

Mode of Transmission: Poliovirus is transmitted through the fecal–oral route or droplets, with 80% of the transmissions in person-to-person with 20% from environmental contact.

Diagnostic Testing: Stool sampling along with environmental testing of sewage for presence of poliovirus. Stool cytology is the hallmark screening measure to detect both wild poliovirus and vaccine-derived poliovirus. For polio eradication to be declared, a region must have no detectable poliovirus for at least 3 years. Surveillance activities target children less than 15 years of age.

Clinical Presentation: Once the poliovirus attacks the central nervous system, specifically the motor neurons along the spinal cord, an inflammatory response leads to meningitis. Polio progresses to various degrees of paralysis. Abortive poliomyelitis presents as flu-like symptoms, fever, fatigue, headache, nausea/vomiting, and sore throat. Paralytic poliomyelitis has three subclassifications: spinal, bulbar, and bulbospinal. Spinal polio present with severe muscle pain and spasms, asymmetrical weaknesses, paresthesia, urinary retention, and loss of reflexes progressing to flaccid paralysis mostly in the lower limbs. Bulbar polio presents with dysphagia, nasal regurgitation, dysarthria, facial paralysis, absent gag reflex, and difficulty breathing. Bulbospinal polio presents with symptoms of bulbar polio and respiratory failure.

Pharmacologic Measures: Oral poliovirus vaccine (OPV) and inactivated poliovirus vaccine (IPV) administration is the gold standard of care.

Medical Countermeasures: Medical countermeasures are hand hygiene, sanitary food preparation, use of clean water, and appropriate coughing and sneezing etiquette.

Source: Centers for Disease Control and Prevention. (2019). *What is polio?* https://www.cdc.gov/polio/what-is-polio-/index.htm; Kew, O., & Nathanson, N. (2010). From emergence to eradication: The epidemiology of poliomyelitis deconstructed. *American Journal of Epidemiology, 172*(11), 1213–1229. https://doi.org/10.1093/aje/kwq320; Ochmann, S., & Roser, M. (2017). *Polio: Our world in data*. https://ourworldindata.org/polio; and Snider, C., Diop, O., Burns, C., Tangermann, R., & Wassilak, S. (2016). Polio surveillance: Tracking progress towards eradication worldwide. *Weekly Epidemiological Record, 91*(15), 193–208.

BOX 17.7. Pandemic Insights from the Past: Influenza A H1n1 2009 Pandemic (swine flu)

Epidemiology: First confirmed case in the United States occurred in April 2009 in California. In June 2009, the World Health Organization declared a pandemic. From April 2009 to April 2010, there were 60.8 million cases of H1N1 and 12,469 deaths. The estimated mortality rate for H1N1 was 0.001%–0.007% of the world's population. There were two waves of infection—April to August 2009 and mid-August to late October 2009. Males and females were equally affected. The majority of individuals infected were of Hispanic or Black descent.

Etiologic Agent: H1N1 virus

Mode of Transmission: Primarily respiratory transmission

Diagnostic Testing: Reverse-transcription polymerase chain reaction (RT-PCR) through nasopharyngeal swab collection

Clinical Presentation: Swine flu presents as an upper respiratory tract infection—fever, cough, malaise, rhinorrhea, sore throat, fatigue, nausea/vomiting, and diarrhea. The development of secondary bacterial infections, bronchitis, pneumonia, acute respiratory syndrome, respiratory failure, and death are possible.

Pharmacologic Measures: H1N1 nasal spray vaccine and H1N1 vaccine. Other potential influenza agents were oseltamivir, zanamivir, and peramivir.

Medical Countermeasures: The medical countermeasures included hand hygiene, droplet and standard precautions, maintaining a distance of greater than or equal to 1 meter or 3 feet, surgical masks and N95 masks with

(continued)

BOX 17.7. Pandemic Insights from the Past: Influenza A H1n1 2009 Pandemic (swine flu)
(continued)

patients. Cohort infected patients in hospital rooms. Hospital visitors were limited. Community mitigation measures included quarantine, isolation, school dismissals, and implementation of social distancing.

Source: Centers for Disease Control and Prevention. (2019). 2009 H1N1 pandemic. https://www.cdc.gov/flu/pandemic-resources/2009-h1n1-pandemic.html; Fineberg, H. (2014). Pandemic preparedness and response—lessons from H1N1 influenza of 2009. The New England Journal of Medicine, 14(370). https://www.nejm.org/doi/pdf/10.1056/NEJMra1208802.

infection; mosquito control measures (long pants and shirt sleeves, insect repellent, treating clothing with permethrin, aerial spraying, elimination of stagnant water sources); and safe sexual practices or abstinence.

Source: Barzon, L., Trevisan, M., Simigaglia, A., Lavezzo, E., & Palu, G. (2016). Zika virus: From pathogenesis to disease control. FEMS Microbiology Letters, 363(18), 1–17. http://doi.org/10.1093/femsle/fnw202; Chakhtoura, N., Hazra, R., & Spong, C. (2018). Zika virus: A public health perspective. Current Opinion in Obstetrics and Gynecology, 30(2), 116–122; Poland, G., Ovsyannikova, I., & Kennedy, R. (2019). Zika vaccine development: Current status. Mayo Clinic Proceedings, 94(12), 2572–2586; and Rawal, G., Yadav, S., & Kumar, R. (2016). Zika virus: An overview. Journal of Family Medicine and Primary Care, 5(3), 523–527.

BOX 17.8. Pandemic Insights from the Past: Zika Virus

Epidemiology: The Zika virus was first isolated in monkeys in 1947 in Uganda's Zika Forest. In 2007, there was an outbreak in the Federal States of Micronesia. In 2013, there was an outbreak in French Polynesia. In 2015, an outbreak occurred in Brazil.

Etiologic Agent: Flaviviridae RNA virus

Mode of Transmission: Skin contact is the most common route of inoculation. The most common nonhuman-to-human vector is the Aedes mosquito. Vertical transmission is possible from pregnant woman to unborn child. Sexual transmission is possible.

Diagnostic Testing: The Zika virus is detectable in the blood within 10 days of infection, with peak viral activity coinciding with symptom onset. Diagnostic testing includes presence of viral RNA or antigen. Nucleic acid amplification (NAAT) assay conducted on serum, plasma, blood, cerebrospinal fluid, urine, or amniotic fluid. Placental tissue can be tested via reverse-transcription polymerase chain reaction (RT-PCR).

Clinical Presentation: Clinical presentation includes nonspecific-flu-like symptoms, rash, low grade fever, malaise, conjunctivitis, and joint pain. Zika infections can also precipitate a Guillain-Barré Syndrome. Congenital Zika infection causes life-threatening conditions such as increased intracranial hydrostatic pressure, skull malformation, subcortical calcification, and ocular lesions.

Pharmacologic Measures: Symptomatic treatment with hydration and acetaminophen. There is no vaccine approved at this time.

Medical Countermeasures: Medical countermeasures include screening for individuals who have lived in or traveled to areas with Zika

BOX 17.9. Pandemic Insights from the Past: The Spanish flu of 1918

Epidemiology: An estimated global death toll of 50 to 100 million. The pandemic occurred during World War I. There were three waves of the pandemic—spring of 1918, fall of 1918 (considered the deadliest wave), and winter of 1918 until spring of 1919.

Etiologic Agent: Influenza type A subtype H1N1 with genes of avian origin

Mode of Transmission: The mode of transmission was through droplets. The virus can be spread through direct contact with infected animals, humans, and environmental surfaces.

Diagnostic Testing: There were no diagnostic tests. Diagnosis was based on syndromic surveillance.

Clinical Presentation: Sudden onset of fever, cough, rhinitis, muscle aches, sore throat, headache, and fatigue. Infected individuals progressed to stages of respiratory distress, cyanosis, nose and mouth bleeding, and death.

Pharmacologic Measures: Pharmacologic measures were limited to supportive measures such as hydration, good nutrition, and cough medications such as heroine hydrochloride, codeine sulfate, opium, and morphine sulfate. Fever control measures included injections of camphor oil in the arms or legs.

Medical Countermeasures: Medical countermeasures consisted of screening travelers; border closures; isolation; quarantine; hand hygiene; restriction of social gatherings; coughing and sneezing etiquette; closure of venues that supported large gatherings (such as theaters, churches); and fumigating mail; gauze masks

(continued)

BOX 17.9. Pandemic Insights from the Past: the Spanish flu of 1918 (*continued*)

were used but were eventually determined to be too porous for protection. Open air hospitals and environments were promoted.

Source: Humphreys, M. (2018). The influenza of 1918. *Evolution, Medicine, and Public Health, 2018*(1), 219–229. https://doi.org/10.1093/emph/eoy024; Morens, D., & Taubenberger, J. (2018). The mother of all pandemics is 100 years old (and going strong!) *American Journal of Public Health, 108*(11), 1449–1454. https://doi.org/10.2105/ajph.2018.304631.

BOX 17.10. Pandemic Insights from the Past: Human Immunodeficiency Virus (HIV)

Epidemiology: The pandemic emerged in the United States in 1981. The pandemic initially presented in the men who have sex with men community and injecting substance users but eventually involved all segments of the population engaging in high-risk behaviors, primarily, unprotected sex and sharing of needles/syringes. Perinatal transmission is possible. Racial and ethnic disparities exist.

Etiologic Agent: Human immunodeficiency retrovirus types 1 and 2

Mode of Transmission: HIV infection is transmitted through direct contact with infected blood, body fluids, or items contaminated with infected blood or body fluids. Breastfeeding can be a mode of HIV transmission.

Diagnostic Testing: Screening at-risk individuals with HIV antibody test

Clinical Presentation: There is a vast constellation of syndromic symptoms that include opportunistic infections, flu-like symptoms, muscle wasting, fever, lymphadenopathy, joint or muscle pain, rashes, diarrhea, and Kaposi's sarcoma.

Pharmacologic Measures: Treatment of opportunistic infections. Antiretroviral therapy for HIV infection. Use of antiretroviral preventive therapy (PrEP).

Medical Countermeasures: The medical countermeasures included safe sex education, needle and syringe exchange programs, screening of at-risk individuals to avoid blood and blood product donation, implementation of Universal Standard Precautions for all patients.

Source: Centers for Disease Control and Prevention. (2014). *Revised case definition of HIV infection— United States, 2014*. https://www.cdc.gov/mmwr/preview/mmwrhtml/rr6303a1.htm; Valdiserri, R., & Holtgrave, D. (2020). Responding to pandemics: What we've learned from HIV/AIDS. *AIDS and Behavior*. https://doi.org/10.1007/s10461-020-02859-5.

BOX 17.11. Pandemic Insights from the Past: Ebola

Epidemiology: Outbreak in the United States in 2014 to 2016. Not endemic in the United States. The incubation period is about to 2 to 21 days. The course of illness lasts from 14 to 21 days.

Etiologic Agent: A RNA filovirus, known as Ebola virus. There are six strains, each named for the region of origin—Zaire, Sudan, Tai Forest, Bundibugyo, Reston, and Bombali. Only four strains cause disease in humans. The mortality rate is about 90%. Primarily occurs in Central Africa. In 2014, Ebola was recognized as an international public health emergency.

Mode of Transmission: The mode of transmission is through direct contact with infected body fluids, often through mucosal contact. Droplet transmission is possible. The host is fruit bats, *Pteropodidae* family. Other documented vectors are primates, antelopes, and porcupines. Ebola virus remains transmittable postmortem.

Diagnostic Testing: Polymerase chain reaction viral test along with antibody testing

Clinical Presentation: Presents as severe viral hemorrhagic fever. Early symptoms are nonspecific—fever, malaise, and diffuse myalgia followed by a maculopapillary rash with petechiae. Symptoms progress to conjunctival hemorrhage, epistaxis, melena, hematemesis, and encephalopathy. Final clinical symptoms are internal and external hemorrhage.

Pharmacologic Measures: No approved antiviral therapy. Supplemental oxygenation. Fluid resuscitation with blood transfusions. One approved vaccine for individuals over the age of 18 as a single dose.

Medical Countermeasures: Medical countermeasures include isolation, quarantine, hand hygiene, personal protective equipment, use of disposable equipment, and travel restrictions.

Source: Centers for Disease Control. (2019). *Ebola virus*. https://www.cdc.gov/vf/ebola/about.html; Fisher-Hoch, S., Platt, G., Neild, G., Southee, T., Baskerville, A., Raymond, R. Lloyd, G., & Simpson, D. (1985). Pathophysiology of shock and hemorrhage in a fulminating viral infection (Ebola). *Journal of Infectious Diseases, 152*(5), 887–894. https://doi.org/10.1093/infdis/152.5.887; and Kelsch, N. (2014). Infection control: Ebola virus. *RDH, 34*(10), 86–104.

END-OF-CHAPTER RESOURCES

SUMMARY POINTS

- A pandemic impacts the entire health of the community and multiple countries at the same time.
- One of the concerns during a pandemic is overstressing the healthcare system to the point of collapse or inability to appropriately and effectively respond to the crisis.
- Genetic reassortment involves the genes from different viruses combining to create a new strain with a new genetic complement.
- In genetic mutation, a gene in an animal virus changes, permitting the virus to infect humans and continue transmission from human to human.
- The mitigation of a pandemic needs advance planning and preparedness.
- The whole-of-society multisector approach involves all governmental levels and industry sectors of society.
- The Pandemic Influenza Preparedness (PIP) Framework goals are to improve and strengthen sharing of influenza viruses with human pandemic potential and achieve efficient and equitable access for all countries in need of life-saving vaccines and medicines during a pandemic.
- The foundational principles of the Emergency Risk Management for Health (ERMH) include a comprehensive risk management, all-hazards approach, multisectoral approach, multidisciplinary approach, community resilience, sustainable development, and ethical basis.
- The six essential component categories of ERMH are policies and resource management, planning and coordination, information and knowledge management, health infrastructure and logistics, health and related services, and community emergency risk management capabilities.
- WHO considers there are four phases of a pandemic—interpandemic, alert, pandemic, and transition.
- The all-hazards phases are preparedness, response, and recovery.
- The prepandemic intervals are investigation and recognition.
- In the pandemic interval of initiation, there is confirmation of human cases of the viral infection throughout the world with demonstrated efficient and sustained human-to-human transmission.
- During the initiation interval, case-based control measures and routine personal protective measures such as hand hygiene are critical to reducing transmission.
- In the acceleration interval, there is a consistent increase in the incidence rate of viral cases.
- The deceleration interval is the consistent decreasing rate of viral cases.
- Preparation interval involves suspending mitigation measures.
- A pandemic is declared as ended when surveillance evidence indicates worldwide that the viral infection is transitioning to a seasonal pattern of transmission.
- A pandemic risk assessment aims to determine the likelihood that an infection will impact the health of individuals and the extent to which the impact will occur.
- The pandemic risk assessment should consist of an interprofessional team with multisector representation.
- Medical countermeasures include vaccines, pharmacologic therapeutic agents (such as antiviral and antibiotics), diagnostics, ventilators, and respiratory protective devices.
- Community mitigation efforts include medication administration and/or nonpharmacologic interventions.
- The Public Health Services (PHS) Act forms the legal foundation of authority for the Department of Health and Human Services (DHHS) to respond to public health emergencies.
- An emergency response to a pandemic begins with the state governor or chief executive of the Indian tribe requesting the president of the United States to declare a national emergency.
- PHS Public Readiness and Emergency Preparedness (PREP) Act authorized the DHHS Secretary to issue declarations that provides immunity from liability for the use of medical countermeasures (MCM), except if there is intentional willful misconduct.

EPIDEMIOLOGY CRITICAL REASONING QUESTIONS

1. Select a pandemic. Utilize the information contained in this chapter to develop a case study that includes epidemiologic data; risk assessment data; activities implemented

during the preparedness, response, and recovery phases; and medical countermeasures and community mitigation strategies implemented.

2. Compare and contrast two pandemics using the following: epidemiologic data; risk assessment data; activities implemented during the preparedness, response and recovery phases; and medical countermeasures and community mitigation strategies implemented.

ADDITIONAL RESOURCES

 SPRINGER PUBLISHING CONNECT™ | A robust set of instructor resources designed to supplement this text is located at http://connect.springerpub.com/content/book/978-0-8261-8514-3. Qualifying instructors may request access by emailing textbook@springerpub.com.

REFERENCES

Centers for Disease Control and Prevention. (2014). Updated preparedness and response framework for influenza pandemics. *Morbidity and Mortality Weekly Report, 63*(RR06), 1–9. https://www.cdc.gov/mmwr/preview/mmwrhtml/rr6306a1.htm

Centers for Disease Control and Prevention. (2016). *Regulations and laws that may apply during a pandemic*. Author.

Centers for Disease Control and Prevention (2019). *Influenza risk assessment tool*. https://www.cdc.gov/flu/pandemic-resources/national-strategy/risk-assessment.htm

Centers for Disease Control and Prevention. (2020). *Vaccine and other medical countermeasures*. https://www.cdc.gov/flu/pandemic-resources/planning-preparedness/vaccine-medical-countermeasures.html

Qualls, N., Levitt, A., Kanade, N., Wright-Jegede, N., Dopson, S., Biggerstaff, M., Reed, C., & Uzicanin, A. (2017). Community mitigation guidelines to prevent pandemic influenza—United States, 2017. *MMWR Recommendations and Reports, 66*(RR-1), 1–34. https://doi.org/10.15585/mmwr.rr6601a1

Reed, C., Biggerstaff, M., Finelli, L., Koonin, L. M., Beauvais, D., Uzicanin, A., Plummer, A., Bresee, J., Redd, S. C., & Jernigan, D. B. (2013). Novel framework for assessing epidemiologic effects of influenza epidemics and pandemics. *Emerging Infectious Diseases, 19*(1), 85–91. https://doi.org/10.3201/eid1901.120124

World Health Organization. (2015). *World Health Organization best practices for naming of new human infectious diseases*. http://www.who.int/classifications/icd/en/

World Health Organization. (2017). *Pandemic influenza risk management: A WHO guide to inform and harmonize national and international pandemic preparedness and response*. Author.

Chapter 18

SOCIAL EPIDEMIOLOGY

Demetrius J. Porche

Health inequalities and the social determinants of health are not a footnote to the determinants of health. They are the main issue.

–Sir Michael Marmont

CHAPTER COMPETENCIES

At the conclusion of this chapter, the reader will be able to:

1. Describe the practice of social epidemiology
2. Discuss social factors influencing the determinants and distribution of health
3. Differentiate the core concepts of the ecosocial theory
4. Describe a syndemic

ESSENTIAL TERMINOLOGY

Essential social epidemiology terms are:

- Biologic expression
- Embodiment
- Health inequality
- Social capital
- Social class
- Social epidemiology
- Social equity
- Social inequality
- Social position
- Socioeconomic status (SES)
- Syndemic

Epidemiology purposefully explores the distribution and determinants of health at all levels, from individual influences to social influences (Galea & Link, 2013). Biological and social processes shape population health. From a population perspective, an individual's risk cannot be considered in isolation of the community or population to which the individual belongs. Social epidemiology strives to provide a framework to examine how social factors, such as social relationships, poverty, racial issues, social inequalities, social capital, and work stress impact the health of individuals and populations (Galea & Link, 2013). Social epidemiologists identify the social characteristics that impact the distribution and pattern of disease occurrence in a population (von dem Knesebeck, 2015) as a means to develop programs that improve the health of individuals, populations, and eventually society as a whole.

Social epidemiology is considered a branch of epidemiology that examines the social distribution and social determinants of health within a population. It is concerned with the social etiology of disease. The social etiology of disease systematically examines the population level variations in the incidence of diseases among people from different social structures to determine risk and vulnerability. Social epidemiologists explore the manner in which membership in social groups or population segments relates to behavioral patterns and to exposures to etiologic agents of disease. An aim of social epidemiology is to identify specific social circumstances that are an antecedent to specific behaviors that lead to specific diseases or risks. Common social phenomena examined by social epidemiologist are socioeconomic stratification, social networks, social support systems, and social resources as related to disease (Berkman & Kawachi, 2014; Kaufman & Oakes, 2017).

The nursing assessment is an important element of epidemiologic data collection. During the nursing assessment, nurses collect information on many of the social and lifestyle factors that impact an individual's health. Additionally, nurses collect data on social networks and family relationships. Nurses must remain aware of the status of the population's health within a community and ensure that they collect specific social health data as a component of the nursing assessment. A comprehensive community assessment provides valuable information about the social factors impacting a community and ultimately the population and individuals who reside within a geographical community or affiliate within a social community.

SOCIAL FACTORS INFLUENCING DETERMINANTS AND DISTRIBUTION OF HEALTH

Social epidemiology has established the linkage of social determinants of health in the explanation of differences in disease between and within populations (Tsai, 2018). As social factors affect disease patterns and distribution within populations and society, there are social concepts that have been determined to impact population health. These social factors that impact health are sometimes expressed biologically. Biological expression is known as the manner in which individuals embody and biologically express experiences of social factors that negatively impact their health. These social factors may be social inequality, SES, social relationships, social capital, work stress, health inequality, and socio-structural factors (Kaufman & Oakes, 2017).

Social Inequality

Social inequality is defined as the unequal distribution of goods, services, and opportunities within a population or society. The opposite of social inequality is social equality. Social equalty is the lack of unjust distribution among social groups (Krieger, 2001). Social epidemiologists frequently use "life chances" as a measure of social inequality. Life chances result in the ability of an individual to have a career or achieve life satisfaction. Some common measures of social inequality "life chances" are education, occupation, and annual or household income (von dem Knesebeck, 2015).

Social inequality impacts an individual's access to necessary resources for their health and welfare. The term *impoverished* means that an individual has a lack of or is denied adequate resources. Human poverty is impoverishment in multiple dimensions such as to a long and healthy life, knowledge, a decent standard of living, and in participation and engagement. Income poverty is considered deprivation of a single resource dimension, income, and is considered a critical measure of human poverty and social inequality (Krieger, 2001).

There are various types of deprivation existing at different levels. Material deprivation refers to a lack of material resources such as food, clothing, housing, home goods, environment, and work. Social deprivation refers to a lack of integration into social networks and institutions. Social exclusion is another term associated with poverty. Social exclusion is a process of marginalization that excludes individuals from full participation in social and community life (Krieger, 2001).

Two other measures associated with social inequality are social class and socioeconomic position. Social class is determined by societal categories based on property, ownership, and connections to production, distribution, and consumption of good, services, and information. Social classes are social groupings that arise from the interdependent economic relationships among individuals within society. Social class is a measure of an individual's location within the economic structure. Socioeconomic position is considered an aggregate concept representing both resource-based and prestige-based measures. The resource-based aspect consists of the material and social resources and assets such as income, wealth, and educational achievements. Prestige-based measures refer to an individual's rank or stature within a social hierarchy judged on an individual's access to and consumption of goods, services, and knowledge (Krieger, 2001).

Socioeconomic Status

SES is a concept that continues to be used in social epidemiology to connote an individual's position in the social hierarchy, determine how the social hierarchy is structured, and explain an individual's consequences related to being in the respective socioeconomic position. SES is another explanation as to an individual's access to goods, services, power, education, healthcare, leisure time, and social relationships. Social epidemiologists are interested in understanding the effect of SES on health outcomes. There remains no one acceptable definition of SES; it is used as a construct to understand an individual's access to resources. Most social epidemiologists explore the relationship between race or ethnicity and SES but do not consider it to be an aspect of the concept. Social epidemiologists use indicators of SES such as but not limited to individual income, household income, educational level, and occupational title to measure SES. Typically, SES is measured as a composite or proxy measure (Oakes & Andrade, 2017).

Composite measures attempt to include several domains of information into a single, measurable, scalable quantity. The typical composite measures attempt to integrate information about educational attainment, annual earned income, and occupational prestige into a single number for each individual. Some established composite measures are the Duncan Socioeconomic Index (SEI), Nam-Powers Occupational Status Score (OSS), and household prestige score (HHP), British Cambridge Social Interaction and Stratification Scale (CAMSIS), National Statistics Socioeconomic Classification (NS-SEC), Capital as a function of Socioeconomic Status (CAPSES), Kuppuswamy (SES) scale, and Udai Pareekh's revised scale (Oakes & Andrade, 2017; Wani, 2019).

Proxy measures are also known as univariate socioeconomic measures. Proxy measures are simple direct measures such as annual income or years of education. Income is a single measure of an individual's ability to purchase desired resources; however, it is considered an imperfect proxy of SES, as income can be volatile and fluctuate over the course of a year. Wealth may be considered a better proxy measure than annual income. Wealth includes an individual's total assets, some of which could be tied up in real estate, automobiles, homes, business ownership, investments, and possibly inheritances. Wealth is considered an accumulated proxy measure of SES. In contrast to annual income, wealth provides a measure of the entire breadth of an individual's financial resources (Oakes & Andrade, 2017).

Another proxy measure of SES is poverty threshold. Poverty threshold is measured as a function of an individual's earned annual income in relation to the adequate established standard of living. The United States establishes a poverty level measure that incorporates family size, head of household's age, and food requirements. Most social epidemiologists consider poverty as a weaker measure of SES. Some poverty metrics used are food stamp or food subsidy program usage and reduced school lunch (Oakes & Andrade, 2017).

Educational attainment is another SES proxy measure. An individual's educational attainment is associated with their ability to secure employment and generate earned income. In general, individuals tend to honestly respond to educational level questions more so than earned income questions (Oakes & Andrade, 2017).

Measuring SES is complex. In summary, measures of SES include elements of education, income, occupation, and family size and relationships. Social epidemiologists conceptualize SES and social class as measures of occupational prestige (most recent occupation); resource-based measures (educational attainment, total earned family income, wealth, and composite SES measures); absolute poverty measures (comparison to federal poverty threshold or levels, school or neighborhood indicators); relative poverty measures (material hardships, food insecurity, income-to-need ratio); and subjective social status measures (individual's perception of categories such as "working class," "middle class," and "upper class"; American Psychological Association [APA], 2015).

Table 18.1 presents other terms used to explore relationships among health outcomes and social concepts (Krieger, 2001).

Social Relationships

Social relationships are defined as the interconnectedness of individuals within a relationship dynamic. Three major components of social relationships are degree of integration into social networks, social interactions that are supportive (received social support), and beliefs and perceptions about the availability of support (perceived social support) (von dem Knesebeck, 2015).

Social Capital

Social capital is the social structures that an individual possesses that act as a resource for the individual to facilitate some opportunity or action. Some aspects of social capital are social networks and relationships, level of interpersonal trust and respect, and civic engagement and recognition (von dem Knesebeck, 2015).

Table 18.1 Social Epidemiology Definitions

Social Term	Definition
Biological expression of social inequality	Manner in which an individual embodies and biologically expresses experiences of economic and social inequality
Caste	A term related to SES, conveys social class, status, or position; conveys place in social hierarchy that is set at birth
Discrimination	Process in which members of a social group are treated differently because of their membership in that respective group
Embodiment	Manner in which an individual biologically incorporates the material and social world into their being and manner of living
Gender	Social construct about culture-bound conventions regarding roles, behaviors, and relationships between and among men and women/boys and girls
Human poverty	Impoverishment in multiple dimensions such as knowledge, decent standard of living, participation, and lack of long and meaningful life
Impoverished	Lack of or denied adequate resources to participate meaningfully in society
Income poverty	Single dimension poverty, deprivation in income
Material deprivation	Deprived of dietary, clothing, housing, home facilities, environment, location, and work
Sex	Biological construct based on biological characteristics that enable sexual reproduction
Social class	Construct or measure like SES; classifies an individual according to social stratification in society; social groups arising from economic relationships—determined by property, ownership, labor, and connections between production, distribution, and consumption of goods, services, and information
Social deprivation	Deprivation of employment, family activities, community integration, recreation, education, and participation in social institutions
Social exclusion	Process of marginalization
Socioeconomic position	Sometimes considered synonymous with social class, connotes an aspect of an individual's occupational prestige, rank, or prestige in social hierarchy

Source: From Krieger, N. (2001). A glossary of social epidemiology. *Journal of Epidemiology and Community Health, 55*, 693–700. https://doi.org/10.1136/jech.55.10.693.

SES, socioeconomic status.

Work Stress

Individuals spend a significant amount of their time within the work environment. The work environment provides a context for social interaction with other individuals. The social aspects of the work environment create opportunities and stressors.

Health Inequality

Health inequality is a measure frequently associated with social concepts and may be considered a characteristic of social concepts. Health inequality is considered the observable differences in health among individuals of different social groups or strata. Two common measures of health inequality are total inequality and social group inequality. Total health inequality is a measure of the total health variation; it measures the univariate distribution of health or disease across all individuals in a population without consideration of other characteristics. In contrast, social group health inequality measures health inequality between social groups. Social group health inequality measures the average health differences between individuals from different social groups or strata (Harper & Lynch, 2017).

Sociostructural Factors

Sociostructural factors are another way to categorize the social variables explored by social epidemiologists who examine the effects of sociostructural factors on health states. Social epidemiologists maintain a central focus on the study of how social structure factors influence the health of individuals and ultimately the population. The basic question remains "How do social conditions produce patterns of health and disease in a population?" Common sociostructural factors in social epidemiology are gender, ethnicity/race, social class, discrimination, social network, income distribution, and social policy. Other social and community factors sometimes considered are work environment, living and working conditions, water and sanitation, healthcare services and access, housing, and agriculture and food production.

SOCIAL CONTEXT OF BEHAVIOR

Most behaviors are not randomly distributed in the population but occur among individuals with similar population demographics and behaviors. Therefore, most behaviors are considered socially patterned and therefore cluster in similar groups within the population. An individual's social environment influences behavior by shaping norms, enforcing patterns of social control, providing access to environmental opportunities to engage in certain behaviors, and impacting the manner in which certain behaviors interact with disease etiology (Berkman & Kawachi, 2014).

ECOSOCIAL THEORY OF DISEASE DISTRIBUTION

The ecosocial theory of disease distribution integrates social, historical, ecological, and biological aspects of health into the determinants of population distribution of diseases. The central epidemiologic question to be answered from an ecosocial theory perspective is "Who and what is responsible for the patterns of health, disease, and well-being in a population related to the present, past, and changing social health inequalities?" (Krieger, 2001).

The core concepts of ecosocial theory are embodiment; embodiment pathways; the cumulative interplay between exposure, susceptibility, and resistance; and accountability and agent. Embodiment refers to the manner in which an individual biologically incorporates the material and social world in which the individual lives. Embodiment pathways are the structures that facilitate embodiment. These consist of societal arrangements of power and property, production patterns, consumption, and reproduction and biological restraints derived from our own physiological biology. The cumulative interplay among exposure, susceptibility, and resistance is expressed also by embodiment. Accountability and agency are expressed by knowledge about embodiment in relation to the social factors affecting an individual.

SYNDEMIC

Disease burden in the form of endemic, epidemic, and pandemics were discussed in Chapter 4. In addition to these previous descriptions of the distribution of disease, pandemic, epidemic, and endemic is proposed, a syndemic. The theory of syndemics was first proposed by Merill Singer (1996) to describe the co-occurrence of synergistically related epidemics that cluster within a population arising from harmful social conditions. A syndemic is considered the aggregation of two or more concurrent or sequential epidemics clustering in a population in which there is the interaction of disease burden (morbidity and mortality) and disease interaction with social forces and conditions. A difference between comorbidity and syndemics is that a syndemic occurrence additively increased the negative health consequences of the disease process.

There are multiple methods of interaction proposed that potentiate a syndemic occurrence. These methods consist of:

- Mutually causal epidemics
- Synergistically interacting epidemics—disease burden is attributed to joint health risk that together exceed the sum of individual health risk in isolation
- Serially causal epidemic—adverse health consequences accumulate serially into a combined health risk (Tsai, 2018)

There is a need for epidemiologists to explore the processes and interrelationships of syndemics, the manner in which health and social conditions foster the development of multiple epidemics intersecting and compounding the effects of each other. In addition, syndemic epidemiologic studies should embrace the manner in which environmental changes are impacting the spread of disease and the interaction among new diseases, known as eco-syndemic.

END-OF-CHAPTER RESOURCES

SUMMARY POINTS

- Population health is not only shaped by biological but also social processes.
- Social epidemiologists identify the social characteristics that impact the distribution and pattern of disease occurrence in a population.
- The social etiology of disease systematically examines the population level variations in the incidence of diseases among people from different social structures to determine risk and vulnerability.
- Common social phenomena examined by social epidemiologist are socioeconomic stratification, social networks, social support systems, and social resources as related to disease.
- Biological expression is known as the manner in which individuals embody and biologically express experiences of social factors that negatively impact their health.
- Social inequality is defined as the unequal distribution of goods, services, and opportunities within a population or society.
- Human poverty is the impoverishment in multiple dimensions such as a long and healthy life, knowledge, decent standard of living, and participation and engagement.
- Social class is determined by societal categories based on property, ownership, and connections to production, distribution, and consumption of good, services, and information.
- Socioeconomic position is considered an aggregate concept representing both resource-based and prestige-based measures.
- Social relationships are defined as the interconnectedness of individuals within a relationship dynamic.
- Social capital is the social structures that an individual possesses that act as a resource for the individual to facilitate some opportunity or action.
- Health inequality is considered the observable differences in health among individuals of different social groups or strata.
- Embodiment refers to the manner in which an individual biologically incorporates the material and social world in which one lives.
- A syndemic is considered the aggregation of two or more concurrent or sequential epidemics clustering in a population in which there is the interaction of disease burden and disease interaction with social forces and conditions.

EPIDEMIOLOGY CRITICAL REASONING QUESTIONS

1. Identify a population of interest in your community. Examine the community in relation to the social epidemiology metric of socioeconomic status. What elements did you use to characterize the population's socioeconomic status?
2. Explore a health condition of interest. Identify the social concepts associated with the health alterations for your identified health condition based on evidence and research findings.
3. Identify a syndemic occurring in the United States. What population is affected most? Describe each of the concurrent or sequential epidemics that have occurred in this population. What are the potential social etiologic factors.

ADDITIONAL RESOURCES

A robust set of instructor resources designed to supplement this text is located at http://connect. springerpub.com/content/book/978-0-8261-8514-3. Qualifying instructors may request access by emailing textbook@springerpub.com.

REFERENCES

American Psychological Association. (2015). *Measuring socioeconomic status and subjective social status.* https://www.apa.org/pi/ses/resources/class/measuring-status

Berkman, L., & Kawachi, I. (2014). The historical framework for social epidemiology: Social determinants of population health. In L. Berkman, I. Kawachi, & M. Glymour (Eds.), *Social epidemiology* (2nd ed., pp. 1–16). Oxford Press.

Galea, S., & Link, B. (2013). Six paths for the future of social epidemiology. *American Journal of Epidemiology, 178*(6), 843–849. https://doi.org/10.1093/aje/kwt148

Harper, S., & Lynch, J. (2017). Health inequalities: Measurement and decomposition. In J. Oakes & J. Kaufman (Eds.), *Methods in social epidemiology* (pp. 91–131). Wiley Publishers.

Kaufman, J., & Oakes, J. (2017). Introduction: Advancing methods in social epidemiology. In J. Oakes & J. Kaufman (Eds.), *Methods in social epidemiology* (pp. 1–21). Wiley Publishers.

Krieger, N. (2001). A glossary of social epidemiology. *Journal of Epidemiology and Community Health, 55,* 693–700. https://doi.org/10.1136/jech.55.10.693

Oakes, J., & Andrade, K. (2017). The measurement of socioeconomic status. In J. Oakes & J. Kaufman (Eds.), *Methods in social epidemiology* (pp. 23–42). Wiley Publishers.

Singer, M. (1996). A dose of drugs, a touch of violence, a case of AIDS: Conceptualizing the SAVA syndemic. *Free Inquiry in Creative Sociology, 24*(2), 99–110. https://ojs.library.okstate.edu/osu/index.php/FICS/article/download/1346/1201.

Tsai, A. (2018). Syndemics: A theory in search of data or data in search of a theory? *Social Science and Medicine, 206,* 117–122. https://doi.org/10.1016/j.socscimed.2018.03.040

Von dem Knesebeck, O. (2015). Concepts of social epidemiology in health services research. *MBC Health Services Research, 15*(357), 1–16. https://doi.org/10.1186/s12913-015-1020-z

Wani, R. (2019). Socioeconomic status scales-modified Kuppuswamy and Udai Pareekh's scale updated for 2019. *Journal of Family Medicine and Primary Care, 8*(6), 1846–1849. https://doi.org/10.4103/jfmpc.jfmpc_288_19

Chapter 19

INFECTIOUS DISEASE EPIDEMIOLOGY

Demetrius J. Porche

All that would be required to prevent the disease [cholera] would be such a close attention to cleanliness in cooking and eating, and to drainage and water supply, as is desirable at all times.
—John Snow

CHAPTER COMPETENCIES

At the conclusion of this chapter, the reader will be able to:

1. Differentiate antigenic shift and antigenic drift
2. Distinguish between infectious and communicable diseases
3. Compare and contrast between an infectious process and colonization
4. Characterize a case as index, primary, or secondary
5. Differentiate the common modes of transmission

ESSENTIAL TERMINOLOGY

Essential infectious disease epidemiology terms are:

- Air-borne transmission
- Colonization
- Communicable disease
- Droplet transmission
- Emerging infection
- Exposed
- Fecal–oral transmission
- Index case
- Infection
- Infectious disease epidemiology
- Perinatal transmission
- Primary case
- Secondary case
- Sociogram
- Vector
- Vehicle

Infectious disease epidemiology is a branch of epidemiology that examines the distribution and determinants of diseases of an infectious nature. Even though infectious diseases are more common in nonindustrialized countries, there remains a significant prevalence of infectious diseases within the industrialized countries. The essence of infectious disease epidemiology is the focus on the interaction between individuals within a population. An area of prime importance for infectious disease epidemiologists is the interaction between cases and contacts. The fundamentals of infectious disease epidemiology are grounded in the interaction between a causative agent, host, and the environment. Modes of transmission are an integral component to understanding infectious disease epidemiology. Breaking the chain of an infectious disease requires a simple intervention of interfering with the infectious agent's mode of transmission. Infectious epidemiology also considers the interaction between individuals within the population group, especially the interaction between infectious cases and potential contacts. Nurses are frequently on the front line of contact with the patient and are essential members of the healthcare team in breaking the chain of infection.

Infectious disease prevention is dependent upon knowledge regarding the etiologic or causative agent, risk factors, host factors, and circumstances that lead to the interaction of these factors. Infectious disease epidemiologists provide recommendations on interventions that can break the chain of infection transmission. A challenge of infectious disease epidemiologists is to remain ahead of etiologic agent changes. A nurses functions as a member of the healthcare team as either a nurse epidemiologist or infection control prevention specialist or practitioner.

ETIOLOGIC AGENT CHANGES

An infectious etiologic agent has the potential to undergo changes that create a renewed ability to infect individuals and populations. An excellent example of infectious etiologic agent changes is the annual changes in the strains of influenza. Infectious agents generally have proteins that are responsible for the antigen production of neutralizing antibodies. Two things can occur that change the antibody resistance to a specific etiologic antigen. These are antigenic drift and antigenic shift. An antigenic drift is the result of point mutations in a gene segment resulting in a minor surface antigen change. An antigenic shift is a major change in one or more surface antigen proteins. Both an antigenic drift and antigenic shift can result in an epidemic or pandemic occurrence since the population will not have any immunity to the changed antigen. Antigenic drifts and shifts can lead to the development of variants that perpetuate an infection within a population and community.

HOST AND POPULATION DYNAMICS

There are multiple host and population level changes that can impact infectious disease epidemiology. Like infectious organisms, humans change and evolve over time, including our immune system and response. Over the past three decades, Straif-Bourgeious et al. report an increase in a population of individuals at high risk for infectious diseases (2014). Some factors that lead to this is a change in lifetime longevity that results in an elderly population that is prone to acquiring infectious diseases. In addition, the elderly are at greater risk of developing life-threatening complications from an infectious illness. Advancements in healthcare treatments have impacted the population's immune status. There are more cancer survivors and organ transplant survivors who may be on immunosuppressive medications. Individuals with infectious diseases such as HIV are living longer and may have compromised immune systems. Also, lifestyle changes increase the risk of exposure to infectious agents. Advances in travel and globalization have increased the number of people who are exposed to different countries and environmental agents than their native habitat. In addition, the ability to make autonomous choices about healthcare has the potential to expose individuals to infectious agents along with personal values and beliefs. Specifically, individuals who do not support, do not believe in, or fear vaccinations and other therapeutics can increase the population of individuals at risk for infectious diseases. Vaccine hesitancy with new vaccines also has the ability to impact the ability to control or eliminate an infectious epidemic or pandemic. Vaccine hesitancy is the delay in acceptance of the vaccination or in receiving the vaccination. In addition, humans can pose a direct intentional threat. Bioterrorism is an intentional act to cause harm to others via the introduction of an infectious agent, such as the anthrax attacks that occur in the United States in 2001 (Straif-Bourgeious et al., 2014).

BASIC INFECTIOUS DISEASE CONCEPTS

Basic infectious disease concepts necessary to understand infectious disease epidemiology are presented in this chapter. The reader is also directed to review companion content in Chapter 6, which is necessary to understand infectious disease epidemiology. Appendix J presents some common infectious agents, incubation periods, and their modes of transmission.

Infection Types

There are different types of infection, depending on the source of the infection. A zoonosis is an infection that is transmitted under natural conditions from a vertebrate animal to a human. Two types of zoonosis are anthropozoonosis and zooanthroponoses. Anthropozoonosis is an infection transmitted from a vertebrate animal to human such as rabies, plague, or anthrax. Zooanthroponoses are infections transmitted from humans to vertebrate animals such as bovine tuberculosis. A nosocomial or hospital-acquired infection is one that originates in a patient while in the hospital or healthcare facility that was not incubating at the time of admission. An opportunistic infection is an infection that occurs as a result of a weakened or compromised immune system, taking the opportunity of causing an infection while the immune system is compromised, such as with histoplasmosis or cryptococcal meningitis in HIV-infected patients.

Infectious Versus Communicable Disease

The terms infectious disease and communicable disease are often used interchangeably. The term infectious specifically refers to an infectious agent or the toxic products of an infectious agent that arise from the transmission of the agent into a susceptible host with the ability to cause an infection. This transmission of the infectious agent can occur through animals, plants, vectors, or inanimate environment. Infectious diseases are caused by an infectious agent, of which the most typical ones are bacteria, virus, fungus, Protozoa, or helminths. The term communicable specifically refers to a disease that can be transmitted from an infected individual to another individual.

A contagious disease is one that can be transmitted through contact. All contagious diseases are potentially infectious but not all infectious diseases are contagious. An infective animal or human is at a stage of an infection in which they are capable of transmitting an infection to others. Noncommunicable is an infection or disease that cannot be transmitted among animals or humans.

Exposed, Infected, Colonized, or Carrier

An exposed person is someone who has been in a situation where effective transmission of an infectious agent could have occurred. A mere exposure does not mean that an individual will have the infectious disease. An infected person is someone who has an established infection with signs or symptoms of infection present. Colonization is the presence of infectious agents in or on a host with the ability to grow and multiply without the overt clinical expression or immune reaction of the host to the infectious agent or development of an infectious process. Patients and healthcare workers can be colonized with infectious agents with the ability to transmit or spread the infection with and without an infectious process being initiated. In the healthcare environment, we are concerned with colonization of organisms such as *Staphylococcus aureus*, *Escherichia coli*, and *Clostridium difficile* (also known as *Clostridioides difficile*). A carrier is an individual who harbors a microorganism in the absence of clinical disease. A carrier

is a person who is capable serving as an infection source or infectious agent of transmission. A carrier can be colonized, incubating the disease in an asymptomatic state, infected but asymptomatic, or convalescing from an acute infection (Straif-Bourgeious et al., 2014).

Two of terms of importance are contamination and infestation. Contamination is the presence of an infectious agent on the body surface or other items such as clothing; bedding; surgical instruments; dressings; or other consumable products such as food, water, or milk. An infestation is the development and reproduction of anthropods on the surface of the body of a person or animal.

Infectious Case Types

Infectious disease epidemiologists characterize the cases to discern the dynamics of disease transmission. As mentioned in Chapter 8, a case is an operational definition for epidemiologic data collection purposes. A case definition does not constitute a diagnostic definition. A case definition should be precise and restrictive to eliminate subjectivity about case identification. It is important to differentiate that a diagnosis is a clinical judgment made by a healthcare provider that directs the selection of appropriate therapeutic interventions.

An index case is considered the earliest documented case of an infection or disease known to occur. An index case can also be the first case identified in an infectious disease outbreak. A primary case is the first case identified that brought the infection to the at-risk population. The primary case may be the index case but is not always. A secondary case is a case resulting from exposure and infection from a primary or subsequent case to the primary case. These case determinations are important to understanding the initial exposures and determining the waves of an infection or infection generations.

Transmission

Modes of transmission are important to understanding the spread and necessary interventions to reduce or eliminate the infectious disease. Modes of transmission are also discussed in Chapter 6. A reservoir can be any person, animal, plant or environmental source in which infectious organisms live and multiply. The infectious organisms may also depend on the reservoir for survival. A source of infection is a person, animal, or inanimate object from which an infection is acquired. A source of contamination is also a person, animal, or inanimate object from which some environmental medium is contaminated. A transmission vehicle is an inanimate object that serves as the source by which an infectious organism is transmitted. A vector is a live organism that transmits an infectious organism.

The modes of transmission are categorized according to the method by which an infectious organism is transmitted from one person or source to another person or source. Table 19.1 presents modes of transmission with the differentiating characteristics.

Exposed contacts are investigated for possible transmission. This is conducted through contact tracing. Contact tracing is presented in Chapter 7.

A reservoir can be considered a homologous or heterologous reservoir. A homologous reservoir is when the reservoir is a member of the same species. A heterologous reservoir is when an infection is derived from a reservoir other than human, such as with rabies. Reservoirs can also be classified as animal, human, or environmental reservoirs.

EMERGING INFECTIONS: DEFINITIONS

Disease emergence is a result of dynamic balances and imbalances within complex ecosystems that consist of humans, animals, pathogens, and the environment (Morens & Fauci, 2020). Morens and Fauci warn that newly emerging and re-emerging infectious diseases have been threatening humans since the Neolithic revolution, 12,000 years ago. Within the past decade, we have experienced unprecedented infectious pandemics—H1N1 (swine flu), chikungunya, Zika, Ebola, severe acute respiratory syndrome coronavirus (SARS-CoV), and Middle East respiratory syndrome coronavirus (MERS-CoV).

Emerging infectious diseases are categorized as newly emerging, re-emerging, or deliberately emerging. A newly emerging infectious disease is one that is novel or new to infecting humans. This could be a zoonotic infection that has been transmitted into humans. A re-emerging infection is one that may have previously been reduced in disease burden, eliminated, or eradicated that begins to emerge again. Deliberately emerging infectious diseases are frequently

Table 19.1 Modes of Transmission Differentiated

Mode of Transmission	Differentiated Characteristic
Droplet	Generated by upper respiratory tract when talking, singing, spitting, sneezing, coughing, suctioning, sputum induction, bronchoscopy; size varies from 1 to 100 µm; droplets fall to the floor at varying speed dependent upon their size; transmission is common within 3 feet of an infectious source
Airborne	Droplet nuclei or dust particle facilitates transmission; droplets are generally less than 5 µm in diameter; transmission may occur over a longer distance from an infection source
Direct contact	Direct body surface contact with physical transfer of organisms
Indirect contact	Transmission occurs through contact with an intermediate object
Fecal–oral route	Organism is excreted by feces; transmission occurs generally through contaminated food, water, milk, drinks, hands, or flies
Skin or mucous membrane	Skin is a natural barrier to infection; intact skin is ineffective in transmission; mucous membranes permit penetration of organisms
Perinatal	Transmission of organisms to newborn during passage through birth canal, cervix, or vagina
Transplacental or vertical	Transmission occurs through the placenta to the fetus
Anthropod-borne	Transmission can be active (multiplication of organisms in anthropod) or passive (anthropod picks up organism and transmits to another person); common anthropods are mosquitos, flies, fleas, ticks, and lice
Soil	Infectious agent resides in the soil, such as hookworm and tetanus mycosis

associated with bioterrorism. There are also accidentally emerging infectious diseases that result from repeated emergences of vaccine derived viruses such as poliovirus. A de-emerging infectious disease is known as one that has been eliminated or possibly eradicated or is in the process of being eliminated or eradicated from the world (Morens & Fauci, 2020).

HEALTHCARE INFECTIOUS DISEASE EPIDEMIOLOGY

Nosocomial or hospital-acquired infections are a major cost of healthcare and a determinant of poor health outcomes. Infectious disease epidemiologists engage in healthcare epidemiology to investigate and eliminate infectious disease that results within and from the healthcare environment. Nurses have an essential role in infection prevention within the healthcare environment. Healthcare provider-to-patient transmission of infection is the primary source of nosocomial or hospital-acquired infections. Nurses' hand hygiene practices are the most effective means of preventing nosocomial or hospital-acquired infections. Healthcare infectious disease epidemiology is presented in Chapter 23.

END-OF-CHAPTER RESOURCES

SUMMARY POINTS

- Infectious disease epidemiology is a branch of epidemiology that examines the distribution and determinants of diseases of an infectious nature.
- An area of prime importance for infectious disease epidemiologists is the interaction between cases and contacts.
- Breaking the chain of an infection requires a simple intervention of interfering with the infectious agent's mode of transmission.
- Antigenic drift is the result of point mutations in a gene segment resulting in a minor surface antigen change.
- Antigenic shift is a major change in one or more surface antigen proteins
- The terms infectious specifically refers to an infectious agent or the toxic products of an infectious agent that arise from the transmission of the agent into a susceptible host.
- The term communicable is specifically referring to a disease that can be transmitted from an infected individual to another individual.
- An exposed person is someone who has been in a situation where effective transmission of an infectious agent could have occurred.
- An infected person is someone who has an established infection with signs of symptoms of infection present.
- Colonization is the presence of infectious agents in or on a host with the ability to grow and multiply without the overt clinical expression or immune reaction of the host to the infectious agent.
- An index case is considered the earliest documented case of an infection or disease known to occur.
- Primary case may be the index case, but is not always the index case.

- Emerging infectious diseases are categorized as newly emerging, re-emerging, or deliberately emerging.

EPIDEMIOLOGY CRITICAL REASONING QUESTIONS

1. Compare and contrast the following— infectious disease, communicable disease, infectious process, colonization, asymptomatic and symptomatic, and exposed and contact.
2. Differentiate among index, primary, and secondary cases.
3. Distinguish among a source of infection, source of contamination, and vehicle and vector.
4. Differentiate the modes of transmission— droplet, airborne, fecal-oral route, skin or mucous membrane (sexual), perinatal, anthropoid-borne.

ADDITIONAL RESOURCES

 SPRINGER PUBLISHING CONNECT™ | A robust set of instructor resources designed to supplement this text is located at http://connect. springerpub.com/content/book/978-0-8261-8514-3. Qualifying instructors may request access by emailing textbook@springerpub.com.

REFERENCES

Morens, D., & Fauci, A. (2020). Emerging pandemic diseases: How we got to COVID-19. *Cell, 182*(5), 1077–1092. https://doi.org/10.1016/j.cell.2020.08.021

Straif-Bourgeious, S., Ratard, R., & Kretzschmar, M. (2014). Infectious disease epidemiology. In W. Ahrens & I. Pigeot (Eds.), *Handbook of epidemiology* (pp. 2041–2119). Springer Science+Business Media.

Chapter 20

GENETIC AND ENVIRONMENTAL EPIDEMIOLOGY

Demetrius J. Porche

Our own genomes carry the story of our evolution, written in DNA, the language of molecular genetics, and the narrative is unmistakable.

–Kenneth R. Miller (American cell biologist and molecular biologist)

A nation that destroys its soils destroys itself. Forests are the lungs of our land, purifying the air and giving fresh strength to our people.

–Franklin D. Roosevelt

CHAPTER COMPETENCIES

At the conclusion of this chapter, the reader will be able to:

1. Describe genetic and environmental epidemiology
2. Differentiate the types of genetic testing
3. Identify common air, water, and soil pollutants
4. Conduct a personal environmental assessment of air, water, and soil pollutants
5. Conduct an exposure assessment

ESSENTIAL TERMINOLOGY

The essential genetic and environmental epidemiology terminology are:

- Genetics
- Genomics
- Gene
- Chromosome
- Genetic epidemiology
- Environmental epidemiology
- Primary pollutant
- Secondary pollutant
- Genetic testing
- Genetic counseling

The Human Genome Project expanded our understanding of the human genetic code that transformed healthcare practice. The Human Genome Project mapped and sequenced the entire human genome. This information further advanced genetic science which impacts both early detection of diseases and the clinical management of diseases. As genetics has advanced so has the understanding of the environment. Genetic and environmental epidemiology provide a scientific base about the genetic distribution and determinants of health at an individual and population level while also considering the larger context of the environmental impact on an individual. As the science in both areas, genetics and environment, continue to evolve, there will be a better understanding of the synergy and dynamic relationship between which genetics and the environment impact each other in the expression of health and disease. Genetic and environmental epidemiologist will have a critical role with advancing the interrelationship between genetics and the environment as etiologic agents of disease within a population.

GENETIC EPIDEMIOLOGY

Genetic epidemiology is considered a newer branch of epidemiology that focuses on the etiology, distribution, and control of diseases in groups of genetically related individuals and those with inherited genetic diseases. Genetic epidemiology attempts to understand the manner in which genetic factors interact with the environment in the context of population diseases and health conditions. The content area of genetic epidemiology consists of the etiology of inherited diseases, the distribution of inherited disorders, and methods to prevent or alter the impact of inherited disorders. Simply stated, genetic epidemiology examines the role of inherited factors in disease etiology (Seyerle & Avery, 2013). There is also a therapeutic aspect of genetic epidemiology that integrates the sciences of genetics and pharmacology (Austin, 2020).

Other public health benefits of combining genetic and epidemiologic data into genetic epidemiology are improving the understanding of disease mechanisms, targeting therapeutic treatments such as for oncologic conditions, and determining dosage and combination pharmacologic regimens (Seyerle & Avery, 2013). Through population-level analysis, genetic epidemiology has facilitated the assessment of genetic bases for diseases such as Tay-Sachs, Huntington's, and cystic fibrosis.

Genetics and genetics epidemiology is a continually developing area of nursing practice. The International Society of Nurses in Genetics describes a genetics nurse as a licensed professional nurse with specialized education and training in the discipline of genetics. Genetic nurses perform risk assessments, analyze the genetic contribution to health conditions, and educate or counsel on the impact of these risks on the healthcare management of individuals, families, and communities. Nurses involved in the practice of genetics and genetic epidemiology obtain detailed family histories and construct a family history pedigree, assess and analyze hereditary and nonhereditary disease risk factors, identify potential genetic conditions or the genetic predisposition to a disease, and provide genetic counseling. Advanced practice nurses provide the same scope of practice as the professional nurse in addition to facilitating genetic testing, genetic test and other clinical laboratory test reports, and prescribing pharmacologic and nonpharmacologic interventions as within their state's scope of practice.

Foundational Genetic Concepts

The basic unit of all life is the cell. A human has trillions of cells that coexist. Within the cell, there is a nucleus where chromosomes are contained. Chromosomes control the function of cells. Each human cell (except gametes) has 46 chromosomes. Of these 46 chromosomes, 44 are autosomes chromosomes and two are sex chromosomes. Females have two X sex chromosomes (XX) and males have an X and Y chromosome (XY) within the cell's nucleus. Chromosomes are composed of deoxyribonucleic acid (DNA) and proteins known as histones. Ribonucleic acid (RNA) is produced from DNA. RNA produces functional proteins for cellular life. Proteins are made up of amino acids, which are considered the basic building blocks of a cell (Macha & Mc Donough, 2011).

A specific component of the DNA that codes for a specific protein is known as a gene. A genome is a complete set of genes that code for all proteins in the body. Each gene in the DNA codes for a specific protein. Both DNA and RNA are capable of carrying genetic information for protein building. The genetic code of an individual is present in both the DNA and RNA. Each individual has a genetic code that synthesizes all their proteins in the body which is necessary for the existence of human life (Macha & Mc Donough, 2011).

Genetic information is transmitted through the sperm and ovum. Sperm are produced through meiotic divisions with each sperm containing either one X or Y chromosome. The ovum carries one X chromosome. If the sperm with an X chromosome enters the ovum, then the zygote will have two XX chromosomes resulting in a female. If the sperm with a Y chromosome enters the ovum, then the zygote will have a X and Y chromosome, resulting in a male (XY). During zygote replication, crossing over may occur, which is when the paternal chromosome may be exchanged with the maternal chromosome and vice versa. Through this process, the DNA contains two strands of DNA that are not similar. An individual has two genes for any given trait. A variant of a gene is known as an allele. Alleles may be dominant or recessive. If the nucleotides in the genes of a trait have a similar sequence on both DNA strands, then this is considered homozygous. If the sequence of nucleotides in the genes of a trait are not similar in sequence on both DNA strands, then the genotype is considered heterozygous. Table 20.1 provides additional foundational genetic terminology to understand genetic epidemiology (Elston et al., 2012; Morris-Rosendahl, 2010).

Table 20.1 Foundational Genetic Terminology

Term	Definition
Recessive	A recessive gene is expressed only if genes are homozygous
Sex chromosome	The chromosome that determines the sex
Somatic chromosome	A nonsex chromosome
X chromosome	The sex chromosome when present in duplicate (XX) is female and single is male (XY)
X-linked	Genes on the X chromosome
Y chromosome	The sex chromosome present only in males (XY)
Allele	One or more alternate forms of a gene or maker at a specific chromosome locus point
Epigenetics	Inherited changes to DNA structure that do not alter the underlying DNA sequencing
Epigenomics	Application of epigenetics to the entire genome
Genetic association	Nonrandom occurrence of genetic markers with a trait
Genotype	Genetic constitution of alleles at one or more pairs of genetic loci; the total of the genetic information contained on the chromosomes
Monogenic disorder	Etiology of disorder is a result of one or more mutations in a single gene
Phenotype	Observable properties of an individual
Dominant gene	A dominant gene is expressed when heterozygous
Locus	Location of an allele on the chromosome

Source: Adapted from Elston, R., Satagopan, J., & Sun, S. (2012). Genetic terminology. *Methods of Molecular Biology, 850,* 1–9. https://doi.org/10.1007/978-1-61779-555-8; Morris-Rosendahl, D. (2010). A glossary of relevant genetic terms. *Dialogues in Clinical Neuroscience, 12*(1), 116–120. https://doi.org/10.31887/DCNS.2010.12.1/dmrosendahl

Genetic Testing

Genetic testing is a surveillance and secondary prevention strategy to identify and confirm the presence of genetically caused diseases or health conditions. Specifically, genetic testing identifies mutations or variants that are changes in an individual's DNA. Genetic testing assists with the identification and diagnosis of medical conditions or provides information about potential genetic risk for a disease. Other reasons for genetic testing include family planning decisions, pregnancy screening of the fetus, carrier testing, management of general health, and guidance for therapeutic and pharmacologic decisions. This information supports the healthcare provider and the individual impacted with the opportunity to formulate a plan of care. Genetic testing is best supported by genetic counseling. The current standard of care is to provide genetic counseling with genetic testing, along with a detailed family history and genogram.

Genetic testing can begin prior to birth through amniocentesis and chorionic villous biopsy. Newborn screening is another surveillance and secondary prevention strategy that can screen infants for diseases such as phenylketonuria (PKU). PKU is a genetic metabolic condition that results from the lack of phenylalanine hydroxylase enzyme. This enzyme is essential for protein formation. Without this enzyme, phenylalanine amino acid levels are elevated in the blood that could result in mental retardation and seizure disorders. Another common disorder that can be detected with early genetic screening is sickle cell anemia. These are just two of many examples demonstrating the benefit of genetic testing and counseling. Nurses are involved in genetic testing education and counseling, in addition to collecting the genetic test samples.

Genetic testing provides information about an individual's genes and chromosomes. There are several types of genetic testing. The most common types of genetic testing are:

1. **Newborn screening:** Screening conducted after birth to identify genetic disorders that have the potential for an early intervention such as phenylketonuria (PKU). All states test for PKU and congenital hypothyroidism.
2. **Diagnostic genetic testing:** Genetic test used to identify or rule out a specific genetic or chromosomal disorder. Diagnostic genetic testing is used to confirm or support a diagnosis based on physical examination and presentation along with signs and symptoms. Diagnostic genetic testing can be conducted before birth or at any point in an individual's life.
3. **Carrier genetic testing:** Carrier tests are used to identify an individual who may carry one copy of gene mutation that, when present in two copies or combination with another gene, may cause a genetic disorder.
4. **Prenatal genetic testing:** Prenatal tests are used to identify changes, mutations, alterations, or gene sequences or chromosomes before birth. Prenatal genetic tests are performed on a fetus considered at risk for genetic abnormalities.
5. **Preimplantation genetic testing:** Preimplantation testing is also known as preimplantation genetic diagnosis (PGD). Preimplantation testing is used to detect genetic abnormalities in an embryo created through reproductive techniques such as in vitro fertilization. A small number of cells are harvested from the embryo and tested prior to uterine implantation.
6. **Predictive and presymptomatic genetic testing:** Predictive and presymptomatic testing is used to identify gene mutations associated with health conditions or disorders that appear after birth, or later in life. This testing can be conducted when there are family members with a genetic disorder as a means to identify the individual's risk of developing a disorder.
7. **Forensic genetic testing:** Forensic testing is used to identify DNA sequences of an individual for legal purposes. Forensic tests are not used to identify genetic mutations associated with disease but to prove an individuals' identity associated with a crime or other event.

Genetic testing can examine both chromosomes and gene expression. Chromosome testing examines the DNA for changes in chromosome structures rather than focusing on genes. Gene expression testing compares normal and disease cells for the level of gene expression known to be associated with the respective disease (Centers for Disease Control and Prevention [CDC], 2020).

In addition, genetic testing can be single gene, panel, or large-scale genetic or genomic testing. Single gene testing examines the DNA for changes in only one gene. Single gene testing is conducted when there is suspicion of a specific condition or syndrome or there is a known genetic mutation that exists within the family. Panel testing examines for multiple genes in one genetic test. For example, an individual could have one genetic test for several oncologic genetic markers. There are two types of large-scale genetic testing. These are exome and genome sequencing. Exome sequencing examines all the genes in the DNA. Clinical exome sequencing is a type of exome testing that examines specifically all the genes related to a specific medical condition in the DNA. Genome sequencing is the largest genetic test conducted that examines all of the individuals DNA, not just the genes in the DNA (CDC, 2020).

An exemplar of the benefit of genetic testing is for breast cancer. The *BRCA1* and *BRCA2* genes are related to the occurrence of breast cancer. Genetic testing and counseling for the presence of these genes can provide vital information for women considered at risk for breast cancer to make informed decisions about changes in lifestyle, estrogen or progesterone hormone avoidance, and prophylactic surgical options. Advances in mental health and gene mapping have resulted in the identification of genes linked to schizophrenia, *DRNBP1* and *NRG1*. The presence of these genes can assist with differential diagnosis of a presenting mental health condition.

Epidemiologic data on the genetic expression of these genes in a population provide vital information to inform a clinician's genetic counseling. Genetic epidemiologic information about population dynamics needs continual surveillance and genetic mapping within populations. This is necessary as humans migrate and reproduce, creating different genetic expressions of gene sequences. Therefore, genetic epidemiologic studies are necessary to continually monitor disease morbidity and mortality data correlated with population-based genetic mapping. It is important to remember that disease etiology is complex and the determination of genetic risk alone may not equate to genetic determinism that the disease or health condition will occur in the individual. There is a complex interaction between genetics and environment that results in the final expression of a disease or health alteration (Seyerle & Avery, 2013).

Pharmacogenetics and Pharmacogenomics

The interaction between genetics and therapeutic drugs involves pharmacogenetics and pharmacogenomics. Pharmacogenetics examines the genetic etiology of an individual's unusual response to a therapeutic drug. Pharmacogenomics examines the linkage between genetic differences in a population to drug responses. Pharmacogenomics examines the genomic underpinnings of a drug's pharmacologic response to improve the understanding of adverse drug interactions and to determine the appropriate pharmacologic combinations to individualized treatments (Seyerle & Avery, 2013). Both pharmacogenetics and pharmacogenomics are transforming the clinical decision-making of drug selection for specific individuals and populations. The collection of population-based epidemiologic research on pharmacogenetics and pharmacogenomics informs healthcare decision-making at the individual, institutional and community level.

ENVIRONMENTAL EPIDEMIOLOGY

The environment is a critical component of the epidemiologic triad. There has long been a connection between the environment and health. Environment is a broad concept that encompasses the setting of human activity and life within geographical spaces, along with the existence of physical, chemical, and biological factors that can impact humans. Environmental epidemiology is considered a specialty or branch of epidemiology. Environmental epidemiology is the study of health-related conditions or diseases in specific populations that are influenced by physical, chemical, biological, and psychosocial factors in the environment.

Environmental health nurses focus on improving the health of an entire population. An environmental health nurse is a professional nurse who focuses on identifying different environmental hazards within the community that impact the health and well-being of individuals, families, and populations. The role of the environmental health nurse involves identifying potential environmental health

hazards, developing programs or initiatives to reduce these environmental health hazards, providing education to populations and entire communities who may be at risk for or impacted by an environmental health hazard, and conducting environmental assessments to explore whether or not environmental risks remain present.

Environmental epidemiology integrates multiple disciplines such as epidemiology, environmental science, and toxicology. Environmental science is considered a broad discipline that examines the interaction between the natural environment and human society. Some consider environmental science as the science that examines the interaction of the epidemiologic triad—agent, host, and environment (Kreis, 2013). Toxicology is the study of adverse health effects from chemicals on all living organisms. Environmental epidemiology is also concerned with the human exposure to toxic agents in the environment.

Environmental epidemiologists study the effects of environmental exposures on the health and disease occurrence within a population. Essentially environmental epidemiologists are concerned in principle with environmental health which consists of all external factors to the human body that impact an individual's and population's health. This approach to environmental health is considered an all-inclusive approach (Brunekreef, 2008). The environmental epidemiologist prioritizes the competing environmental health issues based on epidemiologic data. Epidemiologists propose these health priorities using a diverse set of criteria. These criteria include but are not limited to:

1. Transmission factors
2. Strength of the scientific evidence
3. Population and individual health benefits and threats
4. Societal benefits and implications
5. Political issues
6. Cost-effectiveness of interventions
7. Legal issues
8. Technological issues
9. Quality of life impact
10. Public opinion (Kreis, 2013)

Environmental Exposures

The determination of the health effects of an environmental exposure is dependent upon the specific environmental agent exposure, route of transmission or exposure, host characteristics, and toxicology or infectiousness of the environmental agent. Environmental exposures can occur through inhalation, oral ingestion, or possibly through skin and mucous membrane absorption. Environmental epidemiology considers an exposure as the contact between an agent and the target or host. Environmental epidemiologists use exposure science to understand the relationship of the exposure to host characteristics such as life stage, genetic susceptibility, and stressor or chemical interactions with other risk factors. The target of the exposure in the host is an important element to evaluate in the risk exposure. For example, is the environmental agent target of exposure specific cells, tissues, organs, cell receptor sites, or hormone interruption? Exposure science combined with epidemiologic data provide critical information from risk level, to exposure, to the extent to which the environmental agent causes cellular or end-organ damage.

Appendix C presents a list of hazardous environmental agents, route of entry, and symptoms.

Environmental Assessment

Simply, the environment can be considered everything external to an individual. Inclusive in the environment are all agents that exist in the environment. These agents consist of substances released from all human activities, inclusive of industrial activities. These environmental agents accumulate in the air, water, and/or soil. A comprehensive environmental assessment is an essential component of an epidemiologic investigation with the potential to identify environmental etiologic agents. Nurses conducting a community assessment should integrate an environmental assessment within the comprehensive community assessment.

During an epidemiologic environmental investigation, there should be an assessment of air, water, and soil pollutants associated with or correlated to morbidity and mortality data. A primary pollutant is one that has a direct impact on the environment. For example, chemicals released into the air can have a direct impact on the environment alone or as they react with other chemicals in the air. This interaction of a primary pollutant with another chemical has the potential to cause an environmental impact known as secondary pollutant. Epidemiologic environmental assessment should include both primary and secondary

pollutants correlated with morbidity and mortality epidemiologic data.

Pollutants can be point or nonpoint source pollutants. Point source pollutants result from a single, discrete facility or location that emits the pollutants. Common point source pollutants are factories, wells, automobile engines, or smokestacks. Point source pollutants are easier to monitor and control. The U.S. Environmental Protection Agency (EPA) establishes emission standards for chemical and compound discharges into the environment. Epidemiologic environmental surveillance can consist of sampling point source pollutants. Nonpoint source pollutants result from a diffuse and widespread pollutant source and may originate from multiple sources such as vehicles discharging chemicals in multiple locations, and soil distribution during farming and construction. Surveillance is more challenging with nonpoint source pollution. Point source pollutants can be monitored at the source, but nonpoint source pollutants are monitored at the destination of the pollutant. The common epidemiologic metric for environmental pollutants is micrograms per milliliter or parts per million (ppm).

The environment can be tainted with pollutants other than air, water, and soil contaminants. Some other environmental pollutants to consider in an epidemiologic investigation are prescription drugs, heavy metals, light, and noise.

Air Pollutants

Pollutants that exist in the air are known as air pollutants. There are eight classes of air pollutants—oxides of carbon, sulfur, nitrogen, volatile organic compounds, suspended particulate matter, photochemical oxidants, radioactive substances, and hazardous air pollutants. Table 20.2 presents air pollutants for each of those classes.

Water Pollutants

Water pollutants consist of eight classes. These classes are infectious agents, oxygen-depleting wastes, inorganic chemicals, organic chemicals, plant nutrient pollutants, sediments, radioactive materials, and thermal pollution. Table 20.3 presents water pollutants for each of these classes.

Soil Pollutants

Water pollutants can cross-contaminate the soil and soil pollutants can cross-contaminate the water. Other important soil pollutants to note

Table 20.2 Air Pollutant Classes

Oxides of carbon	Carbon monoxide (CO) Carbon dioxide (CO$_2$)
Oxides of sulfur	Sulfur dioxide (SO$_2$) Sulfur trioxide (SO$_3$)
Oxides of nitrogen	Nitric oxide (NO) Nitrogen dioxide (NO$_2$) Nitrous oxide (N$_2$O)
Volatile organic compounds	Hydrocarbons—methane (CH$_4$), propane (C$_3$H8), octane (C$_8$H$_{18}$) Chlorofluorocarbons—dichlorodifluoromethane
Suspended particulate matter	Dust Soot Asbestos Liquid microdroplets—sulfuric acid, pesticides
Photochemical oxidants	Ozone (O$_3$)
Radioactive substances	Radon
Hazardous air pollutants	Benzene Carbon tetrachloride

Table 20.3 Water Pollutant Classes

Infectious agents	Bacteria Viruses Parasites
Oxygen depleting	Animal manure Plant debris Farm runoff Industrial discharge Urban sewage
Inorganic chemicals	Mineral acids Toxic metals—lead, cadmium, mercury, and hexavalent chromium
Organic chemicals	Oil Gasoline Pesticides Organic solvents
Plant nutrient pollutants	Farm and garden runoff that contains chemicals such as nitrates, phosphates, and ammonium—common chemicals in fertilizers and detergents
Sediments	Soil erosion and deposits into water
Radioactive	Iodine-131— result of nuclear plants Strontium-90—result of nuclear plants
Thermal pollution	Warm water discharge from industrial plants into rivers, lakes, and oceans

are pesticides, which consists of insecticides (to kill insects), herbicides (to kill plants), fungicides (to kill fungi). In addition, soil can absorb other pollutants such as sulfuric acid from rain that converts in the soil to sulfates, and nitric acid from rain that converts into nitrates in the soil.

Air, Water, and Soil Pollution Assessment Tools

The EPA provides on-line assessment tools to assist with identifying environmental pollutants. The EPA developed ExpoBox located at https://www.epa.gov/expobox. This toolbox provides a comprehensive resource to conduct environmental exposure assessments. The ExpoBox is a compendium of exposure assessment tools that links to guidance documents, databases, models, reference materials, and other related resources.

RISK ASSESSMENT

Risk assessment is the quantitative assessment of risk associated with a specific level of exposure to a substance or agent in the population (Brunekreef, 2008). Risk assessment consists of doing a hazard assessment and exposure assessment. A hazard assessment determines the extent to which an agent or substance can potentially harm an individual. An exposure assessment collects information on the specific exposure to a hazardous agent or substance to determine the level of exposure and potential for health alterations (2008).

Exposure Assessment

The methods used to assess an exposure should be valid and reliable. The reliability aspect of an exposure assessment should be accurate and precise. Accuracy is the extent to which the measure is close to the true measurement. Precision is the extent to which the exposure measurement can be repeated with the same or similar results (Brunekreef, 2008). Exhibit 20.1 presents some sample health history questions for environmental exposures used in the clinical setting. Nurses can conduct an environmental exposure assessment within their health history and physical examination. Sometimes the environmental exposure assessment is completed by the individual with their intake assessment documents and reviewed by the nurse during the assessment and physical examination.

EXHIBIT 20.1. Environmental Exposure History Questions

1. Are you currently exposed to any of the following:

   a. Metals (name if known) _____
   b. Dust or fibers (name if known)

   _____
   c. Chemicals (name if known) _____
   d. Fumes (name if known) _____
   e. Smoke (name if known) _____
   f. Radiation (name if known) _____
   g. Biological agents (name if known)

   _____
   h. Loud noise (name if known) _____
   i. Vibrations (name if known) _____
   j. Extreme heat or cold (name if known)

   _____

2. Have you been exposed to any of these in the past:

   a. Metals (name if known) _____
   b. Dust or fibers (name if known)

   _____
   c. Chemicals (name if known)

   _____
   d. Fumes (name if known) _____
   e. Smoke (name if known) _____
   f. Radiation (name if known) _____
   g. Biological agents (name if known)

   _____
   h. Loud noise (name if known) _____
   i. Vibrations (name if known) _____
   j. Extreme heat or cold (name if known)

   _____

3. For each exposure, describe in detail below the following: Where you were exposed, how you were exposed, beginning date of exposure and ending date of exposure (if you do not know specific dates, provide estimated dates).

   _____

4. What was the frequency of your exposure?

   a. Daily
   b. More than daily but not every day of the week
   c. Every workday
   d. Couple of times a month
   e. Couple of times a quarter
   f. Other (explain frequency)

   _____

5. Describe your actions after your exposure; for example, did you wash your skin, remove and clean your clothes?

   _____

(continued)

EXHIBIT 20.1. Environmental Exposure History Questions (*continued*)

6. What type of personal protective equipment (ear protection, face shield, eye goggles, face masks, respirators, gowns, gloves) do you routinely wear at work? When do you wear the personal protective equipment?
7. How often do you practice hand hygiene (wash your hands)? _____
8. Do you smoke at work? If so, what do you smoke? _____
9. Do you vape at work? If so, what do you vape? _____
10. Are you exposed to secondhand tobacco smoke at work?
11. Do you eat at the workplace? What is the location of where you eat?
12. Do you have the ability to remove soiled or contaminated clothing at work? Can you shower at work?
13. Have any family members experienced any symptoms?
14. Has there been a change in the health of any pets in your home or close contact?
15. Do you have any symptoms that you consider to be associated with work?
16. Do your symptoms get better at work, home, on weekends, or on vacations?
17. Do your symptoms get worst at work, home, on weekends, or on vacations?
18. What have you done to alleviate any of your symptoms? Has this been effective? If so, please explain.
19. Have you been exposed to any of the following agents at work, home, or in your leisure activities? Specify where you have been exposed.
20. Have you missed any work because of an illness? How long did you miss? What were your symptoms? Did you seek care from a healthcare provider? If so, what was the diagnosis?

21. Have you ever changed jobs or moved/relocated your place of living due to symptoms? If so, explain when you moved and from where to where you moved.

22. Describe your work conditions—cleanliness, agents in environment, ventilation.

23. Do you live near an industrial plant, commercial business, waste or dump site?
24. Do you have the following in your home?

    a. Smoke detector
    b. Radon detector
    c. Air conditioner
    d. Air purifier
    e. Heating unit (describe type of heating device)
    f. Gas stove
    g. Electric stove
    h. Fireplace
    i. Furnace
    j. Wood stove
    k. Humidifier

25. Have you made any changes in your home environment lately such as new carpet, new furniture, new air fresheners, pets, remodeling?
26. Do you use any pesticides or herbicides in your home, garden, or on pets?
27. What type of drinking water do you use? What is the source of your drinking water?
28. Do you have a garden or fruit trees? What do you eat from your garden or fruit trees?

Source: Thompson, J., Brodkin, C., Kyes, K., Neighbor, W., & Evanoff, B. (2000). Use of a questionnaire to improve occupation and environmental history taking in primary care physicians. *Journal of Occupational and Environmental Medicine/American College of Occupational and Environmental Medicine*, *42*(12), 1188–1194. https://doi.org/10.1097/00043764-200012000-00014

END-OF-CHAPTER RESOURCES

SUMMARY POINTS

- The Human Genome Project mapped and sequenced the entire human genome.
- Genetic and environmental epidemiology provides a science base about the genetic distribution and determinants of health at an individual and population level.
- Genetic epidemiology attempts to understand the manner in which genetic factors interact with the environment in the context of population diseases and health conditions.
- The basic unit of all life is the cell.
- Each human cell (except gametes) have 46 chromosomes.
- Females have two X sex chromosomes (XX).
- Males have a X and Y chromosome (XY).
- A genome is a complete set of genes that code for all proteins in the body.
- Genetic information is transmitted through the sperm and ovum.
- Genetic testing is a surveillance and secondary prevention strategy to identify and confirm the presence of genetically caused diseases or health conditions.
- Genetic testing assists with the identification and diagnosis of medical conditions or provide information about potential genetic risk for a disease.
- Newborn screening is screening conducted after birth.
- Diagnostic genetic testing is used to identify or rule out a specific genetic or chromosomal disorder.
- Carrier tests are used to identify an individual who may carry one copy of gene mutation that, when present in two copies or combination of another gene, may cause a genetic disorder.
- Prenatal tests are used to identify changes, mutations, alterations, or gene sequences or chromosomes before birth.
- Preimplantation testing is used to detect genetic abnormalities in an embryo created through reproductive techniques such as in vitro fertilization.
- Forensic testing is used to identify DNA sequences of an individual for legal purposes.
- Pharmacogenetics examines the genetic etiology of an individual's unusual response to a therapeutic drug.
- Pharmacogenomics examines the linkage between genetic differences in a population to drug responses.
- Environmental epidemiology is the study of health-related conditions or diseases in specific populations that are influenced by physical, chemical, biological, and psychosocial factors in the environment.
- Environmental science is considered a broad discipline that examines the interaction between the natural environment and human society.
- Toxicology is the study of adverse health effects from chemicals on all living organisms.
- Essentially environmental epidemiologists are concerned in principle with environmental health, which consists of all external factors to the human body that impact an individual's health.
- The determination of the health effects of an environmental exposure is dependent upon the environmental agent exposed to, route of transmission or exposure, host characteristics, and toxicology or infectiousness of the environmental agent.
- The target of the exposure in the host is an important element to evaluate in the risks exposure.
- A comprehensive environmental assessment is an essential component in an epidemiologic investigation with potential environmental etiologic agents.
- A primary pollutant is one that has a direct impact on the environment.
- Point source pollutants result from a single, discrete facility or location that emits the pollutants.
- Common point source pollutants are factories, wells, automobile engines, or smokestacks.

EPIDEMIOLOGY CRITICAL REASONING QUESTIONS

1. Differentiate pharmacogenetics and pharmacogenomics.
2. Utilize Exhibit 20.1 to conduct an environmental exposure history on yourself or a family member. What are the three top priority environmental health concerns for you or your family member? What

recommendations would you provide to reduce your environmental exposure risk?

3. Identify the air, water, and soil pollutants of concern in the community where you live, work, and engage in leisure activities using the Environmental Protection Agency website—ExpoBox (https://www.epa.gov /expobox).

ADDITIONAL RESOURCES

 SPRINGER PUBLISHING CONNECT™ | A robust set of instructor resources designed to supplement this text is located at http://connect. springerpub.com/content/book/978-0-8261-8514-3. Qualifying instructors may request access by emailing textbook@springerpub.com.

REFERENCES

Austin, C. (2020). *Genetic epidemiology.* https:// www.geonome.gov/genetics-glossary/ Genetic-Epidemiology

Brunekreef, B. (2008). Environmental epidemiology and risk assessment. *Toxicology Letters, 180,* 118–122. https://doi.org/10.1016/ j.toxlet.2008.05.012

Centers for Disease Control and Prevention. (2020). *Genetic testing.* https://www.cdc .gov/genomics/testing/genetic_testing.htm

Elston, R., Satagopan, J., & Sun, S. (2012). Genetic terminology. *Methods of Molecular Biology, 850,* 1–9. https://doi.org/ 10.1007/978-1-61779-555-8

Kreis, I. (2013). Introduction to environmental epidemiology for health protection. In I. Kreis, A. Busgy, G. Leonardi, J. Meara, & V. Murray (Eds.), *Essentials of environmental epidemiology for health protection: A handbook for field professionals* (pp. 3–7). Oxford University Press.

Macha, K., & Mc Donough, J. (2011). *Epidemiology for advanced nursing practice.* Jones and Bartlett Learning.

Morris-Rosendahl, D. (2010). A glossary of relevant genetic terms. *Dialogues in Clinical Neuroscience, 12*(1), 116–120. https:// doi.org/10.31887/DCNS.2010.12.1/ dmrosendahl

Seyerle, A., & Avery, C. (2013). Understanding genetic epidemiology: The potential benefits and challenges of genetics for improving human health. *North Carolina Medical Journal, 74*(6), 505–508. https://www.ncbi .nlm.gov/pmc/articles/PMC4041482/pdf/ nihms578209.pdf

Thompson, J., Brodkin, C., Kyes, K., Neighbor, W., & Evanoff, B. (2000). Use of a questionnaire to improve occupation and environmental history taking in a primary care physicians. *Journal of Occupational and Environmental Medicine/American College of Occupational and Environmental Medicine, 42*(12), 1188–1194. https://doi .org/10.1097/00043764-200012000-00014

Chapter 21

OCCUPATIONAL EPIDEMIOLOGY

Demetrius J. Porche

It is neither wealth nor splendor; but tranquility and occupation which give you happiness.
–Thomas Jefferson

Your work is going to fill a large part of your life, and the only way to be truly satisfied is to do what you believe is great work, and the only way to do great work is to love what you do. If you haven't found it yet, keep looking, don't settle. As with all matters of the heart, you'll know when you find it.
–Steve Jobs

CHAPTER COMPETENCIES

At the conclusion of this chapter, the reader will be able to:

1. Define the practice of occupational epidemiology
2. Differentiate between the functions of the Occupational Safety and Health Administration (OSHA) and the National Institute for Occupational Safety and Health (NIOSHA)
3. Identify the most frequently cited OSHA standard violations
4. Describe the NIOSHA research area sectors

ESSENTIAL TERMINOLOGY

Essential occupational epidemiology terms are:

- National Institute for Occupational Safety and Health
- Occupational epidemiology
- Occupational health and safety
- Occupational surveillance
- Sentinel health event (occupational)

Occupational health and safety is considered a branch of public health focusing on diseases, health alterations, and injuries within the working population. Occupational health and safety programs implement strategies and regulations that are designed to prevent or reduce the occurrence of occupational disease and injury among the working population. Occupational health and safety integrates multiple professionals such as the industrial hygienist, toxicologist, and epidemiologist. Occupational health exists at the intersection of government regulation, management, and labor relations (Halperin & Howard, 2011).

Occupational epidemiology is a branch of epidemiology concerned with the determination of the distribution and determinants of health, illness, and risk factors within the occupational environment. Occupational epidemiology supports healthcare practice in several areas. Occupational epidemiology contributes to occupational health care by:

- Developing an evidence base that supports healthcare and medical occupational issues such as occupational prevention programs, adjudication of workers compensation, third-party litigation, and insurance settlements
- Establishing occupational health and safety priorities
- Promoting the development of occupational health surveillance protocols
- Educating workers on health, first aid, and safety measures

- Identifying associated factors or etiology of occupational injuries or health alterations
- Facilitating occupational hazard assessments (Guidotti, 2000)

Advances in occupational epidemiology could be supported by:

- Sharing data among workers' compensation and industrial insurance agencies into a centralized data clearing house
- Actuarial analyzing of pooled claim data to inform the development of occupational health and safety programs
- Analyzing occupational injury data with consideration to socio-economic factors of the worker and the community
- Developing health policy and legislation that promotes access to occupational and insurance-related occupational data for the advancement of population level occupational health (Guidotti, 2000)

Occupational health nursing is a specialized area of community and public health nursing practice. Nurses have the knowledge, skills, and ability to integrate nursing knowledge with occupational health knowledge to develop, plan, implement, and evaluate the effectiveness of occupational health programs on employee health outcomes.

OCCUPATIONAL HEALTH AND SAFETY HISTORICAL EVOLUTION

Occupational health and safety concerns evolved into national prominence through the development of several occupational injury events. In March 1911, the Triangle Shirtwaist Fire occurred. This event led to the death of 146 young, mostly female immigrant garment workers who attempted to get out of a burning building but encountered locked doors in a "sweat shop." This event led to the development of state-based occupational safety regulations workers' compensation programs and federal safety legislation.

As well as economic benefits, the New Deal brought funding that supported the development of occupational hygiene programs. After this time, until about the 1960s, there was a lack of interest in occupational safety and health programs. In 1968, there was a mine disaster in Farmington, West Virginia, that killed 78 miners. This led to the passage of the Federal Coal Mine Health and Safety Act. This Act led to the introduction of federal regulation and inspections of the mining industry.

Scientific advances also changed the occupational and safety health concerns. As there was an increase in the use of synthetic organic chemicals in several industries, there were increasing health concerns evolving such as epidemics of bladder cancer, anemia, and leukemia. In addition, there was the association between occupational exposures and environmental contamination of chemicals that would not only impact the health and safety of industrial workers but also the community surrounding the industrial sites (Box 21.1). The signage of the Occupational Safety and Health (OSH) Act was described as the capstone event for occupational safety and health (Halperin & Howard, 2011).

OCCUPATIONAL SAFETY AND HEALTH ADMINISTRATION

The Occupational Safety and Health Administration (OSHA) is an agency within the U.S. Department of Labor. OSHA has the responsibility to improve worker safety and health protection. In 1970, President Nixon signed the OSH Act into law. However, the development of this OSH Act was formulated under the leadership of President Lyndon Johnson, the son-in-law of a miner who died from silicosis. This OSH Act created the agency, OSHA, which became functional in 1971. This was the first time there was uniform national enforcement of OSH throughout the United States.

The OSH Act assisted in shaping the field of occupational epidemiology. Through the OSH Act, industry was provided expert epidemiologic consultation to assist with the assessment of the potential for or occurrence of occupational disease and injury within the workplace. The evaluations that were conducted became known as health hazard evaluation (HHE).

OSHA Standards, 29, CFR 1904, prescribes that employers must maintain records of job-related injuries and illnesses as a means to determine risk factors and causation and to develop prevention programs. This regulation requires employers of 10 or more employees to maintain a record of serious work-related injuries and illnesses. The employer does not need to maintain a list of minor injuries. Minor injuries are those requiring first aid only. Injury records must be maintained at the workplace site for at least 5 years. Employers are also required to post a summary of the injuries and illnesses recorded in the previous year each February through April. Any fatal injury must be reported within

BOX 21.1. Occupational Health Article

Title:	Demonstration of subclinical early nephrotoxicity induced by occupational exposure to silica among workers in the pottery industry
Summary:	Silica exposure has been associated with nephrotoxic effects, which consist of renal dysfunction involving glomerular and renal tubules dysfunction. The purpose of this study was to identify the early signs of subclinical nephrotoxic effects among male Egyptian workers exposed to silica in the pottery industry. A cross-sectional study of 29 occupationally silica-exposed nonsmoking subjects were recruited from a handicraft pottery area in Greater Cairo, Egypt. The nonexposed comparisons group were 35 male nonsmoking subjects recruited from an administrative department in Kasr Al-Ainy Hospital who had a history of unusual exposure to silica during their daily life but without an occupational exposure. A questionnaire was administered to identify demographic and lifestyle characteristics such as smoking habit, detailed occupational history, and medical history with medication history. Workers with an occupational exposure were excluded if they were smokers, had experienced any kidney disease or any disease likely to alter or impair renal function, along with any medication or exposures to agents known to cause renal dysfunction. The comparison group was comparable and matched to sex, age, and socio-economic standards. Each subject provided a single random voided urine sample. Each urine sample was analyzed to assess for total protein (TP) and microalbumin (Malb), and proximal tubule integrity via Υ–GT and alkaline phosphatase (ALP), and lactate dehydrogenase (LDH) located at distal tubular cells, and urinary silicon levels along with urine level of KIM-1. Occupational silicon-exposed male workers had significantly increased levels of TP, Malb, ALP, Υ-GT, LDH, KIM-1, and silicon ($p < .001$, except Malb $p = .03$) compared to the comparison subjects. There was a significant positive correlation between silica-exposed worker duration and urinary silicon levels ($p < .001$). There was no significant correlation between age and urinary measures among silica-exposed workers. This study suggests that occupational silica exposure in the pottery industry affects subclinical glomerular and tubular function with significant positive correlation between renal dysfunction and silica duration of exposure and intensity of exposure.

Source: Mourad, B., & Ashour, Y. (2020). Demonstration of subclinical early nephrotoxicity induced by occupational exposure to silica among workers in pottery industry. *International Journal of Occupational & Environmental Medicine*, *11*, 85–94. https://doi.org/10.34172/ijoem.2020.1886

8 hours. Any injury resulting in any amputation, loss of an eye, or worker hospitalization must be reported within 24 hours.

Regular and periodic workplace inspections were provided for through the OSH Act. The OSH Act let to the development of OSHA, a regulatory agency and the National Institute for Occupational Safety and Health (NIOSH) , a research institute (described later). OSHA strives to ensure that there are safe and healthful working conditions by establishing standards and providing annual training, outreach, education, and consultative assistance to the workplace. OSHA has established several worker rights through the OSHA Standards. Some of these rights are:

- *Safe and healthful workplace:* It is the duty of the employer to provide a workplace free of known dangers and adequate protection from hazards
- *Access to information about hazardous chemicals:* Employers must have a written, complete hazard communication program that labels chemicals, provides training on chemical safety, and has Safety Data Sheets regarding potential workplace chemical hazards
- Process to report injuries and right to view annual injury and illness summary
- Ability to file a complaint or request workplace hazard correction
- Access to training on workplace hazards
- Ability to file a confidential OSHA complaint about an OSHA violation, health hazard, or imminent danger situation that exist in the workplace
- Participation in OSHA inspection by speaking with inspectors and freedom to point out health, safety and hazard concerns
- Freedom from retaliation for exercising safety and health rights

There are several types of OSHA inspections that occur for workplace safety. The types of OSHA inspections are imminent danger, fatality or hospitalization postinspection, worker complaints, targeted inspections for specific hazards or specific industries, and follow-up inspections. OSHA citations can be of several types: willful, serious, other-than-serious, and repeated. Willful violation is when the employer intentionally or knowingly commits a violation with plain indifference to the law. Serious violation occurs when there is substantial probability that death or serious physical harm could result and the employer was knowledgeable or should have known about the hazard (Box 21.2). Other-than-serious violations have a direct relationship to the safety and health of an employee but probably would not cause death or serious harm. Repeated violation is one that is the same or similar to a previous violation by the same employer. OSHA citations from an inspection can result in monetary penalties that may be as high as $70,000 per violation along with requirements for injury or illness prevention program development or industry quality improvements.

OSHA Standard Violations 2019

Violations in OSHA standards are an indication of workplace safety. Each year OSHA publishes the list of most frequently cited OSHA standards violations as a means for the occupational industry to develop program improvements and ameliorate occupational hazards. The ten most common OSHA standards violations (29 CFR) are:

1. Fall protection, construction
2. Hazard communication standard, general industry
3. Scaffolding, general requirements, construction
4. Control of hazardous energy (lockout/tagout), general industry
5. Respiratory protection, general industry
6. Ladders, construction
7. Powered industrial trucks, general industry
8. Fall protection, training requirements
9. Machinery and machine guarding, general requirements
10. Eye and face protection (OSHA, 2020).

NATIONAL INSTITUTE FOR OCCUPATIONAL SAFETY AND HEALTH

NIOSH is responsible for conducting research and making recommendations for the prevention of work-related injuries and illness. NIOSH is considered a nonregulatory agency; however, the guidance and recommendations provided by NIOSH are used by other regulatory agencies for developing and enforcing workplace safety and health programs. OSHA creates and enforces regulations. NIOSH advances the scientific field of occupational safety and health providing the research and evidence to support OSHA's regulations.

BOX 21.2. Occupational Health Article

Title:	Assessment of bone turnover biomarkers in lead-battery workers with long-term exposure to lead
Summary:	Lead exposure can reside within the skeletal system. The rate of bone turnover affects the release of lead into the circulatory system from bone. There has not been an exploration of bone turnover biomarkers (BTM) in lead-battery exposed workers. The purpose of this study was to evaluate the BTM (formation and resorption) in lead-battery workers who have long-term exposure to lead in a lead-battery manufacturing plant. This cross-sectional study included male workers in a lead-battery manufacturing plant who were occupationally exposed to lead for at least 2 years. A total of 176 lead-battery plant workers in Tamil Nadu, India, were recruited along with a group of 80 male office workers with no occupational exposure to lead. The comparison group was matched according to age and socio-economic status. Blood (5 mL) and urine (2 mL) samples were collected using a spot urine collection technique. Blood was analyzed for blood lead levels (BLL) and urine was measured for urinary hydroxyproline (UHYP) and creatinine. BLL is considered a reliable indicator of recent lead exposure. BTM is used to assess early stage osteoporosis. Lead exposed workers had a significantly higher bone formation biomarker and bone resorption biomarkers. Bone resorption biomarker levels were higher among those workers with higher BLL. The duration of lead-battery exposure was significantly associated with bone-specific alkaline phosphatase ($p = .037$), deoxypyridinoline ($p = .016$), tartarate-resistant acid phosphatase-5b ($p = .001$), and urinary hydroxyproline levels ($p = .002$). This study suggests that long-term (greater than 2 years) lead exposure affects bone turnover. This indicates that long-term exposure to lead results in high BLL and altered bone turnover biomarkers.

Source: Kalahasthi, R., Barman, T., & Bagepally, B. (2020). Assessment of bone turnover biomarkers in lead-battery workers with long-term exposure to lead. *International Journal of Occupational and Environmental Medicine*, *11*, 140–147. https://doi.org/10.34172/ijoem.2020.1951

NIOSH has three described epidemiologic roles. NIOSH conducts field epidemiology investigations of individual workplaces with an interprofessional team of experts. These field investigations collect data on occupational diseases and injury, identify potential workplace hazards, measure exposure levels, and identify appropriate occupational control measures to limit exposures. A second epidemiologic role is to conduct large-scale epidemiologic studies of multiple industrial facilities throughout the United States. The purpose of these large-scale epidemiologic investigations are to assess the relationship of occupational exposures to possible adverse health outcomes and to develop a knowledge base about occupational exposure–response–dose relationships. The ultimate goal is to develop evidence-based practices to prevent occupational injuries. A third epidemiologic role is to conduct surveillance of occupational disease and injury in the workplace. NIOSH's goal is to estimate the magnitude and trends of occupational disease and injury, identify the occurrence of new occupational diseases and injuries, detect sentinel health events, and develop prevention health programs. NIOSH has a specific definition of occupational surveillance (Halperin & Howard, 2011). The NIOSH surveillance definition is the systematic collection, analysis, and dissemination of health-related information for the purposes of prevention or control of disease or injury (Centers for Disease Control and Prevention [CDC], 2001). NIOSH's surveillance system extends beyond the collection of morbidity and mortality data to include data on injuries, hazards, and occupational exposures.

NIOSH's occupational surveillance system utilized the concept of Sentinel Health Event—Occupational (SHE-O). NIOSH defines a sentinel health event—occupational as "a disease, disability, or untimely death, which is occupationally related and whose occurrence may: provide impetus for epidemiologic or industrial hygiene studies; or serve as a warning signal that materials substitution, engineering control, personal protection, or medical care may be required" (Rutstein et al., 1983). NIOSH has developed state-based surveillance systems for occupational diseases and injury to provide comprehensive national occupational surveillance systems. Two such systems are the Fatal Assessment and Control Evaluation (FACE) and National Traumatic Occupational Fatality (NTOF) Surveillance System (Halperin & Howard, 2011).

The National Occupational Research Agenda (NORA) establishes the research agenda of NIOSH. The number of workers at risk for an injury or illness, seriousness of the occupational hazard, and potential for new research to improve practice influence NORA research priorities. For the last decade, the ten sectors for NORA research were:

- Agriculture, forestry, and fishing
- Construction
- Healthcare and social assistance
- Manufacturing
- Mining
- Oil and gas extraction
- Public safety
- Services
- Transportation, warehousing, and utilities
- Wholesale and retail trade (NIOSH, 2017)

OCCUPATIONAL INJURIES DATA—2019

Other OSH data sources consist of the Bureau of Labor Statistics Census of Fatal Occupational Injuries (CFOI) and Non-Fatal Occupational Injuries. These censuses produce fatal and non-fatal work injury data that detail the fatal injury, the occupation, equipment involved, circumstances of the event, and other worker characteristics. The purposes of the censuses are to:

- Inform workers of life-threatening hazards associated with various jobs and occupations
- Promote safer work environments through job safety training
- Assess and improve workplace safety standards
- Identify areas for safety research (U.S. Bureau of Labor Statistics, 2012)

According to the United States Bureau of Labor Statistics (2020), there were 2.8 million non-fatal workplace injuries and illnesses in 2019. In 2019, the private industry incidence rate of total recordable cases (TRC) was 2.8 cases per 100 full-time equivalents (FTE) workers, which has remained consistent with 2018 and 2017. Figure 21.1 presents the incidence rates of TRC 2010 to 2019.

In addition to recording the workplace injuries that occur, data are collected on missed time from the workplace due to illness. In 2019, private industries experienced 888,220 nonfatal injuries and illnesses that caused a worker to miss at least 1 day of work. Figure 21.2 presents data on missed work time or days of job transfer or restriction in 2019.

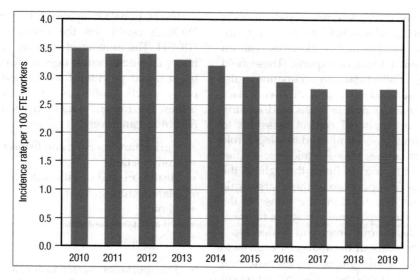

Figure 21.1 Total reportable cases incidence rate, private industry, 2010 to 2019.

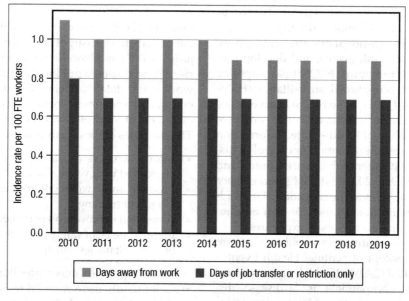

Figure 21.2 Job transfer or job restriction, incidence rate of days from work, private industry, 2010 to 2019.

Occupational epidemiology also tracks types of injuries and illnesses by industry type and occupations. Figure 21.3 presents manufacturing occupational injury data by industry and Figure 21.4 presents occupational injury data by selected occupations. Manufacturing accounted for 15% of all private industry non-fatal injuries and illnesses in 2019. In 2019, 10 occupations accounted for 33.2% of all private industry cases involving days away from work in both 2018 and 2019.

OSH concerns continue to exist. Some OSH concerns that remain in the American workforce are falls, health or humidity illness, repetitive stress injuries, sedentary behaviors, and workplace violence.

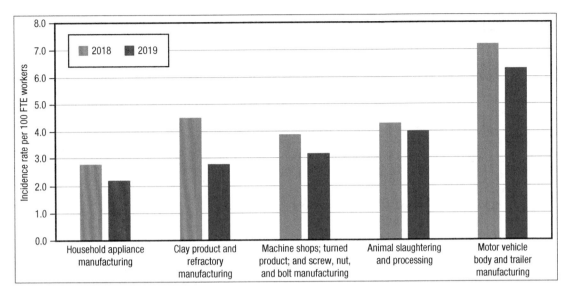

Figure 21.3 Total reportable cases incidence rate, private manufacturing industry, 2018 to 2019.

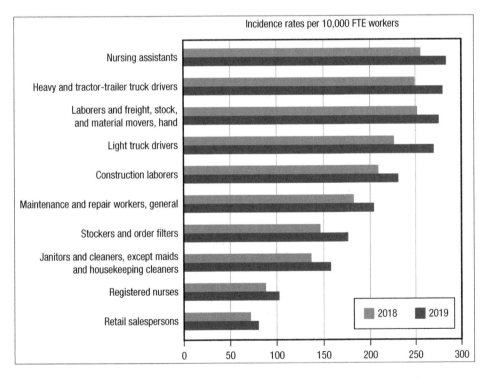

Figure 21.4 Days away from work, incidence rates, selected occupations, private industry, 2018 to 2019.

END-OF-CHAPTER RESOURCES

SUMMARY POINTS

- Occupational health and safety is considered a branch of public health focusing on diseases, health alterations, and injuries within the working population.
- Occupational health exists at the intersection of government regulation, management, and labor relations.
- Occupational epidemiology is a branch of epidemiology concerned with the determination of the distribution and determinants of health, illness, and risk factors within the occupational environment.
- OSHA has the responsibility to improve worker safety and health protection.
- OSHA Standards, 29, CFR 1904, prescribes that employers must maintain records of job-related injuries and illnesses as a means to determine risk factors, causation and develop prevention programs.
- 29, CFR 1904 requires employers of 10 or more employees to maintain a record of serious work-related injuries and illnesses.
- Any fatal injury must be reported within 8 hours.
- Any injury resulting in any amputation, loss of an eye, or worker hospitalization must be reported within 24 hours.
- OSHA strives to ensure there are safe and healthful working conditions by establishing standards and providing annual training, outreach, education and consultative assistance to the workplace.
- Willful violation is when the employer intentionally or knowingly commits a violation with plain indifference to the law.
- Serious violation occurs when there is substantial probability that death or serious physical harm could result and the employer was knowledgeable or should have known about the hazard.
- Other-than-serious violation has a direct relationship to the safety and health of an employee but probably would not cause death or serious harm.
- Repeated violation is one that is the same or similar to a previous violation by the same employer.
- NIOSH is responsible for conducting research and making recommendations for the prevention of work-related injuries and illnesses.
- NIOSH is considered a nonregulatory agency.
- Sentinel health event–occupational (SHE-O) is "a disease, disability, or untimely death, which is occupationally related and whose occurrence may: provide impetus for epidemiologic or industrial hygiene studies; or serve as a warning signal that materials substitution, engineering control, personal protection, or medical care may be required."

EPIDEMIOLOGY CRITICAL REASONING QUESTIONS

1. Explain the difference between OSHA and NIOSHA.
2. Describe the type of data that OSHA examines in the workplace.
3. Identify three of the most frequently cited OSHA standard violations in 2019.

ADDITIONAL RESOURCES

 A robust set of instructor resources designed to supplement this text is located at http://connect. springerpub.com/content/book/978-0-8261-8514-3. Qualifying instructors may request access by emailing textbook@springerpub.com.

REFERENCES

Centers for Disease Control and Prevention. (2001). *Tracking occupational injuries, illness, and hazards: The NIOSH surveillance strategic plan.* NIOSHA, CDC. http://www.cdc.gov/niosh/docs/2001-118/pdfs/2001-118.pdf

Guidotti, T. (2000). Occupational epidemiology. *Occupational Medicine, 50*(2), 141–145. https://doi.org/10.1093/occmed/50.2.141

Halperin, W., & Howard, J. (2011). Occupational epidemiology and the National Institute for Occupational Safety and Health. *Morbidity and Mortality Weekly Report, 60*(4), 97–103.

National Institute for Occupational Safety and Health. (2017). *National Occupational Research Agenda: second decade in review.* By S. Felknor, D. F. Williams, S. C. Soderholm. U.S. Department of Health and Human Services,

Centers for Disease Control and Prevention, National Institute for Occupational Safety and Health, DHHS (NIOSH) Publication 2017-146.

Occupational Safety and Health Administration. (2020). *Top 10 most frequently cited standards: Fiscal year 2019.* https://www.osha.gov/top10citedstandards

Rutstein, D., Mullan, R., Frazier, T., Halperin, W., Melius, J., & Sestito, J. (1983). The sentinel health event (occupational): A framework for occupational health surveillance and education. *Journal of the American Pharmacology Association, 73,* 1054–1062. https://doi.org/10.2105/ajph.73.9.1054

United States Bureau of Labor Statistics. (2012). *Injuries, illnesses, and fatalities: Census of Fatal Occupational Injuries (CFOI).* https://www.bls.gov/iif/oshfat1.htm

United States Bureau of Labor Statistics. (2020). *Employer-reported workplace injuries and illnesses—2019.* USDL-20-2030.

Chapter 22

REPRODUCTIVE AND MATERNAL HEALTH EPIDEMIOLOGY

Demetrius J. Porche

Fight for things you care about, but do it in a way that will lead others to join you.
–Ruth Bader Ginsburg

CHAPTER COMPETENCIES

At the conclusion of the chapter, the reader will be able to:

1. Define reproductive and maternal health epidemiology
2. Differentiate impact, outcome, and process indicators of reproductive and maternal health epidemiology
3. Calculate reproductive and maternal health epidemiology measures

ESSENTIAL TERMINOLOGY

The essential terminology for reproductive and maternal health epidemiology consists of:

- Antenatal care coverage rate
- Cesarean section rate
- Direct maternal death
- Indirect maternal death
- Infant vaccination coverage rate
- Infertility rate
- Lifetime risk of maternal death
- Maternal case fatality rate
- Maternal mortality
- Maternal mortality ratio
- Neonatal mortality rate
- Perinatal mortality rate
- Reproductive health
- Reproductive health epidemiology
- Reproductive health surveillance
- Reproductive processes
- Reproductive rate of infection
- Stillbirth rate
- Unspecified maternal death

Maternal and infant health historically have been public health indicators of a population's health status. Maternal and infant health nursing has early historical roots with nursing leaders such as Lilian Wald. Reproductive health encompasses the broad area of reproductive processes. Reproductive processes consist of the physical, mental, and social well-being associated with the reproductive system. Reproductive health includes the ability to regulate and control fertility, safe birthing processes, safe parenting, infant and child health survival, growth and development, and safety from sexually transmitted infections.

Reproductive epidemiology includes reproductive health surveillance, a component of public health surveillance systems that permit the identification, notification, quantification, and determination of events of reproductive health during a specific period of time in a specific geographical location. Reproductive health surveillance provides the data for reproductive epidemiology, which is the determination of the distribution and determinants of reproductive health. Reproductive health surveillance facilitates the monitoring of trends in health outcomes such as the occurrence and distribution of disease, changes in infectious agents and host factors, as well as the determination of the etiology and natural history of reproductive diseases, the evaluation of reproductive health programs, and the establishment of public health reproductive priority areas (Curtis et al., 2003). Some reproductive and maternal measures used to determine reproductive and maternal health are abortion rates, hypertensive disorder of pregnancy or pre-eclampsia, labor and delivery complications, birth rate, neonatal mortality rate, perinatal mortality rate, maternal mortality rate, infant mortality rate, coverage of antenatal care, low birth weight, and sexually transmitted infection (STI) incidence and prevalence rates.

Nurses who specialize in reproductive health are known as reproductive nurses or fertility nurses. Reproductive health nurses provide care to individuals, couples, and families. Reproductive nurses can practice at both the nurse generalist and advanced practice level. These reproductive health nurses engage in conducting assessments that may involve genetic testing or fertility testing, fertility counseling, patient education about reproductive health, fertilization and embryonic development, and the course of pregnancy. These nurses can also conduct scans, collect blood and urine samples, and perform physical examinations and assist with embryo transfers.

REPRODUCTIVE HEALTH EPIDEMIOLOGY RATES

Reproductive health epidemiology uses several factors: impact, outcome, and process. Impact indicators reflect changes in the primary health event generally expressed as morbidity and mortality data. Perinatal mortality rate would be an impact indicator. Outcome indicators represent changes in the knowledge, skills, attitudes, behaviors, or availability of services resulting from reproductive health programs. An outcome indicator would be a rate of STIs among pregnant women. Process indicators assess the actions taken and implemented as a means to achieve the expected programmatic outcomes. A process indicator would be the rate for screening tests conducted for an STI (Curtis et al., 2003).

Reproductive health formulas for these types of indicators are:

An impact indicator for morbidity such as perinatal mortality rate would be:

$$= \frac{\begin{array}{c}\text{Number of deaths in perinatal period} \\ \text{(22 weeks gestation through 7 days of} \\ \text{life) during the time period}\end{array}}{\begin{array}{c}\text{Total number of births (live births} \\ \text{plus fetal deaths) during the time} \\ \text{period}\end{array}} \times 100$$

An outcome indicator for an STI among pregnant women would be:

$$= \frac{\begin{array}{c}\text{Number of pregnant women} \\ \text{screened for an STI in the time} \\ \text{period who tested positive for the} \\ \text{STI}\end{array}}{\begin{array}{c}\text{Number of pregnant women who} \\ \text{were tested for and STI at deliv-} \\ \text{ery in the time period}\end{array}} \times 100$$

A process indicator such as coverage for screening of an STI before delivery would be:

$$= \frac{\begin{array}{c}\text{Number of women delivering in} \\ \text{the time period who have been} \\ \text{tested for "X" disease during} \\ \text{pregnancy}\end{array}}{\begin{array}{c}\text{Number of live births in the time} \\ \text{period}\end{array}} \times 100$$

Several reproductive health epidemiology rates are commonly used as impact and outcome indicators. The common impact and outcome reproductive health epidemiology rate formulas are presented in the following.

Reproductive and Maternal Health Impact Indicators

Maternal mortality ratio (MMR) measures risk of death due to pregnancy. The MMR formula is:

$$\text{MMR} = \frac{\begin{array}{c}\text{Number of maternal deaths} \\ \text{occurring in a given time} \\ \text{period}\end{array}}{\begin{array}{c}\text{Number of live births in the} \\ \text{given time period}\end{array}} \times 100$$

The maternal mortality rate also measures the risk of death due to pregnancy. The maternal mortality rate formula is:

Maternal mortality rate

$$= \frac{\begin{array}{c}\text{Number of maternal deaths in a} \\ \text{given time period}\end{array}}{\begin{array}{c}\text{Number of women of reproductive} \\ \text{age}\end{array}} \times 100$$

Proportionate mortality is a measure of the percentage of deaths due to pregnancy. The proportionate mortality formula is:

Proportionate mortality

$$= \frac{\text{Number of maternal deaths in given time period}}{\text{Number of deaths to women of reproductive age in the time period}} \times 100$$

Lifetime risk (LTR) of maternal death is a measure of a women's chance of dying from maternal causes over her reproductive life span. The LTR is determined based on the chance of pregnancy (fertility) and risk of death once pregnant. The LTR of maternal death formula is:

LTR of maternal death =

$$\frac{\text{Number of maternal deaths in 1 year}}{\text{Number of women of reproductive age}} \times 35 \text{ years}$$

Maternal case fatality rate is a measure of the proportion of women with obstetric complications who die. This represents several different types of complications such as hemorrhage (ante-partum and postpartum), postpartum sepsis, abortion complications, pre-eclampsia, ectopic pregnancy, and ruptured uterus. The maternal case fatality rate formula is:

Maternal case fatality rate

$$= \frac{\begin{array}{c}\text{Number of women with obstetric complications who die in a facility in a given time period}\end{array}}{\begin{array}{c}\text{Number of women admitted to the facility with an obstetric complication or who develop an obstetric complication while in the facility during the same time period}\end{array}}$$

Cause-specific proportionate maternal mortality is a measure of the percentage of maternal deaths that result from a specific cause. The cause-specific proportionate maternal mortality formula is:

Cause-specific proportionate maternal mortality

$$= \frac{\text{Number of maternal deaths due to specific cause}}{\text{Total number of maternal deaths due to all causes}} \times 100$$

Figure 22.1 presents the most frequent causes of maternal death during pregnancy by time of pregnancy. On the day of delivery, through 6 days postpartum, the most frequent cause of death is hemorrhage. From 43 days to 1 year postpartum, the most frequent cause of death is cardiomyopathy.

The perinatal mortality rate is a measure of the deaths occurring during the perinatal period. The perinatal mortality rate formula is:

Perinatal mortality rate

$$= \frac{\begin{array}{c}\text{Number of deaths during the perinatal period (22 weeks' gestation through 7 days of life) in a specific time period}\end{array}}{\begin{array}{c}\text{Total number of births (live births plus fetal deaths) during the same time period}\end{array}} \times 100$$

The neonatal mortality rate measures the deaths of live infants during the neonatal period. The neonatal mortality rate formula is:

Neonatal mortality rate

$$= \frac{\begin{array}{c}\text{Number of live-born infants who die within <28 days of life in a specific time period}\end{array}}{\begin{array}{c}\text{Number of live births in the specific time period}\end{array}} \times 1,000$$

Low-birth-weight percentage measures the number of infants born at less than 2500 g. The low-birth-weight percentage formula is:

Low−birth−weight percentage formula

$$= \frac{\begin{array}{c}\text{Number of live born infants weighing less than 2500 g in a given time period}\end{array}}{\begin{array}{c}\text{Total number of live births in the same time period}\end{array}} \times 100$$

Stillbirth rate is a measure of the number of infants born dead. The stillbirth rate formula is:

Stillbirth rate =

$$\frac{\begin{array}{c}\text{Number of infants >21 weeks/500 g born dead in a specific time period}\end{array}}{\begin{array}{c}\text{Total number of live births and stillbirths in the same time period}\end{array}}$$

Figure 22.2 presents the trend of stillbirth deaths in the United States. In this figure, the dark purple line shows the rate of early stillbirth, meaning at 20 to 27 completed weeks' of gestation. The light purple line shows the rate

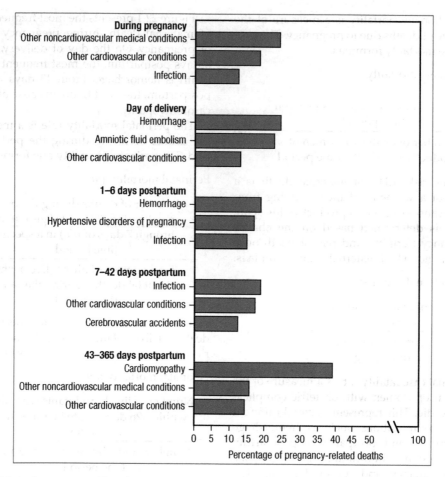

Figure 22.1 Cause-specific pregnancy-related deaths by end of pregnancy time—United States, 2011 to 2015.

Source: From Petersen, E. E., Davis, N. L., Goodman, D., Cox, S., Mayes, N., Johnston, E., Syverson, C., Seed K., Shapiro-Mendoza, C. K., Callaghan, W. M., & Barfield, W. (2019). Vital signs: Pregnancy-related deaths, United States, 2011–2015, and strategies for prevention, 13 states, 2013–2017. *MMWR Morbidity Mortality Weekly Report, 68*, 423–429. https://doi.org/10.15585/mmwr.mm6818e1

of late stillbirth, meaning at 28 or more completed weeks of pregnancy. Figure 22.3 presents the race-specific stillbirth rates. This figure indicates that the stillbirth rate is higher in the non-Hispanic Black population followed by the American Indian or Alaska Native with the lowest stillbirth rate evident in the Asian or Pacific Islander population.

Reproductive Health Outcome and Process Indicators

Some other common reproductive health outcome and process indicators are presented in the following. These epidemiologic metrics are used for healthcare service planning and management activities to ensure appropriate allocation of human, fiscal, and physical resources.

Antenatal care coverage provides a measure of access to care and the provision of antenatal care. The antenatal care coverage formula is:

Antenatal care coverage

$$= \frac{\begin{array}{c}\text{Number of pregnant women who attend at}\\\text{least one antenatal care visit by a provider}\\\text{and deliver in the specific time period}\end{array}}{\begin{array}{c}\text{Number of live births in the specific time}\\\text{period}\end{array}}$$

Infant vaccination coverage provides a measure of access to infant vaccinations and acceptance of the vaccination program by the population. The infant vaccination coverage formula is:

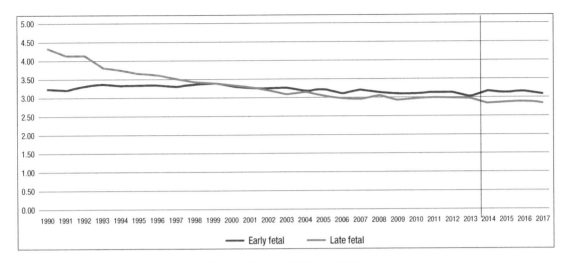

Figure 22.2 Stillbirth rate in the United States: 1990 to 2017.

Note: Starting with 2014 data, the obstetric estimate of gestation at delivery replaced the gestational age measure based on the date of the last normal menses, introducing a discontinuity in early and late fetal mortality rates from earlier years; rates calculated using the different measures are noncomparable.

Source: Centers for Disease Control and Prevention/National Center for Health Statistics, National Vital Statistics System. *Fetal death public-use file, 2017*. https://www.cdc.gov/ncbddd/stillbirth/data.html

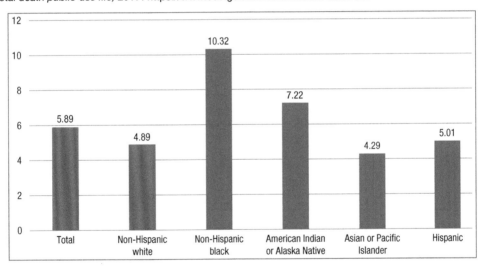

Figure 22.3 Stillbirth rate by race/ethnicity: 2017.

Source: Centers for Disease Control and Prevention/National Center for Health Statistics, National Vital Statistics System. *Fetal death public-use file, 2017*. https://www.cdc.gov/ncbddd/stillbirth/data.html

Infant vaccination coverage:

$$= \frac{\begin{array}{c}\text{Number of children 12 to 23 months of age}\\\text{who were fully vaccinated before their first}\\\text{birthday}\end{array}}{\text{Number of children 12 to 23 months of age}}$$

Referral rate is the number of women who have actual or potential obstetric complications that are referred to another provider, generally for specialized care. The referral rate formula is:

Referral rate

$$= \frac{\begin{array}{c}\text{Number of women with potential or actual}\\\text{obstetric complication referred to another}\\\text{provider}\end{array}}{\begin{array}{c}\text{Total number of women with obstetric com-}\\\text{plications in the same geographic area and}\\\text{time period}\end{array}}$$

Cesarean section rate measures the women who had a cesarean section in a specific geographical area during a specific time period. The cesarean section rate formula is:

Cesarean section rate

$$= \frac{\begin{array}{c}\text{Number of live-born infants deliv-}\\\text{ered by cesarean section in a specific}\\\text{geographical location in a specific}\\\text{time period}\end{array}}{\begin{array}{c}\text{Number of live-borne infants in a}\\\text{specific geographical location in the}\\\text{specified time period}\end{array}} \times 100$$

Figure 22.4 presents the method of delivery rates, including cesarean section rate, from 2016 to 2018 demonstrating that the total cesarean rate remains consistent in 2016 and 2018 at 31.9% but from 2017 to 2018, there was a slight decrease in the total cesarean rate from 32% to 31.9%.

Provider delivery rate is a measure of the proportion of deliveries attended by a specific provider or provider type, such as an obstetrician or nurse midwife. The provider delivery rate can be calculated to compare geographical or facility metrics. The provider delivery rate formula is:

Provider delivery rate

$$= \frac{\begin{array}{c}\text{Number of deliveries by the provider}\\\text{or provider type in the geographic}\\\text{area (or facility)}\end{array}}{\begin{array}{c}\text{All live births during the time period}\\\text{and in the same geographical area as}\\\text{the numerator (or facility)}\end{array}} \times 100$$

Site delivery rate is a measure of the proportion of births by a specific site such as a birthing center, home, or hospital. The site delivery rate formula is:

Site delivery rate

$$= \frac{\begin{array}{c}\text{Deliveries by site type in a specific}\\\text{time period}\end{array}}{\begin{array}{c}\text{All live births during the same time}\\\text{period and in the same geographical}\\\text{area as numerator}\end{array}} \times 100$$

REPRODUCTIVE TRACT INFECTION EPIDEMIOLOGY

Reproductive tract infections consist of STIs, endogenous infections caused by organism overgrowth in the genital tract, and iatrogenic infections associated with medical procedures (Patel et al., 2003). Reproductive tract infections are considered preventable and treatable with primary and secondary prevention measures. The burden of reproductive tract infections can be asymptomatic with some symptoms not being recognizable or differentiated.

The common etiologic agents for reproductive tract infections are bacterial, parasitic, and viral. The common mode of transmission includes mucous membranes during unprotected vaginal, anal, or oral intercourse with an

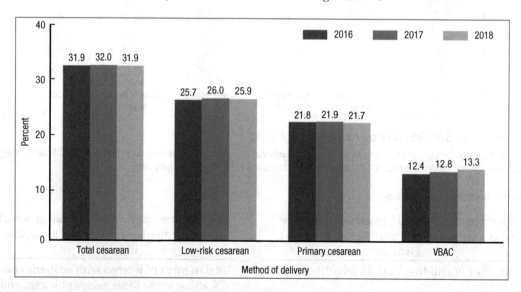

Figure 22.4 Method of delivery, United States, 2016 to 2018.

Note: Low-risk cesarean is cesarean delivery among nulliparous, term, singleton, and cephalic births. VBAC is vaginal birth after cesarean.

Source: National Center for Health Statistics, National Vital Statistics System, Natality. https://www.cdc.gov/nchs/data/nvsr/nvsr68/nvsr68_13-508.pdf

infected individual. Maternal to fetal transmission is possible with reproductive tract infections. Reproductive tract risk and probability of transmission is higher from males to females than females to males. This is often referred to as "biological sexism." Biological sexism exists when the anatomical sex characteristics facilitate efficient transmission of reproductive tract infections. The reproductive tract infections' rate of spread is measured by the average number of new cases resulting from each infected individual. The average number of new reproductive tract infection cases caused by each infected individual is called the basic reproductive rate of infection or R_0 (Patel et al., 2003).

The reproductive rate of infection (R_0) is determined by the average probability that infection is transmitted from an infected individual to a susceptible individual (known as beta, β), the effective mean rate of sexual partner change (c), and the average duration of infectivity of an individual (D). Efficiency of transmission (β) depends on the infectiousness of the pathological agent, infectivity of the individual, host susceptibility, and type of sexual contact. The effective mean rate of sexual partner change is the average number of sexual partners per person per unit of time, heterogeneity in rates of sexual partner change, patterns of sexual contact, and types of preventive or prophylaxis utilized. Duration of infection is the period of time the infected individual is infected with the pathological agent. Duration of infection is affected by early detection and treatment measures. Other factors known to affect the transmission of reproductive tract infections, specifically STIs, are biological, behavioral, medical, social, and economic. Some biological factors are duration of infectivity, presence of reproductive tract or sexually transmitted co-infections, pathogen infectivity strain, age and presence of cervical or other mucosal erosion, immunologic status, and circumcision status. Behavioral factors are the rate of sexual partner change, type of sexual behaviors, use of prophylaxis, and patterns of sexual contact and mixing. Medical factors are access to healthcare services, access to laboratory or diagnostic testing, and availability of treatment. Social and economic factors are migration patterns, ease of travel, educational level, religion, civil unrest, women's position in society, and poverty (Patel et al., 2003). This formula is represented as:

Reproductive tract transmission rate (STI rate)

$$R_0 = \beta c D$$

As the rate of reproductive transmission exceeds 1.0, this determines the rapidity by which an infection can potentially spread through a community.

There is an interactive effect of reproductive tract infections impacting reproductive health. Sequelae from reproductive tract infections can impact an individual's reproductive health. These sequelae result in long-term reproductive health outcomes. Some measures for long-term reproductive health outcomes are reproductive tract infection prevalence, infertility rate, reproductive tract infection cause-specific mortality rate, or congenital syphilis or ophthalmia neonatorum.

Reproductive tract infection target population prevalence is the number of individuals diagnosed with a specific reproductive tract infection or syndrome at a specific point in time per 100,000 persons in the population. The formula for reproductive tract target population prevalence is:

Reproductive tract target population

$$= \frac{\begin{array}{c}\text{Number of reproductive tract} \\ \text{infections by syndromic signs} \\ \text{or symptoms or etiologic} \\ \text{identification}\end{array}}{\begin{array}{c}\text{Number of people in population} \\ \text{segment screened or covered by} \\ \text{case reports}\end{array}} \times 100,000$$

Infertility rate is the proportion of sexually active, noncontracepting individuals in a reproductive age group (typically 15–45 years of age) at risk for pregnancy who have not had any pregnancy in the previous 5 years. The formula for infertility rate is:

Infertility rate

$$= \frac{\begin{array}{c}\text{Number of women of reproduc-} \\ \text{tive age (15–45) not using con-} \\ \text{traceptives (now and within the} \\ \text{past 5 years), not pregnant, and} \\ \text{not pregnant in the last 5 years}\end{array}}{\begin{array}{c}\text{Total number of women of repro-} \\ \text{ductive age at risk for pregnancy} \\ \text{and not using contraception}\end{array}} \times 100,000$$

Figure 22.5 presents the live birth and fertility rates in the United States trending from 1970 to 2018. The number of live births and fertility rate has been decreasing since 2014.

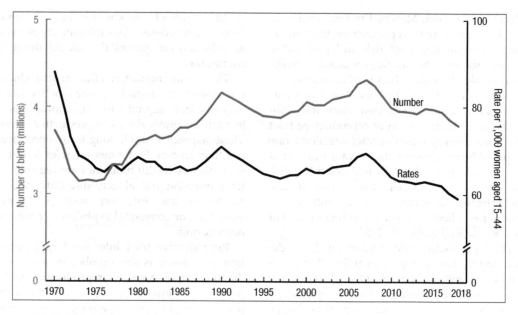

Figure 22.5 Live births and fertility rates, United States, 1970 to 2018.

Source: National Center for Health Statistics, National Vital Statistics System, Natality. https://www.cdc.gov/nchs/data/nvsr/nvsr68/nvsr68_13-508.pdf

Reproductive tract infection (RTI) or STI cause-specific mortality rate is an estimation of RTI or STI related deaths. The reproductive tract infection or STI cause-specific mortality rate formula is:

RTI or STI cause–specific mortality rate

$$= \frac{\text{Number of deaths (male or female) aged 15 to 49 years due to specific RTI or STI}}{\text{Total number of individuals (male or female) aged 15 to 49}} \times 100,000$$

Congenital syphilis or ophthalmia neonatorum rate is the number of infants born infected with syphilis or gonococcal/chlamydial eye infections during a period of time per 100,000 live births. The congenital syphilis or ophthalmia neonatorum infection rate is:

Congenital syphilis or ophthalmia neonatorum infection rate

$$= \frac{\text{Number of cases of infants born with congenital syphilis or ophthalmia neonatorum}}{\text{Number of live births among population represented by the case reports}} \times 100,000$$

Figure 22.6 presents the number of congenital syphilis cases. The cases of congenital syphilis have continued to increase since 2014.

MATERNAL MORTALITY CLASSIFICATIONS

The Tenth Revision of the International Classification of Diseases, known as ICD-10, classifies maternal mortality as the death of a woman temporal to pregnancy, childbirth, or the postpartum period, regardless of the cause (etiology) of the death. Maternal mortality is further differentiated into categories. Direct maternal death is death of a woman resulting from an obstetric implication of the pregnancy state, inclusive of pregnancy, labor, and puerperal mood period. An indirect maternal death is a death of a woman caused by a nonobstetric condition or disease that may exist before the pregnancy and may be aggravated by the pregnancy state, such as cardiac disease, hypertension, or diabetes mellitus. Coincidental maternal death causes are maternal death resulting from coincidental causes of death during pregnancy, childbirth, and the puerperium period such as suicide or homicide. Unspecified maternal death causes are maternal death resulting from an unspecified cause during pregnancy, childbirth, and the puerperium period. Late maternal death is a maternal death from direct or indirect obstetric causes more than 42 days but less than 1 year after pregnancy termination (Patwardhan et al., 2016).

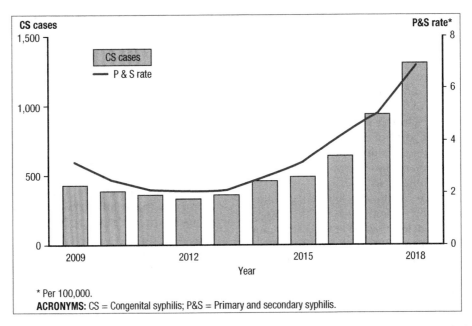

Figure 22.6 Congenital syphilis cases ages 15 to 44 in the United States—2009 to 2018.

*Per 100,000.

CS, congenital syphilis; P&S, primary and secondary syphilis.

In 2018, there were a total of 1,306 reported cases of congenital syphilis, including 78 syphilitic stillbirths and 16 infant deaths, and a national rate of 33.1 cases per 100,000 live births. This rate represents a 39.7% increase relative to 2017 (23.7 cases per 100,000 live births) and a 185.3% increase relative to 2014 (11.6 cases per 100,000 live births). As has been observed historically, this increase in the congenital syphilis rate has paralleled increases in P&S syphilis among all women and reproductive-aged women during 2014 to 2018 (172.7% and 165.4% increases, respectively).

Source: From https://www.cdc.gov/std/stats18/fignatpro.htm#syphilis

REPRODUCTIVE AND MATERNAL DATA SOURCES

The following are some reproductive and maternal data sources:

1. The Pregnancy Risk Assessment Monitoring System (PRAMS) collects state-specific, population-based data on maternal attitudes and experiences prior to, during, and immediately following pregnancy.
2. Harvard School of Public Health Maternal Child Health Data Connect is a comprehensive online database catalogue of maternal child health datasets, interactive tools, and other data sources for healthcare professionals, researchers, policymakers, and students.

3. Centers for Disease Control and Prevention collects surveillance data in the following ways:
   a. Pregnancy Mortality Surveillance System collects pregnancy related mortality data from all states
   b. Sudden Unexpected Infant Death (SUID) and Sudden Infant Death Syndrome (SIDS) collect data on SUID by cause and trends, SUID rates over time, and demographic diversity of SUID.
4. March of Dimes provides an online source of perinatal statistics at the national, state, county, and city level.

END-OF-CHAPTER RESOURCES

SUMMARY POINTS

- Reproductive processes consist of the physical, mental, and social well-being associated with the reproductive system.
- Reproductive health includes the ability to regulate and control fertility, safe birthing process, safe parenting, infant and child health survival, growth and development, and safety from STIs.
- Reproductive health surveillance provides the data for reproductive epidemiology, which is the determination of the distribution and determinants of reproductive health.
- Impact indicators reflect changes in the primary health event generally expressed as morbidity and mortality data.
- Outcome indicators represent changes in the knowledge, skills, attitudes, behaviors, or availability of services resulting from reproductive health programs.
- Process indicators assess the actions taken and implemented as a means to achieve the expected programmatic outcomes.
- Low-birth-weight percentage measures the number of infants born less than 2,500 g.
- Reproductive tract infections consist of STIs, endogenous infections caused by organism overgrowth in the genital tract, and iatrogenic infections associated with medical procedures.
- Biological sexism exists when the anatomical sex characteristics facilitate efficient transmission of reproductive tract infections.
- The effective mean rate of sexual partner change is the average number of sexual partners per person per unit of time, heterogeneity in rates of sexual partner change, patterns of sexual contact, and types of preventive or prophylaxis utilized.
- Duration of infection is the period of time the infected individual is infected with the pathological agent.
- Medical factors are access to healthcare services, access to laboratory or diagnostic testing, and availability of treatment.
- Direct maternal death is death of a woman resulting from an obstetric implication of the pregnancy state, inclusive of pregnancy, labor, and puerperal mood period.
- An indirect maternal death is a death of a woman caused by a nonobstetric condition or disease that may exist before the pregnancy and may be aggravated by the pregnancy state.
- Coincidental maternal death causes are maternal death resulting from coincidental causes of death during pregnancy, childbirth, and the puerperium period.
- Unspecified maternal death causes are maternal death resulting from an unspecified cause during pregnancy, childbirth, and the puerperium period.
- Late maternal death is a maternal death from direct or indirect obstetric causes more than 42 days but less than 1 year after pregnancy termination.

EPIDEMIOLOGY CRITICAL REASONING QUESTIONS

1. During January 1, 2019 to December 31, 2019, there were 311,000 live births in the United States. The Unites States population in 2019 was 382,200,000 people. There were a total of 800 maternal deaths, 250 perinatal deaths (22 weeks' gestation to 7 days of life), and 313,752 low-birth-weight infants born.
   a. Calculate the maternal mortality ratio (MMR).
   b. Calculate the stillbirth death rate.
   c. Calculate perinatal mortality rate.
   d. Calculate low-birth-weight percentage.
2. Describe some determinants of reproductive rate of infection.
3. Differentiate the maternal mortality classifications—direct, indirect, coincidental, unspecified, and late.

ADDITIONAL RESOURCES

| SPRINGER PUBLISHING CONNECT™ | A robust set of instructor resources designed to supplement this text is located at http://connect. |

springerpub.com/content/book/978-0-8261-8514-3. Qualifying instructors may request access by emailing textbook@springerpub.com.

REFERENCES

Curtis, K., Patel, D., & Osisanya, T. (2003). *Public health surveillance applied to reproductive health*. Centers for Disease Control and Prevention.

Patel, D., Burnett, N., & Curtis, K. (2003). *Reproductive tract infections*. Centers for Disease Control and Prevention.

Patwardhan, M., Eckert, L., Siegel, H., Pourmalek, F., Cutland, C., Kochhar, S., & Gonik, B. (2016). Maternal death: Case definition and guidelines for data collection, analysis, and presentation of immunization safety data. *Vaccine, 34,* 6077–6083. https://doi.org/10.1016/j.vaccine.2016.03.042

Chapter 23

CLINICAL AND HEALTHCARE EPIDEMIOLOGY AND EVIDENCE-BASED HEALTHCARE

Demetrius J. Porche

I believe in evidence-based decision making. I want to know what the facts are.
–Hillary Clinton

CHAPTER COMPETENCIES

At the conclusion of this chapter, the reader will be able to:

1. Describe the practice of healthcare epidemiology
2. Determine the existence of nosocomial or hospital-acquired infections
3. Calculate hospital-acquired infection rates
4. Describe evidence-based healthcare practice

ESSENTIAL TERMINOLOGY

Essential clinical and healthcare epidemiologic terms are:

- Antibiogram
- Clinical epidemiology
- Evidence-based practice
- Healthcare epidemiologist
- Hospital-acquired infections
- Hospital epidemiologist
- Nosocomial infections
- Primary care epidemiology

Clinical epidemiology is considered a basic science of medical practice that informs diagnostic, prognostic, and therapeutic clinical decisions related to individual healthcare (Hannaford et al., 2006). Healthcare epidemiology broadens the scope of clinical epidemiology to include various types of healthcare settings not limited to the acute care setting. Healthcare epidemiology is a more comprehensive term to use to designate epidemiology of clinical care in both acute and primary care settings. This chapter provides an overview of healthcare epidemiology, inclusive of clinical infectious hospital-acquired infections, and the basis of healthcare epidemiological data in evidence-based healthcare.

HEALTHCARE EPIDEMIOLOGY

The healthcare epidemiologist is a leader in infection prevention and healthcare epidemiology programs. Healthcare epidemiologists were formally known as hospital epidemiologists. Historically, hospital epidemiologist were primarily focused on infectious disease epidemiology within the hospital setting and nosocomial infections. Hospital epidemiologists were also responsible for the development of patient safety programs and developed occupational health programs in collaboration with employee health for hospital employees (Hierholzer, 1982). Hospital epidemiologists are also referred to as infection preventionists. Nurses can fulfill the role of healthcare epidemiologist, hospital epidemiologist, or infection control preventionist. As the role of the hospital epidemiologist has expanded and changed, so has the focus. Hospital epidemiology focused on nosocomial infections, which are infections that are not present or incubating at the time the patient is admitted to the hospital. However, the healthcare epidemiologist is concerned with not only nosocomial or hospital acquired infections but also hospital acquired injuries or alterations occurring from noninfectious origins. Common hospital-acquired infections are catheter-associated urinary tract infections (CAUTIs), central line-associated bloodstream infections (CLABSIs), ventilator associated pneumonia (VAP), hospital acquired pneumonia (HAP), and surgical site infections (SSIs; Sydnor & Perl, 2011).

The term *healthcare epidemiologist* is currently preferred with the shift and inclusion of healthcare services in the outpatient setting and expansion of the role to other hospital-related conditions. Healthcare epidemiologists engage in various roles that consist of epidemiologist, subject matter expert, continuous quality improvement leader, regulatory compliance, public health liaison, administrator, clinician, outcomes evaluator and researcher (Kaye et al., 2015). A fundamental role of the healthcare epidemiologist is the identification of risk, understanding of risks factors, and development of programs to minimize or eliminate risk.

Healthcare epidemiologists apply epidemiologic science to the healthcare setting. They examine causes and patterns of disease within the healthcare population. The information gathered from healthcare epidemiology is used to develop quality improvement projects, develop evidence-based practice guidelines, and inform areas of research inquiry. Healthcare epidemiologists work within the health care system to develop surveillance systems across departments and healthcare institutions to identify for quality improvement, program development, and policy formulation or changes.

Healthcare epidemiologists are expert clinicians that provide information and education in areas such as but not limited to infectious diseases, infection control and prevention principles, antibiotic stewardship, occupational health and safety, and prevention of hospital or healthcare acquired infections or health conditions, along with regulatory compliance guidance. Nurses' knowledge base about disease processes, disease transmission, pathophysiology, pharmacology, and hospital processes makes the nurse an excellent candidate to serve as a healthcare epidemiologist. Kaye et al. (2015) identify some core competencies for the healthcare epidemiologist. These core competencies are:

- Surveillance systems
- Epidemiologic data management and analysis
- Infectious disease pathogens and transmission
- Infection control and prevention measures
- Outbreak investigation
- Antibiotic stewardship
- Microbiology and laboratory testing—institutional antibiogram
- Quality improvement science
- Provision of care to special populations and in nonacute care settings
- Leadership skills
- Program implementation, assessment, and advocacy
- Outcomes assessment, program evaluation, and research methods
- Public health and emergency preparedness
- Teaching and learning skills for educational purposes

Healthcare epidemiologists remain responsible for the development of infection control and prevention programs. Some essential components of infection control and prevention programs are:

- Surveillance of nosocomial or hospital-acquired infections/injuries
- Outbreak investigation
- Policy and procedure development and implementation of isolation and quarantine measures
- Policy and procedure development and implementation to reduce risks
- Collaboration with occupational or employee health
- Infection control and prevention education and training
- Monitor and surveillance of aseptic, sanitation, and sterile techniques
- Monitor antibiotic utilization and microbiology specimen sensitivities (produce antibiogram)
- Elimination of wasteful or unnecessary procedures that present risks
- Collaboration with quality improvement program
- Consultation and collaboration with local and state public health surveillance programs

The future of healthcare epidemiology will be challenged with emerging infectious diseases and collaborations required across healthcare professions and institutions to detect, diagnose, understand, monitor, and prevent healthcare-associated infections and other health conditions. Healthcare epidemiologists will need to develop and work within local, regional, and national healthcare surveillance systems, possibly extending across country boundaries. Recent pandemics have emphasized the need to have integrated global surveillance systems that promote global harmonization to prevent and control the spread of communicable diseases. Healthcare epidemiologists will be challenged to advocate for the provision of "invasive device-free healthcare" or at least limiting their utilization to prevent healthcare-associated infections and injuries (Gerberding, 2010). Surveillance systems and outbreak investigations are critical components of healthcare epidemiology programs.

NOSOCOMIAL INFECTIONS (HOSPITAL-ACQUIRED INFECTIONS)

Nosocomial infections are infections acquired during hospitalization. Nosocomial infections are most commonly referred to as hospital-acquired infections (HAIs). An HAI is defined as:

- An infection that is acquired during hospitalization and which was not present or incubating at the time of admission to the hospital
- An infection acquired in the hospital that becomes evident after discharge from the hospital
- A newborn infection that is the result of exposure during delivery—cesarean or vaginal birth (Straif-Bourgeois et al., 2014)

An HAI should include an infectious process, not just colonization. There needs to be sufficient time after hospitalization for the infection to occur and present. A true infection is one in which the infection is accompanied by signs and symptoms of an infection such as but not limited to fever, malaise, inflammation, warmth at site to touch, pain, and erythema. The typical time period allocated to determine if an infection is hospital acquired is dependent on the offending organism's incubation period. An infection is classified as an HAI if the patient has been in the hospital for a stay greater than or equal to the offending organism's incubation period. Some institutions use a standard time period of 48 hours or 2 days after hospital admission for the classification of an HAI (Straif-Bourgeois

et al., 2014). Nurses are considered the "last line of defense" for the patient by ensuring asepsis and sterility are maintained appropriately while administering patient interventions.

The calculation of HAIs provides an opportunity to examine the distribution of infections within the hospital. Rates are the common epidemiologic measure used for HAIs. The numerator consists of number of infections, or the number of patients infected. If there is an infection caused by multiple organisms of similar origin at the same site, then this is considered a single infection for the purpose of calculating a rate. If a patient has a previously established HAI, a second HAI would be counted as a case in two instances—the second infection is at a new or different site or there is a new and different organism cultured provided the patient's condition is deteriorating. The denominator for the calculation of HAI consists of the number of patients admitted (or discharged), number of hospital days, or the number of device days.

There are several types of HAI rates calculated. A hospital-wide HAI provides an overall infection rate for the entire hospital. A HAI hospital-wide rate can be calculated for a month, quarter, or year. The formula for a HAI hospital-wide rate is:

Hospital-wide HAI

$$= \frac{\text{Number of HAIs (month, quarter, or year)}}{\text{Number of patients admitted (month, quarter, or year)}} \times 100$$

Generally, a hospital-wide rate calculated with this formula is expressed as per 100 admissions.

HAIs can be calculated for comparison at the unit level of the hospital. These are generally referred to as unit specific rates such as an intensive care unit (ICU) HAI rate. The unit specific rate is generally expressed as per 1,000 hospital days. There can be a rate of infection for the unit, or a rate of patients infected for the unit. The formulas follow:

Rate of infection for the specific unit

$$= \frac{\text{Number of infections on the unit during a specific time period}}{\text{Number of hospital days on unit during a specific time period}} \times 1{,}000 \text{ hospital days}$$

Rate of patients infected for the specific unit

$$= \frac{\begin{array}{c}\text{Number of patients} \\ \text{infected on the unit} \\ \text{during a specific time} \\ \text{period}\end{array}}{\begin{array}{c}\text{Number of hospital} \\ \text{days on unit during a} \\ \text{specific time period}\end{array}} \times 1{,}000 \text{ hospital days}$$

Infections occur as a result of many acute care interventions. HAIs may occur as a result of surgical procedures or the use of acute care devices such as ventilators or intravenous catheters. HAI rates can be calculated for both surgical interventions and devices. The surgical site specific (SSI) rate HAI formula is:

SSI rate

$$= \frac{\begin{array}{c}\text{Number of SSIs in a specific time} \\ \text{period}\end{array}}{\begin{array}{c}\text{Number of patients operated on in a} \\ \text{specific time period}\end{array}} \times 100$$

Device-specific rates are calculated separately for each specific device. The following steps are used to calculate a device-associated infection rate. The method for calculating device-associated infection rates involve five steps. These five steps are:

1. Decide on the time period of analysis: a month, quarter (3 months), 6 months, or a year. This determines the time period of all data collection and the time period for comparison of infection rates.
2. Select the patient population for analysis or the unit/area of the hospital. This determines the population to be included in the numerator and denominator for consistent population comparison.
3. Select the type of infections to be included in the numerator. These infections can be site specific, patient-population specific, or occurring during a specific period of time.
4. Determine the number of device days that should be used in the denominator. Device days are the total number of days of exposure to a device by all patients in the selected population during the specific period of time that they have the device.
5. Calculate the final device-associated infection rate using the multiplier of 1,000 device days. Two exemplars of device-associated infection rate formulas are provided: the VAP rate formula and the CLABSI rate formula:

VAP rate

$$= \frac{\begin{array}{c}\text{Number of VAPs in a specific time} \\ \text{period}\end{array}}{\begin{array}{c}\text{Number of patients on a ventilator} \\ \text{by days}\end{array}} \times 1{,}000$$

CLABSI rate

$$= \frac{\begin{array}{c}\text{Number of catheter-related blood} \\ \text{stream infections in specific period} \\ \text{of time}\end{array}}{\begin{array}{c}\text{Number of patients with intrave-} \\ \text{nous catheter by days}\end{array}} \times 100$$

Device utilization rate (DUR) can be calculated for comparison of device risk over a period of time. The DUR expresses risk based on the amount of time the device is used. The DUR is the proportion of patient days for which a certain device is utilized during the patient's hospitalization. The DUR is calculated for specific devices, just as there are catheter utilization rates and ventilator utilization rates. The DUR calculation method includes five steps which are:

1. Decide on the time period for analysis: a month, a quarter (3 months), 6 months, or a year.
2. Select the patient population for analysis: type of hospital unit or patient population.
3. Determine the number of device days to be used in the numerator. Device days is the total number of days of exposure or use of a device (such as urinary catheter or ventilator) by all patients in the selected population.
4. Determine the number of patient days for the denominator. The number of patient days is the total number of days that all patients are in the hospital unit during the specific time period.
5. Calculate the DUR using the following formula.

The DUR is an indirect measure of patient severity as it indicates the length of time a device is used by patients. The formula for DUR is:

$$\text{DUR} = \frac{\text{Number of device days}}{\text{Number of patient days}} \times 100$$

The last HAI measure for discussion is the standardized infection ratio (SIR). The SIR is a summary measure that compares the HAI occurrence among one or more patient groups to that of a standard population. The SIR is considered an indirect standardization method and is used to examine at an aggregate level the differences of HAI among groups. The formula for SIR is:

$$SIR = \frac{Observed\ (O)\ HAIs}{Expected\ (E)\ HAIs}$$

In this formula, O is calculated as the sum of the number of HAI rates among a group and E is calculated using an appropriate risk-adjusted aggregate data rate.

HEALTHCARE EPIDEMIOLOGY SURVEILLANCE SYSTEM, OUTBREAK INVESTIGATIONS, AND INCIDENT MANAGEMENT

Healthcare epidemiologists generally have the responsibility to establish or consult on the establishment of surveillance systems throughout the healthcare institution. These surveillance systems are used to establish baseline rates, detect and monitor outbreaks, identify areas for risk management and quality improvement, provide evidence to support policy and procedure decisions, assess the impact and effectiveness of interventions, guide antibiotic administration practices, and provide inter-institutional data for benchmarking and comparison. The surveillance system also establishes process measures to monitor interventions and procedures such as vaccination rates among healthcare workers, hand hygiene compliance rates, and compliance with surgical antibiotic prophylaxis. The establishment of a surveillance system must include:

- Clear goals and objectives of the surveillance system
- Standardized case definitions
- Valid and reliable tools/instruments to collect data
- Established and consistent epidemiologic formulas for the calculation of rates (Sydnor & Perl, 2011)

There are various types of surveillance systems employed in the healthcare setting. The surveillance system can be hospital-wide a prevalence survey, a targeted survey, or periodic surveillance. Hospital-wide surveillance is comprehensive in breadth with the application of prospective continuous surveys of all areas in the healthcare facility. Hospital-wide is a labor intensive and expensive surveillance system.

The prevalence survey surveillance focuses on a specific disease or health condition identifying all cases (new and existing) in a specific area of the institution in a specific time period. Targeted surveillance focuses on selected areas of the hospital, selected patient populations, selected procedures, or selected organisms, such as *Clostridium difficile* or vancomycin-resistant enterococcus. Targeted surveillance can be site specific also, such as urinary tract infections. Periodic surveillance systems are conducted during specified time intervals such as monitoring an area for 1 month twice a year (Sydnor & Perl, 2011).

Some other types of surveillance systems are surveillance by objectives, rotating, and outbreak surveillance. Surveillance by objects focuses on specific outcome objectives defined by the healthcare epidemiologist. The objectives could prioritize surveillance based on morbidity data, costs of treatment, length of stay, or frequency of infection occurrence. Rotating surveillance is a period and systematic surveillance plan that focuses on specific units or areas of the healthcare institution at specified periods of time. Lastly, outbreak surveillance systems focus on a cluster of infectious events.

The surveillance system assists the healthcare epidemiologist to determine if there is an outbreak of a specific infection or an increase in specific diseases, health alterations, or injuries in the healthcare facility (Sydnor & Perl, 2011). The healthcare epidemiologist uses the same steps to conduct an outbreak investigation as outlined in Chapter 17.

The surveillance systems also alert healthcare epidemiologists to other incidents occurring within the healthcare environment. Healthcare epidemiologists get involved in incident management, which consists of activities that an organization engages in to prepare for, respond to, and learn from an event or hazard. These events can be institution focused, local such as a flood or fire, or larger events such as responding to the COVID-19 pandemic. The healthcare epidemiologist, as an experienced outbreak investigator, has a vital role in the all-hazards assessments (Banach et al., 2017). Specific activities and areas of responsibility for the healthcare epidemiologist in incident management are:

- **Preparedness:** Propose infection control and prevention training; identify and establish policies and procedures for specific pathogens, environmental decontamination, environmental safety, respiratory etiquette, postmortem care, impact on special populations; develop and implement surveillance systems; develop and implement occupational healthcare such as tracking healthcare workers, provision of personal protective equipment, post-exposure prophylaxis; and development of communication systems for risk management

- **Mitigation:** Monitor adequacy of personal protective equipment stockpile, isolation rooms, hand hygiene product availability; manage healthcare worker exposures; ensure adequate availability of reusable medical equipment; evaluate and recommend strategies based on mode of transmission of the agent
- **Response:** Identify and propose guidance based on the pathogen to include screening/triage, care protocols, isolation, and quarantine; monitor infection control and prevention activities; continue to manage postexposure prophylaxis to healthcare workers, patients, family members, and visitors; advise on postmortem placement, storage, and transfer; ensure open communication with public information officer and incident commander
- **Recovery:** Advise and collaborate on cleanup, garbage and waste disposal; stocking inventory of prophylaxis regimen and personal protective equipment; follow-up on exposures; participate in incident debriefing; conduct a postmortem analysis on infection control and prevention strategies; revise policies and procedures based on postmortem analysis
- **Future Prevention:** Conduct systematic quality improvement projects based on healthcare incident postmortem analysis with appropriate implementation of policies and procedures to improve incident management (Banach et al., 2017)

ANTIBIOGRAM

An antibiogram is constructed collaboratively between the healthcare epidemiologist and clinical laboratory professional. The antibiogram is generated from antibiotic sensitivity surveillance systems. An antibiogram is compiled from individual hospital monitoring of antibiotic sensitivity. The goal of this antibiogram sensitivity surveillance system and report is to estimate the proportion of selected bacteria that are resistant to antibiotics. This information is used by

healthcare providers who are prescribing antibiotics to know what antibiotics the common organisms in the respective healthcare institution are most likely to be sensitive to for therapeutic purposes (Straif-Bourgeois et al., 2014).

PRIMARY CARE EPIDEMIOLOGY

Primary care epidemiology was a term coined to describe the application of clinical epidemiology to primary care practice. Primary care epidemiology applies epidemiologic principles and methods to health care problems encountered within a primary care setting that include but is not limited to disease etiology, diagnosis, and all levels of prevention—primary, secondary, and tertiary. Primary care epidemiology is considered to be at the intersection of individual and community level care. The epidemiologic information gathered at the community level assists with understanding the clinical significance of risk factors and the absolute risk associated with interventions recommended in primary care practice. In addition, individual level information gathered informs population level information from which healthcare providers are responsible for delivering care (Hannaford et al., 2006). With each primary care clinical encounter, potential primary care epidemiology information is collected and documented. This clinical information at the individual primary care level can be used to inform population level epidemiology.

Primary care epidemiology facilitates the description of incidence, prevalence, illness severity and natural history of disease, signs and symptoms, and defined disease and health alterations occurring within a population or community. Primary care is a data source for investigating outbreaks, epidemics, and pandemics. Primary care provides an opportunity to collect epidemiologic data on individuals and entire families on a continuity level of care, as a result of the nature of primary care services. The scope and purpose of primary care epidemiology is influenced by the level of integration of primary care services into the healthcare system. An integrated acute and primary care system maximizes the potential for the provision of comprehensive individual, family, and population-based health oriented to the community. Primary care epidemiology also provides a means to evaluate the adequacy, effectiveness, and efficiency of primary care services (Hannaford et al., 2006).

EVIDENCE-BASED PRACTICE HEALTHCARE

Evidence-based practice is an inclusive term for the multiple healthcare- related disciplines such as but not limited to evidence-based medicine, evidence-based nursing, evidence-based public health, evidence-based dentistry. There are many definitions in the literature about what constitutes evidence-based practice. Regardless of the definition, evidence-based practice must include research evidence, clinical expertise and experience, nonresearch-based evidence, and patient expectations, values, and needs. The evidence-based practice process involves asking the right question; searching for the best evidence; critically appraising the evidence; determining the levels of evidence available; integrating clinical expertise and experience along with the patient's expectations, values, and needs; and evaluating the outcomes of your evidence-based practice decisions and interventions (Melnyk et al., 2010).

The Joanna Briggs Institute (JBI) has developed a framework to guide evidence-based practice that is situated within a context of healthcare evidence. The JBI conceptualizes evidence-based practice as "clinical decision-making that considers the best available evidence; the context in which the care is delivered, client preference and the professional judgment of health professional" (Jordan et al., 2019). The JBI Evidence-Based Healthcare Model proposes there are four major components of evidence-based practice—evidence generation, evidence synthesis, evidence transfer, and evidence utilization. For a thorough description of the JBI Evidence-Based Healthcare Model, the reader is directed to Jordan et al. (2019).

Levels of Evidence (Hierarchy): Joanna Briggs Institute

Evidence synthesis is dependent upon the critical appraisal of each piece of evidence so one must assess the methodological quality and consider the level of evidence. Using the level of evidence for the information based on the study design or type of evidence, epidemiologists can determine a preliminary judgment about the methodological quality and rigor of the evidence (JBI Levels of Evidence and Grades of Recommendation Working Party, 2014). The JBI has developed levels of evidence or evidence hierarchy for various types of studies. The JBI levels are presented here since these levels are congruent with the various types of epidemiologic studies conducted such as effectiveness, diagnostic, and prognostic. The JBI levels of evidence can be found here: https://jbi .global/sites/default/files/2019-05/JBI-Levels -of-evidence_2014_0.pdf (JBI Levels of Evidence and Grades of Recommendation Working Party, 2013).

END-OF-CHAPTER RESOURCES

SUMMARY POINTS

- Clinical epidemiology is considered a basic science of medical practice that informs diagnostic, prognostic, and therapeutic clinical decisions related to individual health care.
- Healthcare epidemiology is a more comprehensive term.
- Healthcare epidemiologists were formally known as hospital epidemiologists.
- Hospital epidemiologists are also referred to as infection preventionists.
- Healthcare epidemiologists remain responsible for the development of infection control and prevention programs.
- Recent pandemics have emphasized the need to have global integrated surveillance systems that promote global harmonization to prevent and control the spread of communicable diseases.
- Nosocomial infections are infections acquired during hospitalization.
- Nosocomial infections are most commonly referred to as hospital-acquired infections or HAIs.
- HAIs should include an infectious process, not just colonization.
- An infection is classified as an HAI if the patient has been in the hospital for a stay greater than or equal to the offending organism's incubation period.
- A hospital-wide HAI provides an overall infection rate for the entire hospital.
- The surveillance system can be hospital-wide, a prevalence survey, a targeted surveillance, or a periodic surveillance.
- The goal of the antibiogram sensitivity surveillance system and report is to estimate the proportion of selected bacteria that are resistant to antibiotics.
- Primary care epidemiology applies epidemiologic principles and methods to healthcare problems encountered within a primary care setting that include but are not limited to disease etiology, diagnosis, and all levels of prevention—primary, secondary, and tertiary.
- Evidence-based practice must include research evidence; clinical expertise and experience; nonresearch-based evidence; and patient expectations, values, and needs.
- The Joanna Briggs Institute Evidence-Based Healthcare Model proposes there are four major components of evidence-based practice—evidence generation, evidence synthesis, evidence transfer, and evidence utilization.
- Evidence synthesis is dependent upon the critical appraisal of each piece of evidence so one must assess the methodological quality and consider the level of evidence.

EPIDEMIOLOGY CRITICAL REASONING QUESTIONS

1. Hospital Dieu has a total hospital bed capacity of 400. During the month of August, there were a total of 30 patients who were determined to have a hospital-acquired infection. Hospital admissions for June were 280, August 320, and July 315. Calculate the hospital-wide acquired infection rate per 100 admissions.

2. Hospital Maxima has four acute care units—intensive care unit, cardiac care unit, surgical intensive care unit, and burn unit. The data presented are for the month of July. The number of hospital-acquired infections per unit were: intensive care unit 10, cardiac care unit 1, surgical intensive care unit 12, and burn unit 4. The number of patients infected on each unit were: intensive care unit 8, cardiac care unit 1, surgical intensive care unit 10, and burn unit 3. The number of hospital days for each unit was: intensive care unit 1,800, cardiac care unit was 1,525, surgical intensive care unit was 2,100, and burn unit was 800. Calculate each unit's specific infection rate for July. Also calculate the rate of patients infected for each unit.

3. Hospital Dieu has a robust surgical service line. The average number of surgeries conducted per month is 2,300. For the month of June, there were a total of 2,180 patients who had surgery. During the month of June, there were a total of 20 surgical site infections. Determine the surgical site infection rate for June.

4. In July, there were a total of 250 central venous catheters placed in patients. The total number of central venous catheter days for July was 875 days. There was a total of eight bloodstream infections in patients who had central venous catheters in place. Calculate the central venous line bloodstream infection rate for July.

ADDITIONAL RESOURCES

 SPRINGER PUBLISHING CONNECT™ | A robust set of instructor resources designed to supplement this text is located at http://connect. springerpub.com/content/book/978-0-8261-8514-3. Qualifying instructors may request access by emailing textbook@springerpub.com.

REFERENCES

Banach, D., Johnston, B., Al-Zubeidi, D., Bartlett, A., Bleasdale, S., Deloney, V., Enfield, K., Guzman-Cottrill, J., Lowe, C., Ostrosky-Zeichner, L., Popovich, K., Patel, P., Ravin, K., Rowe, T., Shenoy, E., Stienecker, R., Tosh, P., Trivedi, K., & The Outbreak Response Training Program Advisory Panel. (2017). Outbreak response and incident management: SHEA guidance and resources for healthcare epidemiologist in United States acute-care hospitals. *Infection Control & Hospital Epidemiology, 38*(12), 1393–1419. https://doi.org/10.1017/ice.2017.212

Gerberding, J. (2010). Healthcare epidemiology: Past and future. *Infection Control & Hospital Epidemiology, 31*(S1), S73–S75. https://doi.org/10.1086/656003

Hannaford, P., Smith, B., & Elliott, A. (2006). Primary care epidemiology: Its scope and purpose. *Family Practice, 23*, 1–7. https://doi.org/10.1093/fampra/cmi102

Hierholzer, W. (1982). The practice of hospital epidemiology. *The Yale Journal of Biology and Medicine, 55*, 225–230.

Joanna Briggs Institute Levels of Evidence and Grades of Recommendation Working Party. (2013). *JBI Levels of evidence.* https://joannabriggs.org/sites/default/files/2019-05/JBI-Levels-of-evidence_2014_0.pdf

Joanna Briggs Institute Levels of Evidence and Grades of Recommendation Working Party. (2014). *Supporting document for the Joanna Briggs Institute Levels of Evidence and Grades of Recommendation.* The Joanna Briggs Institute. https://joannabriggs.org/sites/default/files/2019-05/JBI%20Levels%20of%20Evidence%20Supporting%20Documents-v2.pdf

Jordan, Z., Lockwood, C., Munn, Z., & Aromataris, E. (2019). The updated Joanna Briggs Institute Model of Evidence-Based Healthcare. *International Journal of Evidence-Based Healthcare; 17*(1), 58–71. https://doi.org/10.1097/XEB.0000000000000155

Kaye, K., Anderson, D., Cook, E., Huang, S., Siegel, J., Zuckerman, J., & Talbot, T. (2015). Guidance for infection prevention and healthcare epidemiology programs: Healthcare epidemiologist skills and competencies. *Infection Control & Hospital Epidemiology, 36*(4), 369–380. https://doi.org/10.1017/ice.2014.79

Melnyk, B., Fineout-Overholt, E., Stillwell, S., & Williamson, K. (2010). Evidence-based practice: Step by step. The seven steps of evidence-based practice: Following this progressive, sequential approach will lead to improved health care and patient outcomes. *American Journal of Nursing, 110*(1), 51–55.

Straif-Bourgeois, S., Ratard, R., & Kretzschmar, M. (2014). Infectious disease epidemiology. In W. Agrees & I. Pigeon (Eds.), *Handbook of epidemiology* (2nd ed., pp. 2043–2119). Springer Science+Business Media.

Sydnor, E., & Perl, T. (2011). Hospital epidemiology and infection control in acute-care settings. *Clinical Microbiology Reviews, 24*(1), 141–173. https://doi.org/10.1128/CMR.00027-10

Section V:
Policy and Ethics

Chapter 24

EPIDEMIOLOGY IN HEALTH POLICY AND PROGRAM EVALUATION

Demetrius J. Porche

When you reach the end of your rope, tie a knot in it and hang on.
–Franklin D. Roosevelt

Real change, enduring change, happens one step at a time.
–Ruth Bader Ginsburg

CHAPTER COMPETENCIES

At the conclusion of this chapter, the reader will be able to:

1. Define health policy
2. Differentiate the types of policy
3. Describe the policy development process
4. Discuss the Centers for Disease Control and Prevention (CDC) Policy Process Model
5. Describe the CDC evaluation model
6. Differentiate the types of evaluation
7. Differentiate efficacy, effectiveness, and efficiency

ESSENTIAL TERMINOLOGY

Essential health policy and program evaluation terms are:

- Effectiveness
- Efficacy
- Efficiency
- Health policy
- Monitoring
- Outcome evaluation
- Policy
- Policy analysis
- Policy enactment
- Policy implementation
- Problem identification
- Quality improvement
- Systematic evaluation

Epidemiology provides the data from which to understand the distribution and determinants of health and health alterations within a population. Epidemiologic data can be used as the evidence base to substantiate the development of public health policy. In addition, epidemiologic measures can be used to generate the data necessary to substantiate public health program effectiveness. Essentially, epidemiologic measures serve as evaluative metrics to determine programmatic improvements in population health. Quality improvement metrics can be epidemiologically based for continual quality analysis. Nurses engage in public health policy development, implementation, evaluation, and analysis. Additionally, nurses are involved in policy advocacy for individuals and communities. The continual improvement of nursing practice and healthcare delivery resides within the scope of nursing practice.

WHAT IS HEALTH POLICY?

Policy and political strategies are used by healthcare professionals as a means to improve quality of life; eliminate health disparities; and promote individual, community, and societal changes. Policy development and formulation are population-based interventions used to impact the nation's health (Porche, 2019). Policy development and formulation can occur at the individual, group, aggregate, or institutional level with epidemiologic metrics associated at each level. Epidemiologically based policy is purposeful and goal directed.

An understanding of policy requires an understanding of the various policy definitions. Policy can be implied based on previous actions and behaviors or concrete in the manner of formal written policy. Policy generally provides the principles that govern an action directed toward a specific outcome; provides a stated position on an issue; outlines a plan of action by the government or an organization; or states authoritative statements, decisions, or guidelines outlined by the government or an organization. Health policy is one specific type of policy. Health policy encompasses the broad policy area of individual, group, aggregate, community, or population level health (Porche, 2019).

TYPES OF POLICY

As stated, health policy is one type of policy. There are many classifications of policy. In addition to health policy, Table 24.1 presents the definition of several policy types (Porche, 2019). These policy types are classified but may not be exclusively classified into only one category, depending on the policy intention. Policy intention is the expected or anticipated outcome of the respective policy.

CENTERS FOR DISEASE CONTROL AND PREVENTION POLICY MODEL

A model is a descriptive representation of a complex entity or process in a visual and understandable manner. Models are summative in nature to provide an overview of the specific topic. A model can consist of a narrative description and an associated figure or diagram presenting the relationship between the narrative descriptive statements. A policy model provides a description of the processes of developing, implementing, and evaluating policies or detailing the policy making process (Porche, 2019).

The Centers for Disease Control and Prevention (CDC) provides a nationally accepted policy model that can be applied to population-based community problems. The CDC's policy model is referred to as the CDC's Policy Process Model (Figure 24.1); it provides a systematic manner in which to develop policies that impact public health problems in the community. This policy model consists of five domains that include stakeholder engagement and evaluation. The five processes related steps of the model are problem identification, policy analysis, strategy and policy development, policy enactment, and policy implementation (CDC, 2019).

Table 24.1 Policy Types

Policy Type	Definition
Distributive	An allocative policy that spreads the benefits among the population
Institutional	Policies developed and implemented by an institution that affects only the member constituents of the respective institution
Legal	Policy founded on the laws or officially accepted rules formulated through legislative or executive governmental actions
Organizational	Policies developed by a board of directors that outline the decisions, positions, and official statements of the respective organization
Public	Policy that impacts the general public or citizens
Public health	Policy that impacts the health of the general population
Redistributive	An allocative policy that takes benefits, money, goods, or power from one group and provides it to another group
Regulatory	Regulations or rules that impose restrictions on individuals, groups, or populations
Social	Policy that impacts the general public welfare (human needs of education, housing, and instrumental social support)

Source: From Porche, D. (2019). *Health policy: Application for nurses and other healthcare professionals* (2nd ed.). Jones & Bartlett Learning.

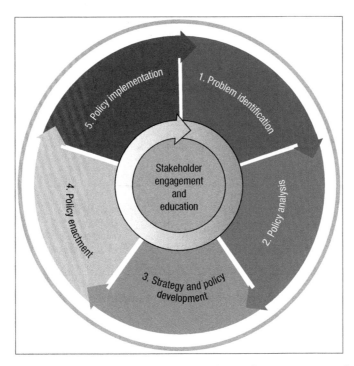

Figure 24.1 Centers for Disease Control and Prevention policy process model.

Source: Centers for Disease Control and Prevention. (2019). *The CDC's policy process. https://www.cdc.gov/policy/polaris/policyprocess/index.html*

Problem identification involves the determination of the root cause of the public health problem. The basis of the problem's root cause can be grounded in population-based epidemiologic data. This step of the process involves the writing of a narrative problem statement that guides the health policy development. The policy identification process clearly outlines the problem in detail with the inclusion of the problem's effect on the population's health. This aspect of the model is aligned with nurses' community assessment. As depicted in the center of the CDC Policy Process Model, stakeholders or groups affected by, interested in, or concerned with the problem should be engaged in the process of identifying the underlying problem, framing the problem accurately, and providing the context of the problem (CDC, 2019). A stakeholder analysis can be included as a component of the problem identification process. Stakeholder analysis should consider both internal and external stakeholders to the problem. Nurses should always conduct a stakeholder analysis as a component of their community engagement strategies. A stakeholder analysis can also be integrated into the comprehensive community assessment. Figure 24.2 presents a stakeholder analysis template. Stakeholders can be classified into one of four quadrants—high support and influence, low support and influence, high support but low influence, and low support but high influence. This stakeholder analysis facilitates a determination about who can influence the policy change or quality improvement initiative and determines their level of support for the project as a means to identify those critical stakeholders to involve in the process.

Some essential steps of the problem identification process are conducting a literature review, analyzing epidemiologic data, conducting surveys, and completing an environmental scan. The final step in the problem identification process is composing a narrative problem statement that provides essential information to frame the problem while illuminating the possible policy solutions. The problem statement should include:

- Who is affected
- How big or the scope of the problem (epidemiologic data)
- What contributes to the problem (etiology and risk factors)
- When and where the problem is likely to occur (epidemiologic data; CDC, 2019).

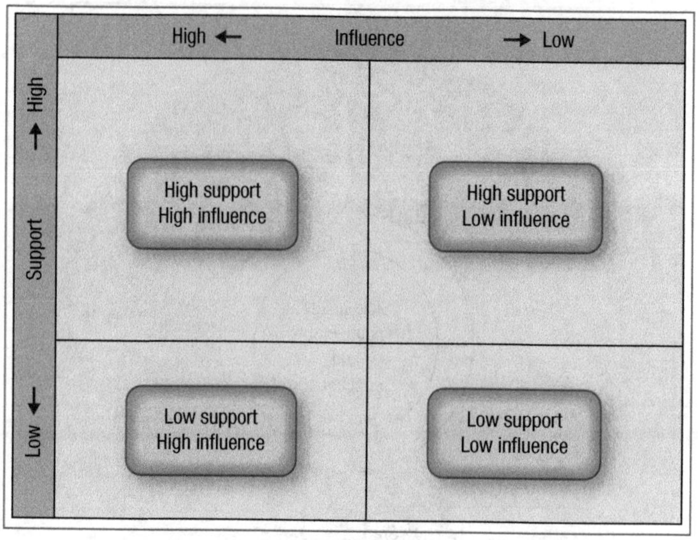

Figure 24.2 Stakeholder analysis template.

Policy analysis consists of identifying possible policy options. Policy analysis in the CDC Policy Process Model is used differently than described in the following. Stakeholders should be engaged in the identification of possible policy solutions. During the problem identification process through the literature review, epidemiologic data analysis, and environmental scan, possible policy solutions are frequently generated as options. The policy analysis process assesses each policy option for potential impact, implementation cost, and feasibility. Each option is ranked based on this assessment (CDC, 2019).

Strategy and policy development involves the planning of how to develop, draft, and enact the proposed policy. The manner in which the policy is drafted will be dependent upon the type of policy solution proposed. For example, if a public health law is proposed as the policy solution, then the process will involve the drafting of a bill to be sponsored and enrolled in the respective legislative or congressional process (CDC, 2019). The strategy aspect of this process also includes the engagement of political processes to generate public support for the respective policy solution.

Policy enactment is the process of securing the authoritative approval of the proposed policy. This process is policy type dependent and will be defined by the type of policy solution proposed. For example, if the policy solution is a proposed state statute, then the respective state legislative process of drafting a bill, sponsoring

the bill in the state legislature, securing legislative approval, and executing the bill into law by the governor's signatory approval defines the authoritative approval process. The stakeholders who may be engaged during this process include individuals affected by the proposed policy, legislators, public officials and administrators, and state and local board members. This process concludes with the approval for policy implementation (CDC, 2019).

Policy implementation involves the implementation of the respective policy and involves more than merely actualizing the policy. Policy implementation includes educating individuals, organizations, and the general public affected by the new policy; developing new or altering existing operational systems to implement the policy; and developing a systematic plan to monitor and evaluate the policy outcomes. The policy implementation process includes the allocation of resources and identification of areas of responsibility for implementation. Epidemiologic data can provide essential information that supports the formative and summative evaluation of the policy implementation and outcome achievement (CDC, 2019).

POLICY ANALYSIS AND EVALUATION

Policy analysis and evaluation both utilize epidemiologic data. Policy analysis in the CDC Policy Process Model describes policy analysis as selecting the appropriate policy action aligned with the problem identification. However, policy analysis in other models and processes, as described in the following, involve the continual analysis of policy for relevancy along with a critical appraisal of the context in which a policy agenda, issue, or policy exists. The policy analysis product is considered a clear description of the problem, identification of policy solutions or alternatives, courses of action with expected outcomes, and the contextual understanding of the problem and policies aligned with the problem (Porche, 2019).

Policy analysis can occur on three levels—macro-, meso-, and micro-level. The macro-level policy analysis encompasses broad global parameters that influence policy such as global economics and globalization. The meso-level policy analysis focuses on the process of policy making and implementation. At the micro-level, policy analysis focuses on the engagement between constituents or consumers and the policy making agency or the policy itself (Porche, 2019).

There are many processes or models for policy analysis such as the substantive model, eightfold path, logical-positivist, participatory policy analysis, forecasting model, and the five "Es" model. These various models include similar processes such as problem identification, identifying potential policy actions, identifying feasibility, and implementation strategies. Porche (2019) proposes the following policy analysis process:

1. First, conduct a problem or issue analysis. A critical step is discerning if the area of concern is a real problem or merely an issue of concern. This is critical to discerning the most appropriate policy solution. To make this discernment, an issue analysis is conducted. Issue analysis consists of twelve steps:
   a. Identification of an area of concern
   b. Background that provides the social, economic, ethical, political, and legal context of the area of concern
   c. Stakeholder and constituents who may be directly or indirectly impacted
   d. Position analysis of the policymakers', stakeholders', and governmental officials' position on the area of concern
   e. Political analysis of the political climate
   f. Statement of concern expressed as a narrative statement that delineates the boundaries of the area of concern

   g. Interaction analysis that outlines the interrelationships of the area of concern to other areas of concern, issues, or problems
   h. Policy identification process that proposes potential policy options and alternatives
   i. Outcome identification to define the desired or expected policy outcomes
   j. Policy recommendation to propose the optimal policy solution
   k. Impact assessment that examines the potential and actual impact the policy may render in relation to the area of concern
   l. A final determination that labels and frames the area of concern as an issue or problem. A problem is something that rises to the level of an actionable agenda item that has political support.
2. Second, if the area of concern is identified as a problem, a problem analysis should be conducted. Much of the information used in the issue analysis will be redundant and usable in the problem analysis process. There are four steps to the problem analysis—sensing, problem search, problem identification, and problem specification.
   a. Sensing analyzes the problem situation as a felt and existing problem
   b. Problem search describes the multiple representations of the problem, stakeholders, and multiple paradigms associated with the problem
   c. Problem definition characterizes the problem as a substantive problem with use of epidemiologic data
   d. Problem specification formalizes the problem through an actionable policy agenda, constituent needs, and assessing the political positions related to the problem.
3. A third step may be conducting a bill or law analysis. A bill or law analysis is a critical appraisal of the components of the bill or law in relation to the areas of strengths, weaknesses, limitations, and opportunities for modification or change of the existing bill or law to impact the identified problem.
4. Lastly, the policy analysis concludes with a summative policy analysis process. This is the concluding systematic process that determines the extent to which existing policy is viable and implementable as a solution to the problem. Porche (2019) proposes the following process:

a. Critical policy review involves an appraisal of existing policies' intentions and directives, outlines issues or problems intended to be resolved by the policy

b. Policy search to identify policies affected by, or related to, the policy being analyzed

c. Historical analysis that reviews historical events that have impacted the issue, problem, and policy over time

d. Authorization analysis determines the process that will be needed to secure approval of the policy

e. Budgetary analysis analyzes the funds necessary to support the approval and implementation of the policy

f. Public health issue or problem analysis involves ensuring steps 2 and 3 are complete

g. Stakeholder or constituency identification of any remaining special interest groups that are or could be impacted by the policy

h. Strengths, weaknesses, opportunities, and threats (SWOT) analysis, which is the conducting of an assessment of the internal strengths and weaknesses of the problem along with the external opportunities and threats

i. PESTEL analysis is an assessment of the political, economic, social, technological, environmental, and legal factors that may affect the policy

j. Gap analysis of the current existing policy and what policy is needed for the future

k. Concluding executive summary of the existing policy analysis along with prioritized recommendations for policy development, formulation, modification, or implementation

Policy evaluation involves determining the extent to which the policy achieves the expected outcome. Policy evaluation is a systematic, empirical assessment of the effects developed from the policy. The metrics for policy analysis may consist of epidemiologic data. As stated earlier, evaluation is a measurement to determine if the expected outcome of a program is being achieved (Porche, 2004). Nurses should remember that regardless of the type of evaluation conducted, evaluation is always an expectation of the nursing process. Systematic evaluation is used to collect information on multiple activities, characteristics, or aspects of a program to discern the program's effectiveness and achievement of expected outcomes. Systematic evaluation informs decision-making about future population-based programs (Porche, 2004).

EFFICACY, EFFECTIVENESS, AND EFFICIENCY OUTCOME EVALUATION

Outcomes evaluation is a type of evaluation that measures the extent to which the desired health effect is achieved as desired. Epidemiologic data measures for outcomes evaluation are measured using morbidity and mortality data along with measures such as quality of life, function status, and patient preferences. Outcomes research can involve the utilization of big epidemiologic data sets to derive the expected outcomes achieved in large population groups.

Epidemiologic evaluation of policy and other healthcare programs frequently evaluate efficacy, effectiveness, and efficiency. These terms are sometimes used interchangeably but should not be used in that manner. Efficacy measures the effect of an agent or intervention under controlled conditions on an expected outcome. Efficacy can also be described simply as the ability to perform under controlled conditions in the expected manner. Effectiveness measures the extent to which something produces the desired result in a "real-life" situation. Effectiveness is a pragmatic measure of achieving a desired outcome. Efficiency is a measure to the extent to which something can be achieved in the least amount of time, expense, or effort.

PROGRAM MONITORING: AN ASPECT OF EVALUATION

Monitoring and evaluation are priority areas in population health. Monitoring and evaluation are related but different concepts. Program monitoring is the systematic documentation of key aspects of performance that indicate the program is functioning as intended or in accordance with planned activities (Porche, 2004). Monitoring ensures that the program is achieving the desired outcomes prior to conducting a summative evaluation.

CENTERS FOR DISEASE CONTROL AND PREVENTION EVALUATION FRAMEWORK

Prevention of disease and health alterations are defining aspects of the scope of nursing practice, along with providing care to the response of individuals to health and illness. The CDC provides an evaluation framework that can also use the integration of epidemiologic evaluation. Figure 24.3 presents the CDC evaluation framework. There are four criteria to be considered for evaluation standards with the CDC evaluation framework—utility, feasibility, propriety, and accuracy. Utility ensures that evaluation information is practical and useful for stakeholders. Feasibility ensures that the evaluation is realistic, prudent, diplomatic, and frugal. Propriety ensures that the evaluation process is conducted in a legal and ethical manner that is best for the welfare of the population. Accuracy ensures that the evaluation methods yield information that is able to determine effectiveness (Porche, 2004).

The CDC evaluation framework incorporates these four criteria in addition to the following process:

1. Engaging stakeholders to ensure their perspectives are integrated into the evaluation process
2. Describing the program in terms of the mission, goals, and expected objectives
3. Focusing on evaluation design
4. Gathering credible evidence
5. Rendering a judgment based on the evaluation evidence
6. Generating lessons learned and ensuring use of findings (Porche, 2004)

STRUCTURE, PROCESS, AND OUTCOME EVALUATION

Donabedian (1966) provided the structure, process, and outcome evaluation framework. Structure evaluates the organizational structure, resources, resource allocation, management and staff qualifications, and adherence to policy, procedures, and legal requirements. Process measures whether the program is being implemented in accordance with the implementation plan and incorporates program monitoring activities. Outcome evaluation measures the extent to which the program achieves the expected goals and objectives (Porche, 2004).

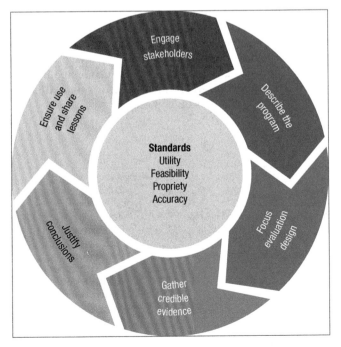

Figure 24.3 Centers for Disease Control and Prevention evaluation framework.

Source: Centers for Disease Control and Prevention. (2017). https://www.cdc.gov/eval/framework/index.htm

Outcome evaluation measures the degree to which the public health program is having an effect on the target population. Several types of outcomes can be used to measure effectiveness. A surrogate outcome is a substitute measure for a direct outcome. For example, the surrogate outcome for diabetes mellitus may be the measured change in glycosylated hemoglobin (HgB A1c) but the direct outcome desired is a reduction in diabetic end organ complications. A composite outcome measure can be used to evaluate population health outcomes and program achievements. A composite outcome measure combines several related outcomes into a single outcome measure. Major cardiovascular event (MACE) is a composite measure that combines any myocardial infarction, cerebrovascular event, and cardiovascular health into one measurement (Ranganathan & Aggarwal, 2020).

Another term sometimes incorrectly used interchangeably with outcome evaluation is impact evaluation. Impact evaluation is the extent to which the public health program achieves the ultimate or overall goal. Both outcome and impact evaluation can provide critical evidence for policy making.

FORMATIVE AND SUMMATIVE EVALUATION

Formative and summative evaluation uses a temporal orientation to evaluation. Formative evaluation is the ongoing evaluation of the program activities and expectations. Formative evaluation culminates into a summative evaluation. The summative evaluation collects data for the purpose of rendering a judgment about whether a program has achieved the expected outcomes (Porche, 2004).

LOGIC MODEL: AN EVALUATION STRATEGY

A logic model is a tool that can be used for planning, describing, managing, communicating, and evaluating a program or intervention. The logic evaluation model provides a visual presentation of how a public health program should function to achieve the desired outcomes by describing the necessary program inputs, activities, outputs, and outcomes. Figure 24.4 presents a simple diagram of the relationships of the logic model components.

Inputs are the resources needed to implement the program or intervention. Inputs can include such resources as financial, human, and supportive. Activities are those actions required to produce the desired outcome. Outputs are the direct, tangible results of an action. Outcomes are the expected results of the program or intervention. Outcomes can be divided into short, intermediate, or long-term. The designation of the outcome as short-term, intermediate, or long-term is dependent upon the length of the program and the expected achievements in relation to time.

The basic structure of a logic model is depicted in Figure 24.5. The basic logic model has two sections, process and outcome. The process section of the logic model contains the inputs (resources), activities (program actions), and outputs (direct product of activities). The outcome section describes the expected effect of the program or intervention as short, intermediate, or long-term outcomes. Programmatic assumptions and contextual factors are sometimes also presented in the logic model. Assumptions are beliefs or theory guiding the development of the program or intervention. Contextual factors include the environmental factors that influence the program's outcomes.

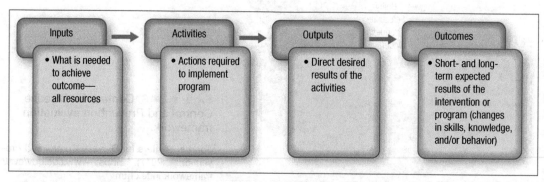

Figure 24.4 Logic model components relationships.

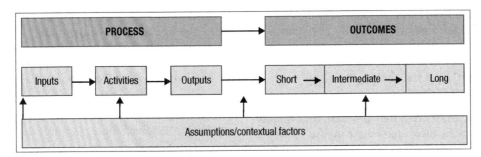

Figure 24.5 Basic logic model components.

Source: Centers for Disease Control and Prevention (CDC). https://www.cdc.gov/dhdsp/docs/logic_model.pdf.

The logic model can be used for program evaluation. Using the logic model for evaluation determines the epidemiologic data to be used to measure short, intermediate, and long-term expected outcomes (The CDC Division for Heart Disease and Stroke, n.d.).

SCREENING PROGRAM EVALUATION (SECONDARY PREVENTION AND SURVEILLANCE)

Screening programs are the cornerstone of secondary prevention and surveillance programs. Screening is essential for the early detection and treatment of health conditions. Public health population-based screening programs can be evaluated for effectiveness based on operational or outcomes measures (Celentano & Szkio, 2018). The operational measures of evaluation would be consistent with Donabedian's process measures. Potential operational screening program metrics could be:

- Number of individuals educated about screening
- Number of individuals consented for screening
- Number of individuals actually screened
- Number of times an individual received screening
- Proportion of the target population screened
- Number of personnel required for screening
- Proportion or ratio of staff required to the number of individual's screened
- Cost of screening program
- Cost per person screened
- Cost per positive screening test
- Proportion of positive individuals screened to those with confirmatory diagnosis
- Predictive value positive of test in target population (Celentano & Szkio, 2018)

Outcome measures for screening program evaluation determine if the expected or desired outcome of the screening program has been achieved. For example, if the expected outcome of the screening test is to identify those asymptomatic individuals with diabetes mellitus to initiate early interventions, then the outcomes measure the extent to which asymptomatic individuals are validly identified to have diabetes mellitus. Some potential screening program outcome measures are:

- Morbidity reduction in the screened population
- Mortality reduction in the screened population
- Case-fatality rate reduction in the screened population
- Case-specific rate reductions (such as age and sex) in the screened population
- Reduction in tertiary disease consequences
- Quality of life improvements (Celentano & Szkio, 2018)

Cost–Benefit Analysis of Screening Program

Screening programs and other population-based health interventions require the allocation of funds to support their implementation. In addition to other evaluative criteria for determining the appropriateness of a screening program, a cost—benefit analysis should be conducted. To conduct a thorough cost–benefit analysis of a screening program, the cost of the screening test along with the cost of the entire follow-up process to discern the validity of the positive screening test into a confirmatory diagnosis of the health condition should be included. This also includes the addition of false-positive results in the cost–benefit analysis. Cost-effectiveness measures the program's effectiveness in relation to the cost expended to implement the screening program.

RESEARCH, EVIDENCE-BASED PRACTICE, AND QUALITY IMPROVEMENT

Research, evidence-based practice, and quality improvement measurements can use epidemiologic data as the measurement metric. These terms are sometimes used interchangeably in an incorrect manner. These terms are distinct and should not be used interchangeably. Research is the process of scientific discovery that results in the generation of generalizable information. Research uses the scientific process to validate and refine existing knowledge or generate new knowledge that is generalizable or transferable. Evidence-based practice applies research and other sources of evidence into practice. Evidence-based practice is a systematic, problem-solving approach that integrates a systematic search for and critical appraisal of the most relevant evidence. Evidence-based practice translates new knowledge such as research into practice. Evidence-based practice can improve quality based on the integration of the strongest evidence into practice. Quality improvement measures changes in quality result from practice changes that are institution specific and nongeneralizable. Quality improvement focuses on using a data-driven systematic approach to improve specific system issue, processes, costs, productivity, and quality outcomes. Quality improvement incorporates existing knowledge and information into the process of improving quality. Evidence-based practice forms the foundation for quality improvement. Quality

improvement processes are cyclic and continually attempt to improve the quality outcomes (Hedges, 2006). Quality improvement efforts continue to drive practice change to achieve better and better results over time.

Plan, Do, Study, Act: Quality Improvement Model

Plan, do, study, and act (PDSA) provides a framework for quality improvement. Figure 24.6 provides the PDSA quality improvement model. Table 24.2 presents the activities to be achieved at each phase of implementing the PDSA quality improvement model. The integration and utilization of epidemiologic data support the rationale for the problem and determination of the effectiveness of the quality improvement intervention.

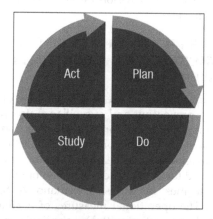

Figure 24.6 Plan, Do, Study, Act model.

Source: Skilled Nursing Facility (SNF) Quality Assurance & Performance Improvement. https://www.snfqapi.com/resources/plan-do-study-act(PDSA)

Table 24.2 PDSA Phase Activities

Phase	Activities
Plan	• Conduct literature review • Collect baseline epidemiologic and other data • Conduct stakeholder analysis, plan with stakeholders, obtain approvals • Plan improvement intervention
Do	• Continue to meet with stakeholders • Implement quality improvement intervention • Collect epidemiologic and other data for quality improvement monitoring
Study	• Evaluate effectiveness of quality improvement intervention—use epidemiologic data as appropriate • Disseminate findings to stakeholders
Act	• Calculate cost–benefit analysis • Decide to adopt, adapt, or abandon use of quality improvement intervention • Identify policy changes needed for continued sustainability • Continue cycle to drive continual improvements in quality

END-OF-CHAPTER RESOURCES

SUMMARY POINTS

- Epidemiologic data can be used as the evidence base to substantiate the development of public health policy.
- Policy development and formulation are population-based interventions used to impact the nation's health.
- Policy generally provides the principles that govern an action directed toward a specific outcome, provides a stated position on an issue, outlines a plan of action by the government or an organization, or states authoritative statements, decisions, or guidelines outlined by the government or an organization.
- Policy intention is the expected or anticipated outcome of the respective policy.
- A model is a descriptive representation of a complex entity or processes into a visual and understandable manner.
- The Centers for Disease Control and Prevention (CDC) Policy Process Model consists of five domains that include stakeholder engagement and evaluation-problem identification, policy analysis, strategy and policy development, policy enactment, and policy implementation.
- Problem identification involves the determination of the root cause of the public health problem.
- Policy analysis consists of identifying possible policy options.
- Strategy and policy development involves the planning of how to develop, draft, and enact the proposed policy.
- Policy enactment is the process of securing the authoritative approval of the proposed policy.
- Policy implementation involves the implementation of the respective policy.
- Policy analysis involves the continual analysis of policy for currency along with a critical appraisal of the context in which an agenda, issue, or policy exists.
- Policy evaluation involves determining the extent to which the policy achieves the expected outcome.
- Policy evaluation is a systematic, empirical assessment of the effects developed from the policy.
- Efficacy measures the effect of an agent or intervention under controlled conditions on an expected outcome.

- Effectiveness measures the extent to which something produces the desired result in a "real-life" situation.
- Efficiency is a measure to the extent to which something can be achieved in the least amount of time, expense, or effort.
- Program monitoring is the systematic documentation of key aspects of performance that indicate the program is functioning as intended or in accordance with planned activities.
- There are four criteria to be considered for evaluation standards with the CDC evaluation framework: utility, feasibility, propriety, and accuracy.
- Structure evaluates the organizational structure, resources, resource allocation, management and staff qualifications, and adherence to policy, procedures, and legal requirements.
- Process measures whether the program is being implemented in accordance with the implementation plan and incorporates program monitoring activities.
- Outcome evaluation measures the extent to which the program achieves the expected goals and objectives.
- Formative evaluation is the ongoing evaluation of the program activities and expectations.
- The summative evaluation collects data for the purpose of rendering a judgment about whether a program has achieved the expected outcomes.
- The logic evaluation model provides a visual representation of how a public health program should function to achieve the desired outcomes by describing the necessary program inputs, activities, outputs, and outcomes.
- Research is the process of scientific discovery that results in the generation of generalizable information.
- Evidence-based practice is a systematic problem-solving approach that integrates a systematic search for and critical appraisal of the most relevant evidence.
- Quality improvement focuses on using a data-driven systematic approach to improve specific system issues, processes, cost, productivity, and quality outcomes.

EPIDEMIOLOGY CRITICAL REASONING QUESTIONS

1. Describe the difference between process and outcome evaluation. Provide an example.
2. Differentiate between efficacy, effectiveness, and efficiency. Provide an example.
3. Identify an area of concern for policy development. Present the epidemiologic data that could be used to support the rationale for the area of concern being a problem. Propose possible policy solutions and epidemiologic data that could be used to evaluate the policy.
4. Identify an epidemiologic policy. Conduct a policy analysis of the epidemiologic policy.
5. Identify an epidemiologic quality improvement project. Use the stakeholder analysis provided in Figure 24.2 to identify the level of influence and support of each stakeholder identified.

ADDITIONAL RESOURCES

A robust set of instructor resources designed to supplement this text is located at http://connect. springerpub.com/content/book/978-0-8261-8514-3. Qualifying instructors may request access by emailing textbook@springerpub.com.

REFERENCES

Celentano, D., & Szkio, M. (2018). *Gordis epidemiology* (6th ed.). Elsevier.

Centers for Disease Control and Prevention. (2019). *The CDC's policy process.* https://www.cdc.gov/policy/polaris/policyprocess/index.html

Centers for Disease Control and Prevention Division for Heart Disease and Stroke. (n.d.). *Evaluation guide: Developing a logic model.* Author.

Donabedian, A. (1966). Evaluating the quality of medical care. *Milbank Memorial Fund Quarterly, 44,* 166–206. https://doi.org/10.1111/j.1468-0009.2005.00397.x

Hedges, C. (2006). Research, evidence based practice, and quality improvement: The 3-legged stool. *AACN Advanced Critical Care, 17*(4), 456–459. https://doi.org/10.4037/15597768-2006-4010

Porche, D. (2004). *Public & community health nursing practice: A population-based approach.* Sage.

Porche, D. (2019). *Health policy: Application for nurses and other healthcare professionals* (2nd ed.). Jones & Bartlett Learning.

Ranganathan, P., & Aggarwal, R. (2020). Study designs: Part 5—Interventional studies (III). *Perspectives in Clinical Research, 11*(1), 47–50. https://doi.org/10.4103/picr.PICR_209_19

Chapter 25

EPIDEMIOLOGIC ETHICAL AND PROFESSIONAL ISSUES

Demetrius J. Porche

I know you won't believe me, but the highest form of Human Excellence is to question oneself and others.

—Socrates

Good actions give strength to ourselves and inspire good actions in others.

—Plato

CHAPTER COMPETENCIES

At the conclusion of this chapter, the reader will be able to:

1. Integrate ethical principles into ethical decision-making processes
2. Demonstrate utilization of personal and professional core values that influence ethical decision-making
3. Engage in ethical and professional epidemiologic behaviors
4. Participate in epidemiologic practice that protects the privacy and confidentiality of individuals, groups, communities, and populations to the extent provided for by law and congruent with core values and ethical principles

ESSENTIAL TERMINOLOGY

Essential ethical and professional issues terminology are:

- Advocacy ethics
- Applied ethics
- Autonomy
- Beneficence
- Bioethics
- Conflict of interest
- Deontology
- Ethical principles
- Ethics
- Fidelity
- Justice
- Nonmaleficence
- Professional ethics
- Utilitarianism
- Values
- Veracity

Epidemiologic and professional issues may arise with the desire to establish the truth in scientific knowledge through epidemiologic research; through epidemiologic practice of conducting surveillance of public health threats; or the implementation of public health interventions to alleviate health risk at the individual, community, or public level. Epidemiologic research is generally funded by external sponsors, while epidemiologic practice occurs as a component of the healthcare system or as an entity of the broader public health system. Dissemination of epidemiologic knowledge is necessary to ensure utilization of epidemiologic findings. The dissemination of epidemiologic knowledge must be in the utmost ethical manner. Epidemiologists have to promote the development of their scientific reputation to advance their professional careers, but most do this in an ethical manner. Meanwhile the public has the right to know their health risks and expect that epidemiologic research is conducted in a manner of scientific rigor while protecting human subjects. Ethical guidelines and principles guide the ethical practice of epidemiology.

DEFINING ETHICS

Ethics is the study of the nature and justification of principles that guide individuals to act in a moral manner, consistent with society's customs, values, beliefs, and norms. Ethics is also defined as the study of the manner in which individuals behave in a situation. Ethics is considered the basis for determining correct action. There are several types of ethics (Porche, 2003).

Professional ethics are the values and standards developed by a profession or discipline over a period of time that identifies the salient and inherent values of the profession or discipline (Callahan & Jennings, 2002). Applied ethics is the practical real-world application of values and principles to ethical issues, situations, or dilemmas. Applied ethics focuses individual behavior and conduct in specific situations based on the values of a profession (2002). Advocacy ethics focuses on representing another individual, group, or population's interest in relation to equality and social justice (Beauchamp & Childress, 2019). The application of ethical guidelines involves ethical values at the individual, team, or profession level.

ETHICAL THEORIES AND PARADIGMS

Ethical theories describe the concepts and conceptual relationships that formulate a cognitive framework that provide the context in which an individual engages in ethical behavior. Ethical behavior is the result of ethical decision-making processes (DMPs) to be described later. Ethical theories assist with the analysis of ethical dilemmas and guide an individual in determining ethical actions. Two classical ethical theoretical frameworks are deontology and utilitarianism.

Deontology

The deontology framework is based on a sense of moral obligation or duty. Deontology states that an action's moral rightness or wrongness depends on the action itself and the motivation behind the action (Beauchamp & Childress, 2019), along with the moral obligation felt toward that action. Moral obligation is an individual's feeling about a sense of duty that requires

action in a particular manner based on values, beliefs, and perspective of societal norms.

Utilitarianism

In contrast, teleology determines rightness or wrongness based solely on the expected outcomes or consequences of an action. Utilitarianism is a theoretical framework of teleology theory. The utilitarian framework proposes that the most ethical action is that which results in the greatest good for the largest number of individuals (Beauchamp & Childress, 2019). Utilitarianism focuses more on the ultimate number of individuals impacted by the action that produces a specific outcome or consequence.

ETHICAL PRINCIPLES

Ethical principles are developed from an individual's guiding ethical theoretical perspective, and personal and professional paradigms regarding moral conduct and societal expectations. Ethical theories along with the moral tone of society facilitate the formulation of ethical principles that guide an individual's ethical behavior. These ethical principles are the foundation of professional codes of ethics, such as the American College of Epidemiology Ethical Guidelines. Ethical principles guide an individual in the critical analysis and reasoning during an ethical dilemma. The most common principles encountered in ethics are beneficence, nonmaleficence, justice, and autonomy (Beauchamp & Childress, 2019). These ethical principles historical roots are defined as follows.

Beneficence is the norms that guide the greatest benefit to an individual, group, or population. Beneficence weighs the benefits of an action against the risks or costs to the individual, group, or population involved (Beauchamp & Childress, 2019).

The nonmaleficence principle focuses on "doing no harm." With nonmaleficence, the epidemiologist focuses on not causing harm to individuals, groups, or populations (Beauchamp & Childress, 2019).

Justice ensures the fair and equitable distribution of benefits, risks, and cost. Justice is known as the ethical principle of fairness (Beauchamp & Childress, 2019).

Autonomy is known as "respect for persons." Autonomy provides individuals with the right to make their own independent decisions. This is also referred to as the right to self-determination. This provides the individuals with the right to make free, uncoerced, and informed decisions. Autonomy is the ethical principle that provides the framework of full disclosure and informed consent (Beauchamp & Childress, 2019) required in the Declaration of Helsinki, the foundation to guide judgments regarding the protection of human subjects.

Other ethical principles considered necessary for ethical decision-making are fidelity and veracity. Fidelity is known as promise keeping. Fidelity ensures that the epidemiologist delivers what was promised. Veracity is known as truth telling. Veracity consists of being honest in delivering information to individuals, groups, populations, or society. Fidelity and veracity are essential for an epidemiologist to develop a trusting relationship within the scientific and general community. Fidelity and veracity are critical for epidemiologic information dissemination.

VALUES CLARIFICATION

Values are beliefs that an individual or social group hold regarding what is relevant and important to their belief system. Values have an emotional aspect. Values are continually formed throughout life as an individual develops personally and professionally, and as the contextual and social situation of the individual changes over time. Some values are permanent, and some values transform and evolve as an individual matures and develops.

Values that typically do not change and form the basis for other values and philosophical perspectives are considered core values. An individual's values comprise the belief system that then structures their paradigm or world view. Value systems create the framework or the individual's paradigmatic worldview about epidemiologic population health (Coletta, 1978).

Values are foundational for ethical decisions. The engagement in moral thought and action, a result of ethical decision-making, evolves from professional and personal life values. The value clarification process promotes clarity regarding an individual's personal and professional values that are foundational to their ethical thoughts and actions.

The value clarification process promotes self-reflection to identify values and one's value system. During this process of self-reflection, the epidemiologist has the ability to analyze and prioritize the values through a DMP of refinement. Raths et al. (1966, 1978) defined a seminal process of values clarification. The process consists of choosing, prizing, and acting. According to Raths, Harmin, and Simon, from this process, a value is that which meets more than two criteria resulting from these three processes.

Choosing consists of three criteria: choosing freely, choosing from alternatives (thoughts and actions), and choosing after thoughtful consideration of the consequences of each alternative. The next process, prizing, consists of two criteria: cherishing and being happy with the choice, and willingness to affirm the choice within a public arena. Lastly, the acting process is defined by doing something with the choice, and repeatedly acting in the same manner to the extent that it forms as a life pattern. Collectively, these three processes define the value clarification process to identify an individual's values which form the basis for that person's personal and professional epidemiologic paradigm to approach ethical situations. This values clarification process can be used by teams/groups, organizations, and associations to identify and clarify their values.

The values clarification process assists each individual or organization to identify core values. Core values are the fundamental beliefs that an individual or organization holds as guiding principles that direct behavior and action. These core values are critical in determining policy ideology, theoretical perspectives, epidemiologic investigative methods, and interpretation of epidemiologic findings. Epidemiologists' ethical practices should continually be grounded in their core values.

ETHICAL GUIDELINES: ETHICAL ROOTS

The roots of ethical guidelines emerged from the Declaration of Helsinki developed by the World Medical Association. The Declaration of Helsinki establishes a set of ethical principles to provide guidance in the conduct of research with human subjects. The Declaration of Helsinki includes principles of safeguarding research subjects, informed consent, minimizing risk, and adhering to an approved research protocol. Informed consent has three critical components which consists of provision of information, understanding of the information, and voluntariness (World Medical Association, 2013).

The Belmont Report was first written by the National Commission for the Protection of Human Subjects of Biomedical and Behavioral Research. The Belmont Report identified three fundamental principles for engaging human subjects into research. These three fundamental principles are:

1. **Respect for persons:** The right to be treated with courtesy and respect, presentation of truthful information, permitting the person to make an independent autonomous decision to participate, and allow for informed consent
2. **Beneficence:** Represents the philosophy of first "Do no harm" while maximizing the benefits of the research
3. **Justice:** Ensure nonexploitive and fair distribution of risks, costs, and benefits (National Commission for the Protection of Human Subjects of Biomedical and Behavioral Research, Department of Health, Education and Welfare, 1978)

ETHICAL DECISION-MAKING PROCESS

Ethical dilemmas arise when there is a conflict in the principles; duties; rights; beliefs; or values of one individual, group, population, or community with another or with societal expectations (Beauchamp & Childress, 2019). Reflective processes, such as values clarification and ethical DMPs, assist with the resolution of ethical dilemmas. The reflective ethical DMP facilitates the generation of solutions or alternatives to the ethical dilemma based on the values identified in the values clarification process.

Ethical DMPs facilitate the selection of an ethical resolution by outlining the steps that promote an understanding of the applicable values to the ethical dilemma and the preferred resolution. Ethical theoretical perspective and ethical principles are used in the ethical DMP to analyze the ethical dilemma. Several DMPs can be used to assist with ensuring that an individual selects the most ethical behavior within the given contextual situation.

Porche (2003) proposed a reflective process with the following steps to gain reasoning about the ethical dilemma:

- Define the ethical dilemma
- Outline the conflicting ethical issues and principles resulting from both sides of the ethical dilemma

- Identify the populations impacted on both sides of the dilemma
- Collect data relevant to both sides of the ethical dilemma
- List alternative options to resolve the ethical dilemma
- Describe the consequences for each option listed
- Analyze each option in relation to the preferred ethical theoretical paradigm, and ethical principles or codes of ethics
- Determine which option would be the best and most ethical resolution
- Draft the action decision that represents the ethical resolution selected
- Ensure that the action is implemented with the ethical intent and context
- Evaluate the implementation and consequences of the ethical resolution
- Consider the impact of the ethical resolution on the population and society (Porche, 2003)

BIOETHICS

Bioethics is the integration of ethics and biology. Bioethics places the ethical question within the context of biology and health-related science. As a critical reflection on the moral dimension of biology, medicine, and healthcare, bioethics embraces an ethical DMP to resolve ethical dilemmas. Forte et al. (2018) proposed the DMP framework that consists of four steps. The DMP framework uses epidemiologic information as a component of the ethical DMP. The first step of the DMP, ethics of accuracy, focuses exclusively on the disease, especially at the probabilistic predictions of risk factors and the disease. Figure 25.1 presents the information utilized in the DMP.

In step one, base rates of incidence, prevalence, mortality, and risk estimations are considered. Accuracy of screening and diagnostic tests are also considered in the first step. The biological and pathophysiologic characteristics of the disease are considered. The second step, ethics of comprehension and understanding, focuses on the person's value and belief system. After there is an accurate understanding about the disease and its potential outcomes, this needs to be reconciled in alignment with the person's values, life goals, expectations, and beliefs. Step two focuses on the consideration of these personal belief systems and personal goals. Step three is considered situational awareness. The third step focuses on the clinical judgment of

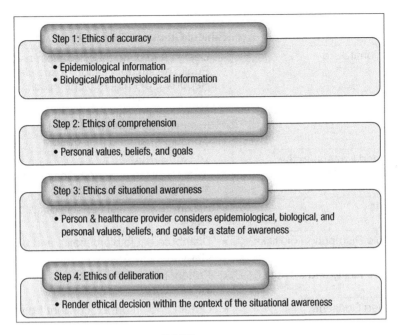

Figure 25.1 Decision-making process (DMP).

Source: Adapted from Forte, D., Kawai, F., & Cohen, C. (2018). A bioethical framework to guide the decision-making process in the care of seriously ill patients. *BMC Medical Ethics*, *19*, 78–85.

the healthcare team. The team's clinical judgment has to be combined with steps one and two, linking the biological aspects of the disease with the person's values, beliefs, and goals to arrive at a state of awareness for both the provider and the person to generate potential ethical options. The last step, the ethics of deliberation, focuses on the mutual goals of care (GOC) aligning with the appropriate treatment and patient's values. It is in step four that the final ethical decisions are rendered for implementation (Forte et al., 2018).

AMERICAN COLLEGE OF EPIDEMIOLOGY ETHICAL GUIDELINES

The American College of Epidemiology (ACE) was incorporated in 1979 to develop criteria for the professional recognition of epidemiologists and address epidemiologists' professional concerns. ACE has developed ethical guidelines (Table 25.1) for use by epidemiologists (ACE, 2000).

ACE recognizes that epidemiology is a set of methods employed by a variety of health and public health-related disciplines and professions. The ACE ethical guidelines are written for

the epidemiologist, not epidemiology. Therefore, healthcare or public health providers whose roles and responsibilities are as an epidemiologist, should embrace their discipline's or profession's ethical guidelines along with the ACE guidelines (ACE, 2000).

CODES OF ETHICS

Codes of ethics are developed by professional disciplines to guide the ethical decision-making for the respective discipline. These ethical codes are grounded in the philosophical paradigm of the discipline and represent the core values that guide the discipline. Ethical codes guide the ethical and moral behaviors for the discipline. Some individual healthcare providers, such as epidemiologists who are nurses may be bound by more than one set of ethical codes or guidelines. For example, a nurse epidemiologist should use both the American College of Epidemiology Ethical Guidelines and the American Nurses Association Code of Ethics for Nurses (ANA, 2015). Nurse epidemiologists that focus on population-based public health should also guide their professional behaviors based on the American Public Health Association's Public Health Code of Ethics.

Table 25.1 American College of Epidemiology Ethical Guidelines

Ethical Guideline	Ethical Guideline Explanation
Maintain Professional Role	• Design and conduct scientific research • Public health application of knowledge • Reporting of epidemiologic results to the scientific community • Maintenance, enhancement, and promotion of health in the community • Consulting and administration
Minimizing Risk and Protecting the Welfare of Research Participants	• Minimize risks • Avoid causing harm to research participants and society
Providing Benefits	• Maximize potential benefits of epidemiologic study
Ensuring Equitable Distribution of Risks and Benefits	• Distribute equitable benefits and burdens of epidemiologic research
Protecting Confidentiality and Privacy	• Protect privacy of individuals and all confidential information
Obtaining Informed Consent	• Obtain prior informed consent from epidemiologic research subjects • Provide information on elements of epidemiologic study such as purpose, sponsors, investigators, scientific methods and procedures, anticipated risks and benefits, anticipated inconveniences or discomfort, and right to refuse to participate or withdraw at any time • Avoidance of manipulation or coercion, participation must be voluntary
Submitting Proposed Epidemiologic Study for Ethical Review	• Epidemiologic studies are reviewed by an independent ethics committee, except if justified to investigate outbreaks of acute communicable diseases or routine public health surveillance
Maintain Public Trust	• Adhere to the highest scientific standards for study design, protocol development and implementation, data collection, transmission, storage, and analysis of data • Appropriate interpretation of data analysis • Dissemination of findings in an ethical manner
Avoid Conflicts of Interest or Partiality	• Maintain honesty and impartiality in the design, conduct, interpretation, and reporting of epidemiologic findings
Communicate Ethical Requirements to Colleagues, Employers, Sponsors, and Confronting Unacceptable Conduct	• Communicate ethical guidelines • Educate epidemiologic students on ethical guidelines • Confront scientific misconduct
Obligations to Community	• Address health problems or conditions requested by the community and impacting the community • Timely reporting of results in an understandable manner to the widest possible community • Advocate for the community but do not impair scientific objectivity • Respect cultural diversity

Source: Adapted from American College of Epidemiology. (2000). *American College of Epidemiology ethical guidelines*. https://www.acepidemiology.org/ethics-guidelines

American Nurses Association Code of Ethics for Nurses

The American Nurses Association Code of Ethics for Nurses provides the foundational values of nursing. This code supports nurses in the consistent practice of respectful, humane, and dignified nursing care. The code consists of the following nine provisions:

1. **Provision 1:** The nurse practices with compassion and respect for the inherent dignity, worth, and unique attributes of every person
2. **Provision 2:** The nurse's primary commitment is to the patient, whether an individual, family, group, community, or population
3. **Provision 3:** The nurse promotes, advocates for, and protects the rights, health, and safety of the patient
4. **Provision 4:** The nurse has authority, accountability, and responsibility for nursing practice; makes decisions; and takes action consistent with the obligation to promote health and to provide optimal care
5. **Provision 5:** The nurse owes the same duties to self as to others, including the responsibility to promote health and safety, preserve wholeness of character and integrity, maintain competence, and continue personal and professional growth
6. **Provision 6:** The nurse, through individual and collective effort, establishes, maintains, and improves the ethical environment of the work setting and conditions of employment that are conducive to safe, quality healthcare
7. **Provision 7:** The nurse, in all roles and settings, advances the profession through research and scholarly inquiry, professional standards development, and the generation of both nursing and health policy
8. **Provision 8:** The nurse collaborates with other health professionals and the public to protect human rights, promote health diplomacy, and reduce health disparities
9. **Provision 9:** The profession of nursing, collectively through its professional organizations, must articulate nursing values, maintain the integrity of the profession, and integrate the principle of social justice into nursing and health policy

Public Health Code of Ethics

The Public Health Code of Ethics applies to all disciplines that practice within the field of public health, including epidemiologists, public health nurses, and nurse epidemiologists. The Public Health Code of Ethics is intended as a set of professional standards and expectations for all public health practitioners. Within this ethical code, there are six core values that must be realized in public health practice. These core values are:

1. Professionalism and trust
2. Health and safety
3. Health justice and equity
4. Interdependence and solidarity
5. Human rights and civil liberties
6. Inclusivity and engagement (American Public Health Association [APHA], 2019)

Public health ethical analysis of a situation should be grounded in the six core values presented and engage four important aspects for an ethical analysis:

1. Determination of the public health goals of the proposed action
2. Identification of the relevant facts and uncertainties of the situation and proposed action
3. Analysis of the meaning and implications of the proposed action for the health and rights of those individuals and communities affected
4. Analysis of how the proposed action aligns with the core public health values (APHA, 2019)

During this ethical analysis, there are eight considerations to be addressed regarding public health interventions, program planning, and policy development. These eight points to consider during ethical analysis are:

1. **Permissibility:** Would the action being considered be ethically wrong even if it were to have a good outcome?
2. **Respect:** Would the proposed action be demeaning or disrespectful to individuals or communities even if it benefited their health?
3. **Reciprocity:** Have we done what is reasonable to offset the potential harms and losses that the proposed action imposes on individuals and communities?

4. **Effectiveness:** Is it reasonable to expect, based on best available evidence and past experience, that the proposed action would achieve its stated health goals?

5. **Responsible use of scarce resources:** Would the proposed action demonstrate good stewardship and deserve the trust that the public has invested in the public health practitioners?

6. **Proportionality:** Would the proposed action demonstrate that public health practitioners are using their power and authority judiciously and with humility?

7. **Accountability and transparency:** Would the proposed action withstand close ethical scrutiny and be justified by valid reasons that the general public will understand?

8. **Public participation:** In deciding on a proposed action, have all potentially affected stakeholders had a meaningful opportunity to participate? If some are to be deliberately excluded from decision-making, is there an ethical justification for doing so? (APHA, 2019).

In addition to the core values, aspects of ethical analysis and eight considerations, there are 12 domains to guide ethical actions. These ethical action guidance domains are meant to inform and enlighten the judgment necessary to be exercised in ethical public health practice. The 12 domains are:

1. Conduct and disseminate assessments focused on population health status and public health issues facing the community
2. Investigate health problems and environmental public health hazards to protect the community
3. Inform and educate the public about health issues and functions
4. Engage with the community to identify and address health problems
5. Develop public health policies and plans
6. Enforce public health laws
7. Promote improved access to social resources conducive to health and healthcare
8. Maintain a competent public health workforce
9. Evaluate and continuously improve processes, programs, and interventions
10. Contribute to and apply the evidence base to public health
11. Maintain administrative and management capacity
12. Maintain capacity to engage with public health governing entities (APHA, 2019)

PRIVACY AND CONFIDENTIALITY

The concept of privacy is rooted in the Fourth Amendment of the U.S. Constitution. The Fourth Amendment protects citizens against searches that violate an individual's reasonable expectation of privacy. Privacy and confidentiality are two concepts frequently used together and incorrectly used interchangeably. In general terms, privacy applies to the individual person and confidentiality to the information or data about the individual person. Privacy refers to the freedom from intrusion into an individual's personal matters or information, whereas confidentiality refers to personal information that is shared with an individual or others that cannot be divulged to a third party without the expressed permission of affected individual. It is important as epidemiologists to remember that acts or behaviors done in a public place or venue would not be considered private; however, there are substantial gray areas as to what can be considered truly "public." As a healthcare provider or member of the public healthcare team, epidemiologists have an implied contract of confidentiality. Box 25.1 provides some strategies for the epidemiologist to consider in relation to privacy and confidentiality.

BOX 25.1. Epidemiological Privacy and Confidentiality Strategies

Privacy Strategies
- Consider the method used to identify and contact individuals
- Ensure privacy in the setting of interaction with an individual
- Minimize the personnel present during the epidemiologic interaction
- Pay attention to the method used to obtain information and the surroundings
- Access minimum amount of information necessary

Confidentiality Strategies
- Destroy information about individuals not involved
- Limit the information obtained in preparation for an epidemiologic investigation
- Shield the individual's identity to protect their information such as data file encryption
- Inform the individual of any potential or known confidentiality risks

ARTIFICIAL INTELLIGENCE AND ETHICAL EPIDEMIOLOGIC ISSUES

The use of artificial intelligence tools is increasing in the healthcare sector. Epidemiologic ethical challenges could arise from the combination of rapidly evolving technologies, engagement of new stakeholders, data quality issues, and a lack of regulatory controls or standards to guide the use of artificial intelligence tools. Artificial intelligence tools, inclusive of apps and biosensors, are being used to generate large data sets. A digital health decision-making framework has been proposed to support ethical considerations with the use of digital health data and artificial intelligence tools. The framework is based on the ethical principles of respect for persons, beneficence, and justice. Four areas to consider are privacy, access and usability, data management, and risks and benefits. Privacy should consider the conveying of personal data collection, terms and conditions and policies supporting privacy, and disclosure of data-sharing practices. Access and usability should consider the diverse populations that the artificial intelligence tools are accessible to, ability to tailor tools for end user, and feasibility of short- and long-term usage. Data management considerations should include protocols for data collection and data storage protection, policy on who can access the data, and use of data security best practices. Lastly, the risks and benefits should consider the evidence used to support the validity and reliability of artificial intelligence tools, the extent to which risks are disclosed, and the extent to which the benefits of articulations of intelligence tools outweigh the risks. As epidemiologists increase the use of digital/artificial intelligence in their practice, this framework can guide ethical decision-making to ensure data privacy and confidentiality (Nebeker et al., 2019).

HEALTH INSURANCE PORTABILITY AND ACCOUNTABILITY ACT, 1996

The Health Insurance Portability and Accountability Act (HIPAA), Privacy Rule, was passed in 1996 as a national set of standards for the protection of certain health information. The goal of the Privacy Rule was to ensure that an individual's health information was properly protected while permitting the flow of health information across healthcare entities and need to provide and promote high quality healthcare to protect the individual's well-being and the public's health. This legislation was an attempt to balance the privacy of individuals with the important need to share health information for individual and population health. This Privacy Rule sets standards for the use and disclosure of an individual's health information known as protected health information (PHI). Healthcare entities that are subject to the Privacy Rule are referred to as covered entities.

The Privacy Rule applies to health plans, health care information/data clearinghouses, and any healthcare provider who transmits health information in an electronic form. This coverage is extended to business associates who perform certain functions or activities for or on behalf of the covered entity as long as this service involves the use or disclosure of PHI. The basic premise is to define and limit the circumstances in which individual's PHI may be used or disclosed to covered entities.

PHI is all individually identifiable health information that is maintained, held, or transmitted by a covered entity or business associates. PHI includes demographic data that identifies the individual or for which there is a reasonable basis to believe that the information can be used to identify the individual. PHI includes common identities such as name, address, birth date, and Social Security number. PHI also includes information related to:

- Individual's past, present, or future physical or mental health or health condition
- Provision of healthcare to the individual
- Individual's past, present, or future payment for the provision of healthcare to the individual

Another aspect of the Privacy Rule is minimum necessary information. A covered entity must make all reasonable efforts to use, disclose, and request only the minimum amount of PHI needed to accomplish the intended purpose for the requested information. The covered entity is required to obtain an individual's written authorization for any use or disclosure of PHI that is not for treatment, payment, or healthcare operations, other than that is permitted by the Privacy Rule. In addition, the individual is required to be provided an acknowledgment of the Privacy Rule receipt.

It is critical for healthcare providers and epidemiologists to be knowledgeable about the utilization of PHI for epidemiologic purposes. Epidemiologists should be knowledgeable regarding the data that can be accessed and disclosed within the parameters of the HIPAA Privacy Rule.

CONFLICTS OF INTEREST

Conflicts of interest can be avoided through transparency. A conflict of interest exists when an individual has a conflict between personal or private interests and the responsibilities associated with their position of authority or their professional role. Conflicts of interest are not limited to financial benefits.

Conflicts of interest can be actual with tangible outcomes and can exist if others perceive that there is a conflict of interest. Several types of conflicts of interest exist: objective, subjective, potential, actual, or apparent. An objective conflict of interest involves a financial relationship. A subjective conflict of interest is based on emotional ties or a relationship. A potential conflict of interest occurs when an individual has an interest that may influence the individual's judgment and decisions in the future that may not be actualized. An actual conflict of interest occurs when an individual has an interest that impacts their judgment and engagement in an activity that is directly related to the area of the conflict. An apparent conflict of interest occurs when there is no actual conflict of interest but other persons who are considering the situation perceive that there is an actual conflict of interest (Velasquez, 2017). An individual's employment position, profession, personal relationships, and personal obligations and responsibilities influence conflicts of interest.

Engagement in a conflict of interest activity is considered unethical behavior. Conflict of interest prevention is considered the best strategy to resolve conflicts of interest, whether it is an actual or perceived conflict of interest. The following strategies are recommended to avoid conflicts of interest:

- Maintain role clarity
- Act in accordance with rules and regulations
- Follow the letter and intent or spirit of the policy
- Recognize potential conflicts of interest early
- Identify primary and secondary constituents of a potential conflict of interest
- Examine and reflect on any potential conflict of interest
- Review policies governing potential conflicts of interest

- Discuss potential conflicts of interest with individuals whose span of authority encompasses the area of potential conflict
- Secure an opinion regarding the potential conflict of interest prior to engaging in an activity that may be determined to be a conflict of interest (Porche, 2019).

ETHICAL COMPETENCE

Ethical competence is the quest for knowledge and action that defines what is right from what is wrong (Menzel, 2016). An ethically competent individual is capable of knowing the boundaries of their knowledge and expertise as to do no harm. Ethical competence is considered a fundamental competence to all health care providers and public health practitioners, including epidemiologist. Figure 25.2 provides the interrelated competencies necessary for ethical competence. The interrelated ethical competencies are:

1. **Ethical reasoning:** The ability to reason through difficult complex ethical dilemmas that require the consideration of more than one principle, value, virtue, or law at the same time while giving consideration to the situation for the purpose of arriving at an ethical decision
2. **Public ethics and values action:** Acting on personal, professional, and humanitarian values
3. **Promotion of organizational ethical practices and behaviors:** Public health providers should lead in an ethical manner while developing and implementing organizational structures, systems, and processes that promote ethical practice
4. **Commitment to high ethical standards:** Personally and professionally holding yourself and others accountable to the highest ethical standards

EPIDEMIOLOGIC ETHICAL ISSUES

Epidemiology, like other health-related and public health disciplines has several potential areas for the emergence of ethical situations. Epidemiology as a discipline grew out of medical and public health science and shares some overlapping areas of ethical concern. Additionally, epidemiologic findings have clinical, public health, and policy implications

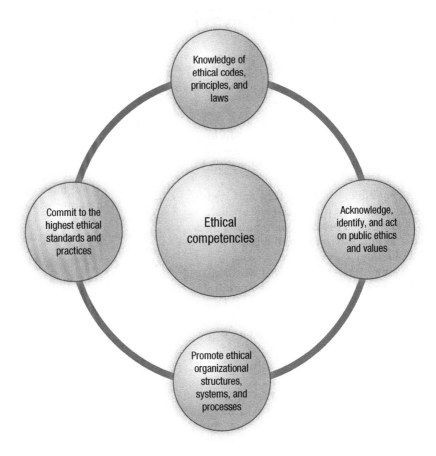

Figure 25.2 Interrelated ethical competencies.

expanding the nature and potential for ethical concerns. The ultimate goal of the ethical conduct of epidemiology is to generate scientific knowledge to impact the distribution and determinants of health conditions within a population, rendering the population and public healthier. Epidemiologists are required to balance the risk and benefits of research and epidemiologic practice, while balancing the rights of the individual and general welfare of the public and society. Box 25.2 presents some potential epidemiologic ethical issues that can arise.

BOX 25.2. Potential Epidemiologic Ethical Issues

- Data falsification and fabrication
- Privacy and confidentiality versus monitoring and surveillance
- Duty to warn
- Benefit and risk determination
- Conflict of interest
- Individual, personal, professional, and community obligations conflict
- Informed consent
- Search and seizure
- Data encryption and data transfer
- Mandatory/compulsory versus voluntary screening

END-OF-CHAPTER RESOURCES

SUMMARY POINTS

- Ethical guidelines and principles guide the ethical practice of epidemiology.
- Ethics is the study of the nature and justification of principles that guide individuals to act in a moral manner consistent with society's customs, values, beliefs, and norms.
- Professional ethics are the values and standards developed by a professional or discipline over a period of time that identifies the salient and inherent varies of the profession or discipline.
- Applied ethics is the practical real-world application of values and principles to ethical issues.
- Advocacy ethics focus on representing another individual, group, or population's interest in relation to equality and social justice.
- Ethical behavior is the result of ethical decision-making processes (DMPs).
- Deontology states that an action's moral rightness or wrongness depends on the action itself and the motivation behind the action along with the moral obligation felt toward that action.
- Moral obligation is an individual's feeling about a sense of duty that requires action in a particular manner based on values, beliefs, and perspective of societal norms.
- Teleology determines rightness or wrongness based solely on the expected outcomes or consequences of an action.
- Utilitarianism focuses more on the ultimate number of individuals impacted by the action that produces a specific outcome or consequence.
- Beneficence weighs the benefits of an action against the risks or costs to the individual, group, or population involved.
- Nonmaleficence principle focuses on "doing no harm."
- Justice ensures the fair and equitable distribution of benefits, risks, and costs.
- Autonomy provides individuals with the right to make their own independent decisions.
- Fidelity is known as promise keeping.
- Veracity is known as truth telling.
- Values are beliefs that an individual or social group hold regarding what is relevant and important to their belief system.

- The value clarification process promotes self-reflection to identify values and value system.
- The Declaration of Helsinki established a set of ethical principles to provide guidance in the conduct of research with human subjects.
- Ethical dilemmas arise when there is a conflict in the principles, duties, rights, beliefs, or values of one individual, group, population, or community with another or with societal expectations.
- Bioethics is the integration of ethics and biology.
- Bioethics places the ethical question within the context of biology and health-related science.
- Privacy refers to the freedom from intrusion into an individual's personal matters or information.
- Confidentiality refers to personal information that is shared with an individual or others that cannot be divulged to a third party without the expressed permission of affected individual.
- Public health information (PHI) is all individually identifiable health information that is maintained, held, or transmitted by a covered entity or business associates.
- A conflict of interest exists when an individual has a conflict between personal or private interests and the responsibilities associated with their position of authority or professional role.
- Ethical competence is the quest for knowledge and action that defines what is right from what is wrong.

EPIDEMIOLOGY CRITICAL REASONING QUESTIONS

1. Integrate your personal, discipline specific, or professional ethical principles with the American College of Epidemiology Ethical Guidelines into a personal code of ethics for your epidemiologic practice.
2. Complete the three-step values clarification exercise:
   a. First, select eight to ten value words below that are most important to your personal and professional practice of epidemiology. Feel free to identify a value word that is not listed:

Truth	Control
Curiosity	Flexibility
Efficiency	Love intelligence
Productivity	Persistence
Initiative	Sincerity
Power	Happiness
Excitement	Relationships
Happiness	Wisdom
Honor	Perspectives
Obedience	Commitment
Innovation	Recognition
Creativity	Learning
Loyalty	Honesty
Clarity	Discipline
Peace	Fairness
Conflict	Order
Respect	Collaboration
Empathy	Sympathy
Family	Independence
Autonomy dependability	Excellence
Risk-taking	Perfection
Freedom	Beauty
Justice	Service
Equality	Profitability
Equity	Self-control
Diversity	Success
Purposefulness	Harmony
Dedication	Simplicity
Friendship	Fairness
Caring	Stewardship
Originality	Fulfillment

_____   _____

Value: _____   Value: _____

Value: _____   Value: _____

Value: _____   Value: _____

Value: _____   Value: _____

Value: _____   Value: _____

b. Second, from the selected list of eight to ten value words, narrow the list to only three to five values words.

Value: _____   Value: _____

Value: _____   Value: _____

Value: _____

c. Third, write your three to five value words in order of priority, with the highest priority value listed first.
   i.   Priority Value 1: _____
   ii. Priority Value 2: _____
   iii. Priority Value 3: _____
   iv. Priority Value 4: _____
   v.   Priority Value 5: _____

d. Fourth, write an outcome statement for each priority value word, such as "integrity—doing the right thing."

   Value:_____

      Outcome Statement: _____

e. Fifth, write specific behaviors that demonstrate the value and outcome statement, such as "always telling the truth." Write at least two to five behaviors for each value and outcome statement.

   Value:_____

      OutcomeStatement:_____

      Behaviors of the Value: 1)_____

                              2)_____

                              3)_____

f. The above five steps have facilitated your identification of your core personal and professional values related to the practice of epidemiology. In this final step, compose a statement that integrates your core ethical values. For example, "As an epidemiologist, I will curiously pursue truth, justice, and fairness in a decisive manner to influence the health and welfare of diverse populations." This serves as your guiding core values statement that clarified the values important to you in the practice of epidemiology.

   Core Value Statement: _____
   _____
   _____
   _____

3. Determine the values of your epidemiologic team.
   a. Identify the top three to five values that reflect the purpose of your team.
   b. What is the alignment of the team's values with the individual team members' values?

c. What is the extent to which the team values reflect the institution's values?

d. What are potential areas of ethical dilemma that may develop as a result of individual and team value conflicts or lack of alignment?

e. What are the behavior observations that align with the team member and team's values? Complete the table below:

Team Member Values	Team's Values	Behavioral Observations that Exemplify Values

ADDITIONAL RESOURCES

 SPRINGER PUBLISHING **CONNECT™** | A robust set of instructor resources designed to supplement this text is located at http://connect. springerpub.com/content/book/978-0-8261-8514-3. Qualifying instructors may request access by emailing textbook@springerpub.com.

REFERENCES

American College of Epidemiology. (2000). *American college of epidemiology ethical guidelines.* https://www.acepidemiology.org/ethics-guidelines

American Nurses Association. (2015). *Code of ethics for nurses with interpretive statements.* American Nurses Publishing.

American Public Health Association. (2019). *Public health code of ethics.* Author.

Beauchamp, T. L., & Childress, J. F. (2019). *Principles of biomedical ethics* (8th ed.). Oxford University Press.

Callahan, D., & Jennings, B. (2002). Ethics and public health: Forging a strong relationship. *American Journal of Public Health, 92*(2), 169–176. https://doi.org/10.2105/ajph.92.2.169

Coletta, S. (1978). Value clarification in nursing: Why? *American Journal of Nursing, 78*(12), 2057. https://www.jstor.org/stable/3462144

Forte, D., Kawai, F., & Cohen, C. (2018). A bioethical framework to guide the decision-making process in the care of seriously ill patients. *BMC Medical Ethics, 19*, 78–85. https://doi.org/10.1186/s12910-018-0317-y

Menzel, D. (2016). Ethical competence. In A. Farazmand (Ed.), *Global encyclopedia of public administration, public policy, and governance.* Springer. https://doi.org/10.1007/978-3-319-31816-5_2458-1

National Commission for the Protection of Human Subjects of Biomedical and Behavioral Research, Department of Health, Education and Welfare. (1978). *The Belmont report.* United States Government Printing Office.

Nebeker, C., Torous, J., & Bartlett Ellis, R. (2019). Building the case for actionable ethics in digital health research supported by artificial intelligence. *BMC Medicine, 17*, 137–143. https://doi.org/10.1186/s12916-019-1377-7

Porche, D. (2003). *Public and community health nursing practice: A population-based approach.* Sage.

Raths, L., Harmin, M., & Simon, S. (1978). *Values and teaching* (2nd ed.). Charles E. Merrill.

World Medical Association. (2013). *WMA declaration of Helsinki – Ethical principles for medical research involving human subjects.* https://www.wma.net/policies-post/wma-declaration-of-helsinki-ethical-principles-for-medical-research-involving-human-subjects/

Velasquez, M. G. (2017). *Business ethics: Concepts and cases* (8th ed.). Pearson Education Limited.

Section VI:
APPENDICES

INTEGRATED POPULATION AND COMMUNITY ASSESSMENT FRAMEWORK: COMMUNITY ASSESSMENT AND EPIDEMIOLOGIC DATA ELEMENTS

Demetrius J. Porche

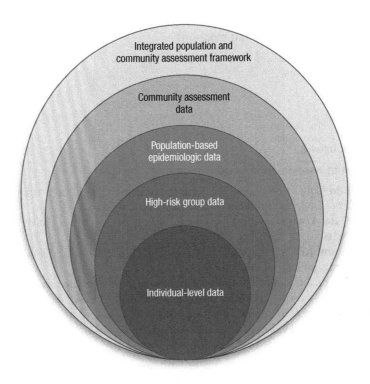

INTEGRATED POPULATION AND COMMUNITY ASSESSMENT FRAMEWORK

I. Dimensions of a Community

  a. Location or Geography
    i. Community boundaries
    ii. Placement of healthcare services
    iii. Geographic features
    iv. Climate
    v. Plants and animals
    vi. Interaction of man and environment

  b. Population/People
    i. Population statistics/demographics
    ii. Population density
    iii. Composition of population
    iv. Population growth or decline
    v. Cultural characteristics
    vi. Social class
    vii. Population mobility (i.e., immigration and naturalization rates)

  c. Social Systems
    i. Welfare and social services available
    ii. Political parties—majority and minority party leadership
    iii. Recreational systems
    iv. Legal/governmental structure and divisions
    v. Communication systems and medium

  d. Relationships
    i. Healthcare systems
    ii. Family
    iii. Economic
    iv. Educational
    v. Religious
    vi. Major industries

II. Community Health Assessment Process

  a. **Phase I—Data Collection:** Collection of information that will determine what the community comprises. Collect population level epidemiologic data
  b. **Phase II—Data Analysis:** Compilation of all data to develop a list of assets, deficits, and possible deficits
  c. **Phase III—Community Diagnosis:** Listing of healthcare assets, deficits, and possible deficits as identified through data analysis
  d. **Phase IV—Proposed Community Level Interventions:** Provide recommendations for identified concerns based on community assets, deficits, and possible deficits
  e. **Phase V—Potential Outcomes:** Expected outcomes from proposed interventions
  f. **Phase VI—Report:** Development of formal report

III. Purpose of Community Assessment

  a. Determine strengths (assets), weaknesses, and needs of communities
  b. Develop a database of community resources and assets
  c. Guide program planning
  d. Provide comprehensive contextual assessment for nurse practitioner practice
  e. Identify at risk populations
  f. Develop primary, secondary, tertiary, and quaternary prevention programs
  g. Reduce the burden of epidemics and pandemics

IV. Community Assessment Processes

    a. Community assets mapping

        i. Leads development of policies and activities based on capacities, skills, and assets of all citizens

        ii. Community development takes place best when local community people are committed to investing in the community

        iii. Builds from the inside out, not top down

        iv. Key to neighborhood regeneration is to locate all the available assets, and begin connecting these assets in a manner that multiplies their power and effectiveness

        v. Assets of a community

            1. Individuals

            2. Associations

            3. Formal and informal groups

            4. Institutions and businesses

            5. Physical assets

            6. Public health and healthcare infrastructure

    b. Windshield Survey

        i. Ride throughout the community at different times of the day, evening, and night

        ii. Scan the community

    c. Traditional Needs-Based Assessment Process

        i. Assess the following aspects of a community:

            1. Housing

                a. How are neighborhoods alike or different in age, type of architecture, materials of construction?

                b. How are houses spaced (e.g., grassy areas, vacant lots)?

                c. What is the general condition of housing?

            2. Zoning

                a. What is the political district?

                b. What is the parish/county seat?

                c. What is the zip code?

                d. What is the police, fire district?

            3. Space use

                a. How is the land used (e.g., open space, residential, agricultural, industrial)?

                b. What is the quality of the space (e.g., flowers, broken pavement)?

                c. Is open space public or private? Used by whom?

                d. What effect does the geography of the community have on its life (e.g., any natural river, valleys)?

                e. Are there any landfills, waste management centers?

                f. Is there any evidence of pollution (e.g., air, water)?

            4. Boundaries

                a. What signs tell you where the community begins and ends? Are the boundaries natural or political, economic, cultural, or ethnic?

                b. Does the community have an official or unofficial local name? Is the name displayed or verbally used by residents or others?

                c. Is there evidence of different neighborhood groups within the community?

            5. Common areas

                a. What are the hangout places where people gather?

                b. Do hangout places differ by age, sex, socioeconomic status, or other factors?

                c. Are common areas territorial or open to strangers?

                d. Are there different types of individuals in different common areas?

6. Transportation

   a. How do people get in and out of the community?
   b. How do streets, roads, and methods of transportation appear to affect the community life? Are potential accidents or problem areas visible?
   c. Is public transportation available?
   d. Do street names reveal history or other community characteristics?
   e. What are the primary modes of transportation that you see?
   f. Are appropriate safety precautions taken for the respective modes of transportation?

7. Service centers

   a. Do you see social agencies, health facilities, recreation centers, and signs of activities at the school?
   b. Are there offices of doctors, dentists, spiritualists, massage therapists?

8. Stores

   a. Where do residents shop?
   b. How do they travel to shops?
   c. Are there differences in shopping among different neighborhoods in the community?
   d. What kind of goods are available to local residents?

9. Street scene

   a. Who do you see on the streets – mothers, babies, teenagers, the unemployed, the homeless, elders, salespersons?
   b. Are they typical of people you would expect to see on the streets at the time you see them?
   c. Are the people you see dressed as you would expect to see them; if not, how do they differ from what you would expect?
   d. Do you see animals, such as stray cats or dogs, pedigreed pets, watch dogs?

10. Community growth and dynamics

   a. Do you see signs of community growth such as real estate signs, new construction (home/industrial), remodeling, street repair, political posters, neighborhood meeting posters?
   b. Do you see signs of community decline such as trash, abandoned cars, real estate signs concentrated in certain neighborhoods, abandoned houses, mixed zoning usage, and so forth?
   c. Is there evidence of graffiti?

11. Race/ethnicity

   a. What evidence do you see of racial characteristics of the people (e.g., genetic characteristics of people, skin color, hair type)?
   b. Is there evidence of diversity and inclusion in the community?
   c. What evidence do you see of the ethnic characteristics of the people (e.g., food stores, churches, private schools, information in a language other than English)?

12. Religion

   a. What denominations are the churches?
   b. Do you see evidence of religious homogeneity or heterogeneity?
   c. What other institutions or agencies are associated with the religious institutions (e.g., schools, community centers)?

13. Politics

   a. Do you see any political campaign posters?
   b. Do you see any evidence of party affiliations? A predominant party affiliation?

14. Media/communications

    a. Do you see TV antennas or presence of satellite dishes?

    b. What kinds of magazines, newspapers are available to the residents?

    c. Which media seem most important to residents (e.g., radio, TV, print)?

    d. What is the quality of internet service provided? Who are the major providers of internet services?

15. Community personality

    a. How does the community affect your senses (e.g., hearing, smell, feeling)?

    b. Does the community give you a good feeling or uncomfortable feeling? Can you pinpoint any particular reasons for this feeling?

    c. How were you greeted by the local residents—friendly or treated as an outsider?

    d. What was the local dialect?

d. Primary and secondary data collection

1. Primary data are data collected by the practitioner through surveys or other research methods

2. Secondary data are data accessed from a primary source such as published reports or articles

3. Population profile

    i. How many people live in the community?

    ii. What are the age, gender, and race distribution?

    iii. What family types (e.g., single-parent, nuclear, extended, nontraditional) are there?

    iv. Which family type predominates?

    v. Number of children in foster care?

    vi. What ethnic or cultural groups exist within the community? How do they affect community life?

    vii. Does the community have refugee/migrant populations?

    viii. What efforts have the community made to incorporate these new members?

    ix. What subcultural groups can you identify in the community? How do they impact on community life?

    x. What child rearing practices predominate? Do you see differences in child rearing ideas among community groups?

    xi. What beliefs, customs or practices do families have surrounding pregnancy and childbirth?

    xii. What social classes are represented in the community (lower, middle, upper)? Which one predominates?

    xiii. What is the population density such as population density per square mile?

    xiv. What are the marriage and divorce rates?

    xv. What is the birth rate?

    xvi. How has the population characteristics changed in the past decade?

4. Housing

    i. What kind of housing is available in the community?

    ii. Does the community support temporary or transient housing opportunities?

    iii. What is the average cost for housing?

    iv. How often do people in the community move (within or into and out of the community)?

    v. How well are the homes maintained?

    vi. Is there a noticeable difference in the quality of housing in different parts of the community?

    vii. Does the community provide programs or sponsor volunteer programs to enable low-income persons to improve or maintain marginal housing?

5. Transportation

   i. Are there major highways that make the community accessible?
   ii. How do people travel within the community (e.g., taxi, Uber/Lift, bus, train, airplane, private car, volunteer transportation, horse and buggy, bicycle)?
   iii. Does the cost of transportation affect community members?

6. Economic system

   i. What occupational groups (e.g., retail, industrial, farming, service, government, tourism, healthcare, unemployed) are represented in the community? Which ones predominate?
   ii. How does the occupation of members of the community affect their lives?
   iii. Do most people work within the community? Or do many travel to other communities for employment?
   iv. Is unemployment a current, past, continuing, or occasional problem for the community? For what reasons would unemployment affect the community?
   v. In what ways are local industries influential in local life?
   vi. Is the industrial/economic base of the community growing, remaining stable, or declining?
   vii. What are typical (median, average) income levels of persons living within the community?

7. Community history

   i. What was the settlement date of the community?
   ii. What important events or factors affect the development of the community?
   iii. Who were important persons in the growth of the community?

8. Protective systems: Police

   i. What are your chances of becoming a crime victim in the community?
   ii. What types of criminal activity are prevalent? How many full-time, part-time police does the department have? Are these numbers adequate?
   iii. What is the police response time?
   iv. Do the police have adequate equipment and training to do their job? Does the community support the department financially?
   v. Does the police department sponsor crime prevention programs? What are they?
   vi. Are there security systems in the houses? Are there bars on the windows?
   vii. Is there police patrol?
   viii. Are there neighborhood watch programs?
   ix. Are geographic crime maps available and updated regularly?

9. Protective systems: Fire

   i. How serious a concern is fire in this community? Industrial? Home? Particular areas of the community?
   ii. How many full-time, part-time, volunteer firemen does the department have? Are these numbers adequate?
   iii. What is the fire department response time?
   iv. Does the fire department have adequate equipment and training to do its job? Does the community support the department financially?
   v. Is there a central water supply for firefighting?
   vi. Does the department offer fire prevention education?
   vii. What methods or programs are used? Are there any universal signals used for fire and rescue (children's bedrooms have special signs)?

10. Protective systems: Emergency health

    i. Types of situations EMS most often responds to in the community

    ii. How many full-time, part-time, and volunteer personnel does the EMS department have?

    iii. What is the response time?

    iv. Does the EMS department have adequate equipment and training to do the job?

    v. Are the ambulances up to date?

    vi. How is the EMS system activated?

    vii. Does the community support the department financially?

    viii. Does EMS sponsor education and safety programs? What are they?

    ix. Is there a 911 system? What other emergency alert systems exist in the community for special populations such as the elderly, demented, mentally challenged?

11. Food supply system

    i. What restaurants are within the community?

    ii. How often do people in the community tend to eat out? Would you say that menus available in restaurants may significantly affect the health of members of this community? How?

    iii. What grocery stores (chain or locally owned), specialty food stores, fresh, or locally grown sources are available in the community?

    iv. Does the cost of food affect the availability of food or certain types of food for members of the whole community or subgroups in the community?

    v. How does the community provide for persons unable to afford, purchase, or prepare their own food?

    vi. Do you see evidence of differences in diet preferences among community subgroups? What differences exist?

    vii. What is the typical diet like within the community?

12. Religious/ethnic groups

    i. What religious groups are there? What belief systems do they represent?

    ii. What ethnic groupings influences are there?

    iii. How significant is the role of religion or ethnicity in the community?

    iv. How many people in the community have church/religious affiliations?

    v. How does religion impact on health decisions?

13. Other community decisions

    i. How is death typically handled by members of the community? What rituals, burials rites, or resources are used to manage the care of deceased persons?

    ii. Are there subgroups within the community in which death is handled in a different manner than the methods used by the majority of the community? What methods do these groups use?

14. Community culture

    i. What are the predominate cultural beliefs of the community? Are they representative of the entire community?

    ii. What cultural groupings are there in the community?

    iii. What belief systems do they represent?

    iv. How significant is the role of culture in the community?

    v. What are the intercultural and intracultural variations?

    vi. What are the cultural values and beliefs about health, wellness, healthcare, research, family, and parenting?

    vii. Does the community have planned cultural events such as blessing of boats, crops, fairs, festivals?

15. Educational systems

    i. How many schools (public or private) are there in the community (e.g., junior high, elementary, middle school, senior high, junior colleges, local colleges, universities, and special schools). If education beyond high school is not available in the community, what schools are accessible within the region?

    ii. What grade levels or specialized focus do these schools include?

    iii. How many students (adult/child) attend the schools?

    iv. What is the average daily attendance? What are the dropout rates? What are the graduation rates? What are the reasons for absences?

    v. What are the average test scores on standardized national examinations?

    vi. What is the typical class size? Student: teacher ratio? What types of programs do schools offer? Is there a latchkey program? How many children use it? How is the program paid for? Are there special programs for adults?

    vii. What recreational activities are there?

    viii. Do schools offer advanced placement or programs for gifted children?

    ix. What percentage of students from this school system go to college?

    x. What types of vocational options are there for students who do not elect to apply to college?

    xi. How do schools address special education needs of children (e.g., learning disabled, hearing impaired, visually impaired, children needing to learn English as a second language)?

    xii. How do schools address the health concerns of their children?

    xiii. Is there a school nurse? What responsibilities does the nurse have? How much time do they spend in the schools?

    xiv. Who pays the school nurse's salary?

    xv. What are the significant health needs, concerns, or issues of students in this school system? What community agencies are involved in meeting the needs of students in the school or school-age population of the community?

    xvi. What state and federally funded programs based on economic needs are the schools in your community eligible to receive? What makes the school eligible or ineligible for such programs?

16. Healthcare system

    i. What Western-type (allopathic) health care facilities/programs/personnel are there in the community?

    ii. Who is available within the community to provide Western-type healthcare (e.g., physicians, nurses, dentists, psychologists, physical therapists, other)?

    iii. What hospitals are most often used by members of the community. Which is the closest?

    iv. What kinds of in-patient care are available within the community?

    v. What kinds of out-patient services are available within the community?

    vi. What emergency/urgent care facilities are included within or easily accessible to the community?

    vii. What extended care facilities are included within or easily accessible to the community?

    viii. What residential care facilities are included within or easily accessible to the community?

    ix. Does the community have access to a hospice program? What agency(ies) provides these services? Who is eligible to use them?

    x. Are respite and adult day care services available? Who provides them?

    xi. What official health department services/programs are conducted within the community?

    xii. How is prevention and monitoring of communicable diseases managed within the community?

xiii. Are there public health systems in place for contact tracing?

xiv. What is the relationship of integrated public, private, and community-based healthcare services?

xv. What is the status of integrated healthcare records within the community and across population healthcare agencies?

xvi. How are environmental or sanitation problems addressed?

xvii. What are the services to mothers and children provided through official agency programs?

xviii. What programs are available for people with special problems such as HIV infection and other chronic diseases?

xix. What traditional healthcare facilities, programs, and personnel exist within the community (e.g., folk healers or practitioners, spiritual healers, other)?

xx. Is there evidence that Eastern-type medicine such as acupuncture, acupressure, massage, meditation is used by members of the community?

xxi. Do members of the community rely on folk or home remedies? What are they?

xxii. Does the community use such healthcare practitioners as chiropractors, homeopathic healers, nurse practitioners, physician assistants?

xxiii. Are there veterinarians for care of community animals?

xxiv. What kinds of animals play a role in community life?

xxv. How do animals affect the well-being of community members?

xxvi. Are there integrated healthcare systems of physicians and veterinary providers?

xxvii. How do members of the community typically pay for healthcare? What resources are there for those who are unable to pay for healthcare? How many citizens are underinsured or uninsured for healthcare?

xxviii. Do those who live in the community perceive barriers to healthcare options of their choice? Do you identify barriers not identified by community members?

xxix. What kind of health education programs are available to those who live in the community? Who provides the programs? What issues have been addressed recently? Who pays for the program?

xxx. What type of self-help or mutual assistance programs exist within the community?

17. Communication system

i. What newspapers (local or regional) are read by community members?

ii. Are local or regional newspapers available electronically?

iii. What radio stations with what type of programming are typically used as a source of entertainment or information by community members?

iv. What TV, satellite, or internet stations (local, regional, national, cable) are most often used as a source of entertainment or information by community members?

v. Are community bulletin boards used to share information or buy and sell goods and services within the community?

vi. Where are bulletin boards located? Are the bulletin boards electronic?

vii. Do you see displays, posters, digital monitors in store fronts that tell you about life in the community?

viii. What did you learn about the community by information posted in store fronts?

ix. What libraries (general use or specialty type) are available to community members? How many people use library services and what kinds of services does the library provide? Are community library resources available electronically?

    x. What informal communication systems (gossip centers) do you identify in the community?

    xi. What are the patterns of linear communication chains (horizontal and vertical communication) within the community?

    xii. Who are the major advertisers within the community?

18. Government and political system

    i. What political parties dominate decision-making in the community?

    ii. How effective is community decision-making through the political process?

    iii. What issues have most affected the community in recent years (e.g., housing, transportation, health, water and sewage, police and fire, group homes, other)?

    iv. What government structure is used by the community?

    v. Does the community have an emergency disaster plan?

    vi. Who is responsible for it? What types of emergencies does it address? Has it been used? If so, how did it work?

    vii. What are the major public health policies developed specific to this community?

    viii. What are the governmental priorities that are addressed by the community budget?

19. Recreational system

    i. Does the community have any recreational programs in place for members of the community?

    ii. Are there any recreational parks nearby for community members?

    iii. What recreational activities do community members take part in?

    iv. Are there any movie theaters in the community?

    v. Are there any health fitness clubs in the community?

    vi. Are there any senior citizen recreational programs available for members of the community?

    vii. What are the primary hobbies of the citizens?

    viii. What is the number of walking tracts or neighborhood fitness trails? Are there community pools, baseball fields, or basketball courts?

    ix. What is the number of people exercising?

    x. Are there bars? How many? What types?

    xi. Are there pet parks? What facilities exist for pet lifestyle?

20. Environmental system

    i. What environment issues affect the community life (personal or industrial)?

    ii. What agencies, policies, or programs affect environmental issues in the community?

    iii. What is the source of water supply for the community? Are sources adequate for current and future use?

    iv. How is the water supply tested and kept free from contaminants?

    v. How does the community dispose of its wastes (e.g., sanitation systems, trash removal, recycling programs/facilities, landfills, cost, industrial or hazardous wastes)?

    vi. Does the disposal of waste constitute an economic or environmental concern for the community?

    vii. What is the air quality? Are there contaminants (e.g., natural, industrial, energy production related, or transportation related) which affect the community? How is air quality monitored?

    viii. What energy sources are used by the community (e.g., gas, electric, nuclear, or other)?

    ix. Does the cost or availability of energy affect individual consumers or industrial growth? How does the community provide for low-income persons who cannot pay for adequate energy supplies?

      x. Does the community have or need vector control programs (e.g., insects, rodents, mosquitoes, other)?

      xi. What is the topography of the land?

      xii. Are there potential environmental hazards such as rivers that may flood, hills with potential for rockslides?

      xiii. What is the climate? Average temperature, precipitation?

      xiv. What are the common natural disasters? What are the associated health problems connected with the natural disasters?

21. Health status and wellness

      i. What are the major causes of mortality, by age, race, and gender?

      ii. What is the infant mortality rate?

      iii. What is the perinatal mortality rate?

      iv. What is the maternal mortality rate?

      v. What are the common communicable diseases and their rates?

      vi. What is the percent of low birth weight infants?

      vii. How adequate is prenatal care?

      viii. What are the major causes of morbidity by age, race, and gender?

      ix. What are the types of disability?

      x. What is the level of tobacco, alcohol, and drug use? Types of drugs used?

      xi. What are the major biological, psychological health alterations?

      xii. What is the average life expectancy, for males and females?

      xiii. What is the teen pregnancy rate?

      xiv. What is the level of violence—child abuse, elder abuse, and partner abuse?

      xv. What are the major acute illnesses—are they seasonal?

      xvi. What are the major chronic illnesses?

      xvii. What are the leading causes of morbidity and mortality statistic by population demographics?

      xviii. What epidemics or pandemics have affected the population within the last 3, 5, and 10 years?

      xix. What are the major findings of genetic, social, environmental, and occupational epidemiologic studies in the community?

      xx. What health disparities exist?

e. Community-based associations

      i. What are the trade/labor, professional, neighborhood, religious, and special interest associations within the community?

      ii. What is the mission of the respective associations?

      iii. What services are provided by the respective associations?

f. Community-based institutions

      i. What are the community-based institutions within the community (institutions immersed within the community to meet the community's needs) such as community-based AIDS service organizations?

      ii. What is the mission of these institutions?

      iii. What services are provided by these institutions?

      iv. What is the power base of the institution?

e. Integrating the Epidemiological Approach into Community Assessment

  i. Epidemiology concepts

    1. The study of the distribution and determinants of disease frequency in man

    2. Utilizes the epidemiologic triad relationship between host–agent–environment when considering multiple health-related associations and causation

    3. To determine the relationships that exist between the host, agent, and environment, it is necessary to identify measurable variables through data collection

    4.   An agent is an animate or inanimate factor which must be present or lacking for a disease or condition to occur

    5.   A host is a living species capable of being infected or affected by an agent

    6.   Environment is everything external to a specific agent and host

ii.   Epidemiology dimensions—Who, where, when, why, and how

    1.   The who dimension encompasses the host factors

    2.   The where and when dimensions describe the environment

    3.   The why and how dimensions are the relationship between the agent, host, and environment

iii.   Variables used are:

    1.   **Person:** Who is affected

        a.   Age, ethnicity, income, occupation, education, health status, cultural norms, and values

    2.   **Place:** Where affected

        a.   Physical, biological, social, resources, and services

    3.   **Time:** When affected

        a.   Time of year, time of day, trends over time

iv.   Epidemiologic measures of disease occurrence

    1.   Epidemiologic measures should be integrated as critical data elements in all population assessments. This information should be integrated and considered within the context of the community assessment data.

        a.   **Counts:** Actual number of cases

        b.   Rates

            i.   Incidence rates

           ii.   Prevalence rates

          iii.   Disease specific rates

          iv.   Gender specific rates

           v.   Race specific rates

          vi.   Age specific rates

        c.   Ratio

            i.   Odds ratios

           ii.   Relative risk

        d.   Diagnostic and Screening Test

          iii.   Test validity

              1.   Sensitivity

              2.   Specificity

          iv.   Population dynamics

              1.   Test predictive value positive

              2.   Test predictive value negative

           v.   Reliability

        e.   Immunization rates

        f.   R-Naught

END-OF-APPENDIX RESOURCES

REFERENCES

Helvie, C. (1998). *Advanced practice nursing in the community*. Sage.

Porche, D. (2004). *Community and Public Health Nursing Practice: A population-based approach.* Sage Publications.

MORBIDITY AND MORTALITY FORMULAS

Demetrius J. Porche

INCIDENCE RATE

$$\frac{\text{Number of new cases of a disease in an at-risk population during a specific period of time}}{\text{Number of persons at-risk of developing the disease during the specific period of time}} \times 10^n$$

SEX-ADJUSTED INCIDENCE RATE

Male Sex-Adjusted Incidence Rate

$$\frac{\text{Number of men with new cases of disease or condition in the at-risk population during the specific period of time}}{\text{Total number of men at-risk of developing the disease during the specific period of time}} \times 10^n$$

Female Sex-Adjusted Incidence Rate

$$\frac{\text{Number of female with new cases of disease or condition in the at-risk population during the specific period of time}}{\text{Total number of females at-risk of developing the disease during the specific period of time}} \times 10^n$$

PREVALENCE RATE

$$\frac{\text{Number of cases of a disease present (new and old cases) in an at-risk population during a specific period of time}}{\text{Number of persons at-risk of developing the disease during the specific period of time}} \times 10^n$$

MATERNAL AND INFANT RATES

Maternal (Puerperal) Mortality Rate

$$\frac{\text{Number of deaths from puerperal causes in a year}}{\text{Number of life births in same year}} \times 10^n$$

Infant Mortality Rate

$$\frac{\text{Number of infant deaths during year}}{\text{Number of live births in same year}} \times 10^n$$

Neonatal Mortality Rate

$$\frac{\text{Number of deaths in a year of children younger than 28 days of age}}{\text{Number of live births in same year}} \times 10^n$$

Fetal Death Rate

$$\frac{\text{Number of fetal deaths during year}}{\text{Number of live births in same year}} \times 10^n$$

Perinatal Mortality Rate

$$\frac{\text{Number of fetal deaths 28 weeks or more and infant deaths younger than 7 days of age during the year}}{\text{Number of live births and fetal deaths 28 years or more gestation in the same year}} \times 10^n$$

MORTALITY RATES

Survival Rate

$$\frac{\text{Number of cases alive at the end of a specific time period}}{\text{Number of cases alive at the start of the time period}} \times 10^n$$

Case Fatality Rate

$$\frac{\text{Number of deaths due to a specific disease}}{\text{Number of cases of specific disease}} \times 10^n$$

Proportional Mortality Rate

$$\frac{\text{Number of death from specific cause in specified time period}}{\text{Total deaths in same time period}} \times 10^n$$

Cause-Specific Death Rate

$$\frac{\text{Number of deaths in a year due to specific cause}}{\text{Average (mid} - \text{year) population}} \times 10^n$$

Crude Death Rate

$$\frac{\text{Number of deaths in the year}}{\text{Average (mid} - \text{year) population}} \times 10^n$$

HAZARDOUS ENVIRONMENTAL AGENTS, ROUTES OF ENTRY, AND SYMPTOMS

Demetrius J. Porche

Agent	Route of Entry	Symptoms
Metals		
Arsenic	Absorbed by ingestion, inhalation, and permeation of skin or mucous membranes.	Initial signs and symptoms of arsenic ingestion include burning lips, throat constriction and dysphagia, followed by excruciating abdominal pain, hemorrhagic gastritis, gastroenteritis, severe nausea, projectile vomiting, profuse "rice water-like" diarrhea, with hypovolemia resulting in hypotension and an irregular pulse. Muscle cramps, facial edema, bronchitis, dyspnea, chest pain, dehydration, intense thirst, and fluid-electrolyte disturbances are also common. A garlic-like odor of the breath and feces may occur. Hypotension and tachycardia are common early signs. Fever and tachypnea may occur.
Arsine	Inhalation or through cuts and breaks in the skin.	Acute poisoning causes severe vomiting and diarrhea, muscular cramps, facial edema, and cardiac abnormalities. Shock is also possible. Chronic arsenic exposure can affect the skin, respiratory tract, heart, liver, kidneys, blood and blood producing organs, and the nervous system. Death may occur quickly following a massive or concentrated exposure.
Beryllium	Inhalation, ingestion, or skin contact	Pulmonary and systemic granulomatous disease. Nodular skin lesions in patients with chronic beryllium disease. Acute chemical pneumonitis, tracheobronchitis, conjunctivitis, dermatitis, and chronic granulomatous pulmonary disease with systemic manifestations. Acute beryllium disease consists of respiratory tract irritation and dermatitis, sometimes with conjunctivitis. Respiratory tract symptoms range from mild nasopharyngitis to a severe chemical pulmonitis, which may be fatal.
Cadmium	Ingestion or inhalation of dust or fumes.	Symptoms of acute poisoning after inhalation include chest pain; cough (with bloody sputum); difficulty breathing; sore throat, "metal fume fever" (shivering, sweating, body pains, headache); dizziness; irritability; weakness; nausea; vomiting; diarrhea; tracheobronchitis; pneumonitis; and

(continued)

Agent	Route of Entry	Symptoms
		pulmonary edema. After acute ingestion, symptoms include abdominal pain, burning sensation, nausea, vomiting, salivation, muscle cramps, vertigo, shock, unconsciousness, and convulsions. Chronic exposure (by inhalation or ingestion) results in kidney damage, gastrointestinal symptoms, loss of sense of smell, nasal discharge, nose and throat irritation, lack of appetite, weight loss, nausea, tooth discoloration, bone defects, liver damage, anemia, pulmonary emphysema, chronic bronchitis, bronchopneumonia, and death.
Chromium	Inhalation, ingestion, or skin absorption.	Irritation to the upper respiratory tract, severe nasal irritation. Ingestion of hexavalent chromium may cause intense gastrointestinal irritation or ulceration and corrosion, epigastric pain, nausea, vomiting, diarrhea, vertigo, fever, muscle cramps, hemorrhagic diathesis, toxic nephritis, renal failure, intravascular hemolysis, circulatory collapse, peripheral vascular collapse, liver damage, acute multisystem shock, coma, and even death, depending on the dose.
Lead	Inhalation or ingestion of dust.	Acute exposure produces symptoms in the nervous, hematologic, renal, gastrointestinal, and cardiovascular systems. Symptoms include anorexia, vomiting, malaise, and convulsions; may cause permanent brain damage and reversible renal injury.
Mercury	Vapor inhalation or skin absorption.	Symptoms include weakness, chills, metallic taste, nausea, vomiting, abdominal pain, diarrhea, headache, visual disturbances, dyspnea, cough, and chest tightness. Chronic mercury exposure may cause rashes, and corneal and lens changes with visual impairment.
Nickel	Inhalation of dust or fumes.	Asthma, urticaria, erythema multiforme, contact dermatitis, and hand eczema. Acute toxicity from nickel inhalation includes sore throat and hoarseness.
Zinc oxide	Inhalation of dust or fumes.	Metal fume fever (zinc chills, brass founder's ague, etc.) from the inhalation of zinc oxide fumes. Symptoms include fever, chills, muscular pain, nausea, and vomiting. Fever can develop after exposure to zinc oxide fume. Tachycardia and/or dyspnea may be present.
Hydrocarbons		
Benzene	Vapor inhalation or skin absorption.	The major toxic effect on the central nervous system. Symptoms include dizziness, weakness, euphoria, headache, nausea, vomiting, tightness in chest and staggering. With severe exposure symptoms include blurred vision, tremors, shallow and rapid respirations, ventricular dysrhythmias, paralysis, and unconsciousness. Toxicities from inhalation of benzene include irritation of conjunctiva and visual blurring, mucous membranes, dizziness, headache, unconsciousness, convulsions, tremors, ataxia, delirium, tightness in the chest, irreversible brain damage with cerebral atrophy, fatigue, vertigo, dyspnea, respiratory arrest, cardiac failure and ventricular arrhythmias, leukopenia, anemia, thrombocytopenia, petechiae, blood dyscrasia, leukemia, bone marrow aplasia, fatty degeneration and necrosis of heart, liver, adrenal glands, fatal overdose.

(continued)

Agent	Route of Entry	Symptoms
Toluene	Vapor inhalation or skin absorption.	Vapors irritate eyes and upper respiratory tract. Symptoms include dizziness, headache, anesthesia, and respiratory arrest. Liquid irritates eyes. If aspirated, causes coughing, gagging, distress, and rapidly developing pulmonary edema. If ingested, causes vomiting, griping, diarrhea, and depressed respiration. Kidney and liver damage may follow ingestion. Toluene embryopathy is characterized by microcephaly, central nervous system dysfunction, attention deficits and hyperactivity, developmental delay with greater language deficits, minor craniofacial and limb anomalies, and variable growth deficiency.
Xylene	Vapor inhalation or skin absorption.	Vapor irritates eyes and mucous membranes and may cause dizziness, headache, nausea, and mental confusion. Liquid irritates eyes and mucous membranes. Swallowing or absorption through skin would cause poisoning. Prolonged contact with skin may result in dermatitis. Repeated, prolonged exposure to fumes may produce conjunctivitis of the eye and dryness of the nose, throat, and skin. Direct liquid contact may result in flaky or moderate dermatitis. Inhalation of vapors may cause central nervous system excitation then depression, characterized by paresthesia, tremors, apprehension, impaired memory, weakness, nervous irritation, vertigo, headache, anorexia, nausea, and flatulence, and can lead to anemia and mucosal hemorrhage.
Formaldehyde	Inhalation	Conjunctivitis, corneal burns; brownish discoloration of skin; dermatitis, urticaria (hives), pustulovesicular eruption. Inhalation results in rhinitis and anosmia (loss of sense of smell), pharyngitis, laryngospasm; tracheitis and bronchitis, pulmonary edema, cough, chest tightness, dypsnea (difficult breathing), headache, weakness, palpitation (rapid heartbeat), gastroenteritis (inflammation of the stomach and intestines). Burning in mouth and esophagus, nausea and vomiting, abdominal pain, diarrhea, vertigo (dizziness), unconsciousness, jaundice, albuminuria, hematuria, anuria, acidosis, convulsions.
Trichloroeth-ylene	Ingestion, inhalation, or skin exposure.	Acute inhalation produces rapid coma and may result in death.
Carbon disulfide	Vapor inhalation or skin absorption.	Conjunctivitis, epithelial hyperplasia of cornea, and eczematous inflammation of eyelids.
Ethylene oxide	Inhalation	Inhalation causes nausea, vomiting, neurological disorders, and even death.
Polychlo-rinated diphenyls	Inhalation, ingestion or skin absorption.	Abdominal pain, anorexia, nausea, vomiting, jaundice, with rare cases of coma and death, may occur. Neurological symptoms such as headache, dizziness, depression, nervousness. Other symptoms such as fatigue, loss of weight, loss of libido, and muscle and joint pains.
Gases		
Ammonia	Inhalation	Vapors cause irritation of eyes and respiratory tract. Contact with skin can cause burns and vesication. Systemic absorption becomes extensive; coma may occur preceded by hypertonic contractions and convulsions.

(continued)

Agent	Route of Entry	Symptoms
Hydrochloric acid	Inhalation or skin absorption.	Inhalation of fumes produces nose, throat and laryngeal burning and irritation, pain and inflammation, coughing, sneezing, choking, hoarseness, dyspnea, bronchitis, chest pain, laryngeal spasms, and upper respiratory tract edema, as well as headache and palpitations. Contact with fumes or liquid can produce corrosive burns. Dermal exposure also results in irritation, pain, dermatitis, and ulceration. Contact with refrigerated liquid can produce frostbite. Eye contact with fumes is extremely irritating. Contact with liquid produces pain, swelling, conjunctivitis, corneal erosion, and necrosis of conjunctiva and corneal epithelium with perforation or scarring.
Hydrofluoric acid	Inhalation, ingestion, or contact (skin, eyes) with vapors or dusts.	Irritation of eyes, nose, and throat; pulmonary edema; skin and eye burns; nasal congestion; and bronchitis.
Sulfur dioxide	Inhalation direct contact with skin or mucous membrane.	Acute symptoms include respiratory tract irritation, cough, burning, lacrimation, conjunctival injection, difficulty in swallowing, and oropharyngeal erythema occurring after substantial exposures. Vomiting, diarrhea, abdominal pain, fever, headache, vertigo, agitation, tremor, convulsions, and peripheral neuritis can also be experienced.
Chlorine	Inhalation	Burning of eyes, nose, and mouth; lacrimation; rhinorrhea; coughing; choking; substernal pain; nausea; vomiting; headache; dizziness; syncope; pulmonary edema; pneumonia; hypoxemia; dermatitis; eye and skin burns.
Ozone	Inhalation	Irritation of eye, nose, throat, skin.
Nitrogen oxides	Inhalation	Usually, no symptoms occur at the time of exposure, with the exception of a slight cough, fatigue, and nausea. Fatigue, uneasiness, restlessness, cough, hyperpnea, and dyspnea appear insidiously, with adult respiratory distress syndrome developing gradually.
Asphyxiants		
Carbon monoxide	Inhalation	Rapidly fatal cases of carbon monoxide poisoning are characterized by congestion and hemorrhages in all organs. Headache, dizziness, and blurred vision.
Hydrogen sulfide	Inhalation	Eye irritation, painful conjunctivitis, photophobia, tearing and corneal opacity. Respiratory symptoms include rhinitis with anosmia, tracheobronchitis, pulmonary edema. Death from rapid respiratory paralysis.
Cyanide	Inhalation of vapor or aerosol, skin absorption.	Massive doses can produce a sudden loss of consciousness and prompt death from respiratory arrest without warning. Ingestion can produce a bitter, acrid, burning taste, followed by a feeling of constriction or numbness in the throat. Salivation, nausea, and vomiting are common. Anxiety, confusion, vertigo, giddiness, and often a sensation of stiffness in the lower jaw. Hyperpnea and dyspnea. Odor of bitter almonds may be noted on the breath or vomitus. A bright pink coloration of the skin due to high concentrations of oxyhemoglobin in the venous return may be confused with that of carbon monoxide poisoning. The skin color appears red. Death from respiratory arrest.

(continued)

Agent	Route of Entry	Symptoms
Pesticides		
Organophos-phates-para-thion	Inhalation, ingestion, or skin absorption.	Headache, giddiness, nervousness, blurred vision, weakness, nausea, cramps, diarrhea, and discomfort in the chest. Sweating, miosis, tearing, salivation and other excessive respiratory tract secretion, vomiting, cyanosis, papilledema, uncontrollable muscle twitches followed by muscular weakness, convulsions, coma, loss of reflexes, and loss of sphincter control. Cardiac arrhythmias, various degrees of heart block, and cardiac arrest may occur. Acute emphysema, pulmonary edema, pink froth in the trachea and bronchi, and considerable congestion of the organs are found at autopsy.
Chloradane	Ingestion by eating foods high in fat such as meats, fish, and dairy products.	Can cause seizures and liver damage; possible carcinogen.
Heptachlor	Ingestion by eating foods high in fat such as meats, fish, and dairy products.	Can cause seizures and liver damage; possible carcinogen.
Dichlorodi-phenyltrichlo-roethane (DDT)	Ingestion through meat, fish, and dairy products. Can occur through inhalation and dermal contact.	High doses can cause vomiting, tremors or shakiness, and seizures; possible carcinogen.
Other Chemicals		
Acrylamide	Ingestion	Requires high level exposure to produce symptoms that impact the nervous system such as muscle weakness, numbness in hands and feet, sweating, and unsteadiness.
Bisphenol A (BPA)	Oral, inhalation, and transdermal	Known as an endocrine disruptor impacting hormones. Linked to coronary artery disease, angina, heart attack, hypertension, and peripheral artery disease.
Dioxins	Ingestion through food such as meats, fish, shellfish, dairy products.	Skin lesions, patchy darkening of skin, altered liver function, long-term exposure can cause immune system, nervous system, endocrine system, and reproductive problems.
Styrene	Exposure by inhalation, ingestion, or dermal absorption.	Irritation of skin, eyes, and upper respiratory tract; acute exposure can cause gastrointestinal problems; human carcinogen.
Chloroform	Exposure by inhalation, ingestion, and dermal contact.	Initial symptoms are excitement, nausea, and vomiting, followed by ataxia, dizziness, drowsiness, convulsions, and coma. Progressive nervous system problems leading to severe paralysis.

END-OF-APPENDIX RESOURCES

BIBLIOGRAPHY

Centers for Disease Control and Prevention, National Biomonitoring Program. (2016). *Insecticides/Pesticides*. at https//www.cdc.gov/biomonitoring/insecticides_pesticides.html.

National Institute of Environmental Health Sciences. (2019). *Environmental agents*. https://www.neihs.nih.gov/health/topics/agents/index.cfm

Porche, D. (2003). *Public and community health nursing practice: A population-based approach*. Sage.

EPIDEMIOLOGIC STUDY MANUSCRIPT COMPONENTS

Demetrius J. Porche

There are four components to an epidemiologic study manuscript, excluding the abstract. The following is a typical outline for an epidemiologic study manuscript:

I. **Abstract:** 250 to 350 words

II. **Introduction**

    a. State of knowledge/science on the topic
    b. Epidemiology of the topic
    c. What is not known on the topic; gap in the literature
    d. Epidemiologic research problem
    e. Purpose, goals, objectives, or aims of the epidemiologic study

III. **Methods**

    a. Study design
    b. Target population description
    c. Sampling method and strategies
        i. How cases are defined and selected
        ii. How cohort is defined and selected
    d. Subject assignment
        i. How randomization is completed (if appropriate)
    e. Study variables
        i. Exposures, risk factors: What are these? How and when measured?
        ii. Outcomes; expected outcomes: How and when measured?
    f. Outcome measurement psychometrics
        i. Reliability measures
        ii. Validity measures
    g. Epidemiologic and statistical data analysis
    h. Data management plans
    i. Strategies to control for biases
    j. Human subjects protection

IV. **Results**

    a. Sample demographics
        i. Group comparisons as appropriate
    b. Present major findings
    c. Identification of confounders, covariance, effect modifiers

V. Discussion

a. Explain the meaning of the findings/results
b. Discuss the findings/results within the context of the existing knowledge/state of science
   i. Supports
   ii. Contradicts
   iii. Expands

c. Recommendations
   i. Program development
   ii. Practice implications
   iii. Policy
   iv. Future research

d. Present strengths and limitations of study

CRITICAL APPRAISAL TOOLS TEMPLATES

Demetrius J. Porche

CASE-CONTROL

Citation:

Study Design: Level of Evidence:

Introduction/Background	Comments/Appraisal
• Rationale provided for study • Significance of study provided • Current state of science or evidence clearly articulated • Problem statement or area identified • Research purpose clearly stated	

Design	Comments/Appraisal
• Research question clearly defined and focused? • Cases clearly defined? • What is the case definition? • Were cases incident or prevalent? • How were cases selected? • What proportion of eligible cases were included in study? • Controls clearly defined? • Were controls adequate? • How were controls selected? Selection procedure clearly defined? • Were controls independent of exposure? • What proportion of controls were included in study? • How were exposures ascertained? • Exposure was clear, specific, and measurable. How was exposure measured? • What was the potential for exposure misclassification? • Was exposure determination similar for cases and controls? • Sample recruitment and selection was appropriate? • Study variables clearly identified? How were study variables measured? • Level of significance established • Data management and analysis plan clearly described	

Results/Findings	Comments/Appraisal
• How comparable were the cases and controls? • Were potential confounders equally distributed between cases and controls? • Were potential confounders adjusted for? How were the confounders adjusted for? • Sample size appropriate based on power analysis? • What was the strength of association between the exposure and outcome? • How accurate was the estimate of association between the exposure and outcome (confidence intervals or p-values)?	

Bias/Confounders	Comments/Appraisal
• What was the potential for recall bias? What research strategies were used to reduce recall bias? • Did the researcher identify all potentially critical confounders? • What was the potential for selection bias and information bias?	

Implications of Findings/Results	Comments/Appraisal
• What is the potential application of findings to practice? • Were all the clinically important outcomes considered? • How do the study findings fit within the existing state of science and available evidence? • Were the recommendations supported by the study findings?	

Strengths	Comments/Appraisal
• What are the major strengths of the study design? • What are the major weaknesses of the study design?	

Limitations	Comments/Appraisal
• What are the major limitations of the overall study design? • What are the major limitations of the sampling method? • What are the major limitations of the measurement methods? • What are the major limitations of the data management and analysis methods?	

Ethical/Legal	Comments/Appraisal
• Did the research consider human subjects protection? • How were the human subjects rights protected? • Any ethical concerns identified? • Any potential conflicts of interest identified? • Any legal concerns identified?	

COHORT DESIGN

Citation:

Study Design:

Level of Evidence:

Introduction/Background	Comments/Appraisal
• Rationale provided for study • Significance of study provided • Current state of science or evidence clearly articulated • Problem statement or area identified • Research purpose clearly stated	

Design	Comments/Appraisal
• Research question clearly defined and focused • Cohort identified • How was the exposed cohort selected? • Was there clear and defined selection criteria for inclusion of the exposed cohort? • What proportion of eligible subjects were included in exposed cohort? • How was the nonexposed cohort selected? • Was there clear and defined selection criteria for inclusion of the nonexposed cohort? • What proportion of the eligible subjects were included in the nonexposed cohort? • What was the exposure? • Was the exposure specific and measurable? • What was the potential for misclassification of the exposure? • How long was the cohort followed? Was this time period adequate?	

Results/Findings	Comments/Appraisal
• What measures were implemented to reduce attrition? What was the rate of attrition? • Was there a difference in those who were lost to attrition and those who remained in the cohort study? • What were the primary and secondary study outcomes? How were the outcomes measured? Was the measurement valid and reliable? • Any surrogate outcome measures identified? How were the surrogate outcomes measured? Surrogate measurement was valid and reliable? • What was the comparative analysis of the exposed and nonexposed cohort? • Sample size appropriate based on power analysis; rationale for sample size estimation appropriate? • What was the strength of association between the exposure and outcome? • How accurate was the estimate of association between the exposure and outcome (confidence intervals or p-values)?	

Bias/Confounders	Comments/Appraisal
• What was the potential for recall bias? What research strategies were used to reduce recall bias? • Was there potential for selection bias? What strategies were used to reduce selection bias? • Did the researcher identify all potential confounders? • What was the potential for information bias? What strategies were used to reduce information bias? • Was there potential for historical or maturation bias? What strategies were used to reduce historical or maturation bias?	

Implications of Findings/Results	Comments/Appraisal
• What is the potential application of findings to practice? • Were all the clinically important outcomes considered? • How do the study findings fit within the existing state of science and available evidence? • Were the recommendations supported by the study findings?	

Strengths	Comments/Appraisal
• What are the major strengths of the study design? • What are the major weaknesses of the study design?	

Limitations	Comments/Appraisal
• What are the major limitations of the overall study design? • What are the major limitations of the sampling method? • What are the major limitations of the measurement methods? • What are the major limitations of the data management and analysis methods?	

Ethical/Legal	Comments/Appraisal
• Did the research consider human subjects protection? • How were the human subjects rights protected? • Any ethical concerns identified? • Any potential conflicts of interest identified? • Any legal concerns identified?	

RANDOMIZED CONTROLLED TRIAL EXPERIMENTAL STUDY DESIGN

Citation:

Study Design:
Level of Evidence:

Introduction/Background	Comments/Appraisal
• Rationale provided for study • Significance of study provided • Current state of science or evidence clearly articulated • Problem statement or area identified • Research purpose clearly stated	

Design	Comments/Appraisal
• Research question clearly defined and focused? • Does the randomized controlled trial (RCT) meet criteria for an experimental study—manipulation, randomization, control group? • Was there random assignment to treatment group? How was randomization achieved? • Were there established criteria for inclusion in the treatment and control group? • Was there a protocol to guide the intervention/treatment? Data collection time intervals were adequate? • What was the sampling method? Was the method appropriate for RCT? • Was an intent to treat analysis conducted? • What type of blinding occurred in the study? • Outcome measurements were valid and reliable?	

Results/Findings	Comments/Appraisal
• What measures were implemented to reduce attrition? What was the rate of attrition? • Was there a difference in those who were lost to attrition and those who remained in the study? • Sample size appropriate based on power analysis; rationale for sample size estimation appropriate? • What is the strength of the findings related to the intervention/treatment and outcome? • What was the comparative analysis of the intervention and control group? • What were the primary and secondary endpoints in the study? • How large was the treatment/intervention effect? What is the estimated treatment effect?	

Bias/Confounders	Comments/Appraisal
• What was the potential for recall bias? What research strategies were used to reduce recall bias? • Was there potential for selection bias? What strategies were used to reduce selection bias? • Did the researcher identify all potentially confounders? • What was the potential for information bias? What strategies were used to reduce information bias? • Was there potential for historical or maturation bias? What strategies were used to reduce historical or maturation bias? • Were there any indications to stop the RCT early? • Were there reported adverse events? • Were there revisions in the intervention protocol?	

Implications of Findings/Results	Comments/Appraisal
• What is the potential application of findings to practice? • Were all the clinically important outcomes considered? • How does the study findings fit within the existing state of science and available evidence? • Were the recommendations supported by the study findings?	

Strengths	Comments/Appraisal
• What are the major strengths of the study design? • What are the major weaknesses of the study design?	

Limitations	Comments/Appraisal
• What are the major limitations of the overall study design? • What are the major limitations of the sampling method? • What were the major limitations associated with the intervention protocol? • What are the major limitations of the measurement methods? • What are the major limitations of the data management and analysis methods?	

Ethical/Legal	Comments/Appraisal
• Did the research consider human subjects protection? • How were the human subjects rights protected? • Any ethical concerns identified? • Any potential conflicts of interest identified? • Any legal concerns identified?	

DIAGNOSTIC STUDY

Citation:

Study Design:
Level of Evidence:

Introduction/Background	Comments/Appraisal
• Significance of study provided • Rationale for needed screening or diagnostic test • Research purpose or question clearly stated? • Current screening and diagnostic test available? • Explanation of psychometrics, sensitivity, specificity, predictive value positive and predictive value negative of current screening and diagnostic test?	

Design	Comments/Appraisal
• What was the study design? • What were the sampling methods used? Were the methods adequate? • Was there a comparative analysis with a "gold" standard test?	

Results/Findings	Comments/Appraisal
• What are the major findings? • What are the sensitivity results? • What are the specificity results? • What are the predictive value positive results? • What are the predictive value negative results? • Was the test evaluated in an appropriate population? • Was there a reference standard applied to the subjects? • How are the test results interpreted? Was a cut-off score determined?	

Implications of Findings/Results	Comments/Appraisal
<ul><li>What is the potential application of findings to practice?</li><li>Were all the clinically important outcomes considered?</li><li>How does the study findings fit within the existing state of science and available evidence?</li><li>Does the test meet the criteria for a good screening test?</li><li>Were the recommendations supported by the study findings?</li></ul>	

Strengths	Comments/Appraisal
<ul><li>What are the major strengths of the study design?</li><li>What are the major weaknesses of the study design?</li></ul>	

Limitations	Comments/Appraisal
<ul><li>What are the major limitations of the overall study design?</li><li>What are the major limitations of the sampling method?</li><li>What were the major limitations associated with the intervention protocol?</li><li>What are the major limitations of the measurement methods?</li><li>What are the major limitations of the data management and analysis methods?</li></ul>	

Ethical/Legal	Comments/Appraisal
<ul><li>Did the research consider human subjects protection?</li><li>How were the human subjects rights protected?</li><li>Any ethical concerns identified?</li><li>Any potential conflicts of interest identified?</li><li>Any legal concerns identified?</li></ul>	

SYSTEMATIC REVIEW

Citation:

Study Design:
Level of Evidence:

Introduction/Background	Comments/Appraisal
<ul><li>Rationale provided for study</li><li>Significance of study provided</li></ul>	

Design	Comments/Appraisal
• Was review question clearly and explicitly stated? Was the systematic review question focused? • What was the systematic review question? • Was the search strategy presented? • Was the search strategy comprehensive and exhaustive? Were all relevant studies included? • What databases were searched? What were the limitations of the search strategy? Was the gray literature included? • What were the inclusion and exclusion criteria? Are these criteria justified? • Was study selection reproducible? • How was validity and quality assessed? • Was the validity and quality assessment conducted in a manner that was reproducible? • Was the methodological quality of each study rated and stated? • For a meta-analysis, were the study results pooled together for analysis? What were the meta-analysis methods? What statistical modeling was used in the meta-analysis? • Was the criteria for appraising the studies presented? Was the criteria appropriate? • Was the critical appraisal of each study conducted by two or more independent reviewers? • What were the methods used to minimize errors in data extraction? • Was there an assessment for heterogeneity? What method was used? • Were the methods used to combine and synthesize studies presented? Were the methods appropriate?	

Results/Findings	Comments/Appraisal
• Were the study populations similar or different? How? • Was the exposure measured the same in each study? If not, how was each measured? How did they differ in measurement? • Was each intervention or outcome measured in the same manner in each study? If not, how was each measured? How did the measurement differ in each study? • What were the consistent measurements among each study? • What were all measurements cited from all studies? • Was a cost–benefit analysis completed? What were the findings? • What are the overall findings of the systematic review?	

Bias/Confounders	Comments/Appraisal
• Was there potential for selection bias? What strategies were used to reduce selection bias? • Was there any evidence of publication bias? How was publication bias assessed?	

Implications of Findings/Results	Comments/Appraisal
• What is the potential application of findings to practice? • Were all the clinically important outcomes considered? • How does the study findings fit within the existing state of science and available evidence and practice? • Were the recommendations supported by the study findings?	

Strengths	Comments/Appraisal
• What are the major strengths of the study design? • What are the major weaknesses of the study design?	

Limitations	Comments/Appraisal
• What are the major limitations of the overall study design? • What are the major limitations of the sampling method?	

Ethical/Legal	Comments/Appraisal
• Did the research consider human subjects protection? • How were the human subjects rights protected? • Any ethical concerns identified? • Any potential conflicts of interest identified? • Any legal concerns identified?	

SUMMARY OF EPIDEMIOLOGICAL RESEARCH FINDINGS TABLE

Demetrius J. Porche

The *Summary of Epidemiological Research Findings* should be used to summarize original epidemiologic studies (see following table). A comprehensive completion of this summary of epidemiological research findings facilitates the synthesis of evidence among multiple epidemiologic studies.

Article Citation	Research Design and Methods	Research Variables, Measurement Tools/Instruments or Methods, Psychometrics, Sensitivity, Specificity, Predictive Value Positive, Predictive Value Negative, Reliability	Setting, Sampling Method, Sample, Population Dynamics	Data Analysis Methods, Epidemiology Data Analysis Methods	Major Findings/Results	Study Strengths	Study Limitations	Practice Application	Evidence Level

EPIDEMIOLOGICAL RESOURCES

Demetrius J. Porche

INFORMATION AND DATA SOURCES

The following provides a list of potential data sources:
1. Administration on Aging (http://www.aoa.gov/) provides data on elderly.
2. Agency for Healthcare Research and Quality (AHRQ) provides data on quality of healthcare services (http://www.ahrq.gov/).
3. Agency for Toxic Substances and Disease Registry (http://www.atsdr.cdc.gov/) provides information and data on the identification, planning, research, monitoring, and evaluation of the toxic effects of materials on the population.
4. Centers for Disease Control and Prevention (http://www.cdc.gov/) coordinates the activities of several agencies to promote the health of the nation.
5. Centers for Medicare and Medicaid Services (http://www.cms.hhs.gov/) provides information and data on Medicare, Medicaid, and Children Health Insurance programs.
6. Food and Drug Administration (http://www.fda.gov/) provides information and data on human and veterinary drugs and drug research, food and food additives, medical devices, and other biological materials such as vaccines.
7. Health Resources Services Administration (http://www.hrsa.gov/) provides information and data on quality healthcare services, access to healthcare, health disparities, and healthcare workforce.
8. Indian Health Services (http://www.ihs.gov/) provides information on the health of Native Americans and Alaskan Natives.
9. National Institutes of Health (http://www.nih.gov/) consists of institutes and centers that conduct and support health related research.
10. Substance Abuse and Mental Health Services Administration (http://www.samhsa.gov/) provides information and data on the prevention, treatment, rehabilitation, and research related to substance use and mental illness.
11. U.S. Census Bureau (http://www.census.gov/) provides information on the demography of the United States population.

NATIONAL SURVEYS AND DATA COLLECTION/SURVEILLANCE

1. Air Data surveys air quality.
2. Fatal Analysis Reporting System provides data on fatal traffic accidents.
3. HIV/AIDS Surveillance System collects data on the rates of HIV infection and AIDS cases.
4. Medical Expenditure Panel Survey collects data on healthcare cost.
5. National Crime Victimization Survey collects data on crime victims.
6. National Electronic Injury Surveillance System collects data on consumer product related injuries.
7. National Health Care Survey collects information on different healthcare settings that influence health policy changes.

8. National Health Interview Survey collects information on health status, access to care, disability, and illness of the noninstitutionalized U.S. population.
9. National Health and Nutrition Examination Survey collects information on the health and nutritional status of the population.
10. National Hospital Discharge Survey collects data on the characteristics of inpatients discharged from the hospital.
11. National Immunization Survey collects data on U.S. childhood, teenage, and adult immunizations.
12. National Program of Cancer Registries collects data on cancer morbidity and mortality.
13. National Vital Statistics collects data on births, marriages, divorces, and deaths.
14. National Youth Risk Behavior Survey collects data on youth risk behaviors.
15. STORET collects data on water quality.
16. U.S. Renal Data System collects data on end stage renal disease.

EPIDEMIOLOGIC ASSOCIATIONS AND ORGANIZATIONS

1. American College of Epidemiology (https://www.acepidemiology.org)
2. American Epidemiological Society (https://www.americanepidemiologicalsociety.org/)
3. American Public Health Association (https://www.apha.org/apha-communities/member-sections/epidemiology)
4. Association of Professionals in Infection Control and Epidemiology (https://apic.org/)
5. Canadian Society for Epidemiology and Biostatistics (http://www.cseb.ca/resources.php)
6. Centers for Disease Control and Prevention (http://www.cdc.gov/)
7. European Centre for Disease Prevention and Control (http://ecdc.europa.eu/en/Pages/home.aspx)
8. European Epidemiology Federation (http://www.iea-europe.org/)
9. International Clinical Epidemiology Network (http://www.inclen.org/)
10. International Epidemiology Association (http://www.ieaweb.org/)
11. International Genetic Epidemiology Society (https://www.genepi.org/)
12. International Society for Environmental Epidemiology (https://www.iseepi.org/)
13. International Society for Pharmacoepidemiology (https://www.pharmacoepi.org/)
14. Netherlands Epidemiological Society (https://www.epidemiologie.nl/index.php?id=6&L=4)
15. Society for Clinical Trials (www.sctweb.org)
16. Society for Epidemiological Research (https://epiresearch.org)
17. Society for Healthcare Epidemiology of America (http://www.shea-online.org/)
18. Society for Veterinary Epidemiology and Preventive Medicine (https://www.svepm.org.uk/)

EPIDEMIOLOGY JOURNALS

1. *American Journal of Epidemiology*
2. *American Journal of Infection Control*
3. *American Journal of Public Health*
4. *Annals of Epidemiology*
5. *Biostatistics and Epidemiology*
6. *Cancer Epidemiology*
7. *Cancer Epidemiology Biomarkers and Prevention*
8. *Clinical Epidemiology*
9. *Clinical Epidemiology and Global Health*
10. *Clinical Practice and Epidemiology in Mental Health*
11. *Emerging Infectious Diseases*
12. *Emerging Themes in Epidemiology*
13. *Epidemics*
14. *Epidemiologic Methods*
15. *Epidemiological Research International*
16. *Epidemiology*
17. *Epidemiology and Infection*

18. *Epidemiology and Psychiatric Sciences*
19. *Epidemiology Reviews*
20. *Ethnicity and Disease*
21. *European Journal of Epidemiology*
22. *Eurosurveillance*
23. *Genetic Epidemiology*
24. *Global Health, Epidemiology, and Genomics*
25. *Infection Control and Hospital Epidemiology*
26. *Infection Ecology and Epidemiology*
27. *Influenza Research and Treatment*
28. *International Journal of Epidemiology*
29. *International Journal of Molecular Epidemiology and Genetics*
30. *Journal of Clinical Epidemiology*
31. *Journal of Epidemiology*
32. *Journal of Epidemiology and Community Health*
33. *Journal of Epidemiology and Global Health*
34. *Journal of Exposure Science and Environmental Epidemiology*
35. *Journal of Virus Eradication*
36. *Morbidity and Mortality Weekly Report (MMWR)*
37. *Ophthalmic Epidemiology*
38. *Pediatric and Perinatal Epidemiology*
39. *Parasite Epidemiology and Control*
40. *Pharmacoepidemiology and Drug Safety*
41. *Social Psychiatry and Psychiatric Epidemiology*

EPIDEMIOLOGY SOFTWARE AND TOOLS

1. ActivEpi (http://www.activepi.com) is an educational resource for learning epidemiology.
2. Birtha (https://www.ehdp.com/birtha/) is a software program to analyze birth data such as birth rates, cesarean rates, teen birth rates, fertility rates, prenatal care rates, and birth outcomes.
3. CDC Wonder (https://wonder.cdc.gov) is a free online resource for analysis of public health data; includes databases, reports and references, and data query systems.
4. CI*Rank (https://surveillance.cancer.gov/cirank/index.html) provides ranked, age-adjusted cancer incidence and mortality rates by state, county, and U.S. region.
5. Cytel (https://www.cytel.com) is a comprehensive software for the design, analysis, and execution of clinical trial research.
6. EpiCal 2000 (http://www.brixtonhealth.com/epicalc.html) is a free statistical calculator.
7. EpiData (http://www.epidata.dk) is an epidemiology software program that assists with data entry and analysis.
8. EpiGram (http://www.brixtonhealth.com/epigram.html) is a software program that produces diagrams such as contract tracing and social network diagrams.
9. Epigram (https://www.ehdp.com/epigram/) assists with the analysis and dissemination of age-adjusted rates, leading causes of death, years of productive life lost, and other mortality data.
10. Epi Info™ (https://www.cdc.gov/Epiinfo/) is a software program that facilitates survey development, data entry, and data analysis. Can produce epidemiologic statistics, maps, and graphs.
11. Epitools (https://cran.r-project.org/web/packages/epitools/epitools.pdf) provides assistance with epidemiologic analysis and graphics.
12. Evidence-based medicine calculators (https://ebm-tools.knowledgetranslation.net/calculator) provides calculators to assist with odds ratio, diagnostic test, prospective study, case control, and randomized controlled trials.
13. G*Power (https://download.cnet.com/G-Power/3000-2054_4-10647044.html) is a software program to assist in analyzing types of power and computing sample size.
14. MapWindow (https://www.mapwindow.org) is a free open-source geographic information system.

15. MedTrend (https://www.ehdp.com/medtrend/) is an analysis software to analyze hospital discharge data.
16. NCHHSTP AtlasPlus (https://www.cdc.gov/nchhstp/atlas/index.htm) analyzes HIV infection, viral hepatitis, sexually transmitted infections, tuberculosis, and social determinants of health data to create maps, charts, and tables.
17. NetEpi (https://sourceforge.net/projects/netepi/) are open-source tools for epidemiology and public health practice.
18. Oncogram is a software program for analyzing cancer registry data.
19. OpenClinica (https://www.openclinica.com) is a software program to manage open clinical trials.
20. OpenEpi (https://www.openepi.com/BriefDoc/About.htm) is an open-source project that assists with epidemiologic computing with a collection of epidemiologic calculators.
21. PopTrend (https://www.ehdp.com/poptrend/) is a software program for analyzing population data and demographic trends.
22. PregData (https://www.ehdp.com/pregdata/) is a software program for analyzing pregnancy data such as births, fetal deaths, and abortions.
23. QuickCalcs (https://www.graphpad.com/quickcalcs/) is a web-based program for quick data analysis.
24. Real Statistics Using Excel (https://www.real-statistics.com) is a practical guide that provides information on how to conduct statistical analyses using Excel with additional software that extends Excel's ability to conduct statistical analyses.
25. Statulator (http://statulator.com/) is a software program for statistical analysis and result interpretation.
26. Survey Documentation and Analysis (https://sda.berkeley.edu) consists of a set of programs that facilitate web-based survey analysis and documentation.
27. Vitalnet (https://www.ehdp.com/vitalnet/) is a health data analysis software program for analyzing data sets.

EPIDEMIOLOGIC DATA PRESENTATION

Demetrius J. Porche

GENERAL PRINCIPLES

Data presentation should include at a minimum the following elements:

- **Title:** Labels the data presentation in terms of what, where, and when
- **Data space**: Area where data are organized and displayed
- **Footnotes:** Explanation of abbreviations, data sources, units of measurement, or other needed explanations
- **Text:** Narrative explanation that summarizes the main patterns or findings of the data

Data are presented as variables. These variables can be either numeric or descriptive. Numeric variables are expressed as numbers. Descriptive variables are presented as a narrative explanation. Variables are presented as nominal, ordinal, interval, or ratio. Nominal variables have discrete and exclusive categories such as alive or dead, present or absent. Ordinal scale variables are ranked and do not necessarily have equal spacing between ranks, such as cancer stages. Interval scales are presented in equally spaced units without a true zero point, such as birth date. Ratio scale presents data in equally spaced units with a true zero point, such as days of illness duration.

Line Listing

A line listing (Appendix Table H.1) organizes information being collected during surveillance or an outbreak investigation. A line listing organizes data into rows and columns in a table. Each row is a record or observation and generally represents one person or one case. Each column contains a variable or information about one characteristic. The first column generally contains the identifying information of the record or case.

Table

A table presents data arranged in rows and columns (Appendix Table H.2). Tables are used to demonstrate patterns, exceptions, differences, and other relationships. Some recommended strategies for constructing a table include:

- Clear and concise title that designates person, place, and time or what, where, and when
- Tables are numbered
- Each row and column should contain units of measurement
- Totals for rows and columns should be presented, if appropriate
- Missing or unknown data for each row or column should be identified as such
- Footnotes should explain all abbreviations, codes, or symbols
- Columns should be used for crucial data comparison
- Numbers are more easily compared down a column than across a row
- Data should be organized by magnitude
- Column of numbers should be aligned on the decimal point
- Data should be rounded to two statistically significant numbers

Graph

A graph displays numeric data in visual form (Appendix Figure H.1). Graphs typically have two scales or axes, one horizontal and one vertical, that intersect at a right angle. The horizontal axis is known as the x-axis and typically displays the independent variable values. The vertical axis is known as the y-axis and typically presents the dependent variable or the frequency measure in epidemiology. Graphs can be:

- **Arithmetic:** Scale line graph that displays patterns or trends over a variable; this graph has a set distance along any axis variables, x-axis generally portrays time
- **Semilogarithmic-scale graph:** Used to display variables with a wide range pf values

Some general guidelines for graph construction are:

- Arithmetic scale should use equal numerical units with equal distances on axes
- A zero level is not necessary unless there is interval data
- Use prominent symbols to plot data
- Ensure that overlapping data points are distinguishable
- Clearly indicate scale divisions and scaling units

Histogram

A histogram displays frequency distribution of a continuous variable (Appendix Figure H.2). There are adjoining columns that represent the number of observations. The area of each column represents the proportion of the number of observations in the interval. Epidemic curves are frequently presented as histograms. Some general guidelines for constructing a histogram are:

- Cases or frequency counts are on the y-axis
- There should be no gaps between the bars
- Use separate, equally scaled epidemic curves for different groups

Population Pyramid

A population pyramid presents the count or percentage of a population by age and sex (Appendix Figure H.3). A population pyramid is produced by constructing histograms for each sex turned sideways.

Scatter Diagram

A scatter diagram displays the relationship between two continuous variables, with the x- and y-axes each representing a variable (Appendix Figure H.4). The shape of the scatter plot can provide some suggestion about the positive or negative correlation of the two variables. A compact pattern from the upper left to lower right indicates a negative or inverse correlation. A compact pattern of points from the lower left to the upper right indicates a positive relationship. Widely scattered points or an inconsistent pattern may suggest little or no correlation.

Bar Chart

A bar chart displays categories of a variable in a comparative manner in which the frequency of the event is represented on opposite axes (Appendix Figures H.5 and H.6). A bar chart is separated by spaces unlike a histogram. The bars can be displayed vertically or horizontally.

Pie Chart

A pie chart displays the data into "slices" or segments that display the proportion of each component. A pie chart displays the proportion of a single variable's frequency distribution.

Maps

Maps are used to display the geographic location of epidemiological events (Appendix Figure H.7). A spot map uses dots or other symbols on the map to display a case or event. An area map is also known as a choropleth map. An area map displays the rates of a disease or health event by shading the map locations to indicate a category or rate.

Appendix Table H.1 Sample Line Listing

ID	Data collection date	Age	Race	Sex	Type of Diagnostic Test	Test Results	Fever	Cough	Shortness of Breath
1XZ22	12/20/20	64	W	M	Nasal Swab	Positive	Present	Present	Not present

Appendix Table H.2 Table Sample

TABLE. Number[a] and outcomes of assisted reproductive technology procedures in which at least one embryo was transferred, by female patient's reporting area of residence[b] at time of treatment—United States and Puerto Rico, 2017

Patient's Reporting Area of Residence	No. of ART Clinics[c]	No. of ART Procedures Performed	No. of ART Embryo-Transfer Procedures[d]	No. of ART Pregnancies	No. of ART Live-Birth Deliveries	No. of ART Singleton Live-Birth Deliveries	No. of ART Multiple Live-Birth Deliveries	No. of ART Live-Born Infants	ART Procedures per 1 Million Women Aged 15–44 years[e]
Alabama	5	969	736	400	326	265	61	391	1,020
Alaska	0	162	136	87	73	58	15	88	1,109
Arizona	15	2,956	2,428	1,334	1,095	876	219	1,321	2,197
Arkansas	1	607	468	234	199	146	53	253	1,051
California	68	24,179	19,425	10,779	8,852	7,789	1,063	9,926	2,983
Colorado	8	2,350	2,116	1,408	1,184	1,013	171	1,355	2,066
Connecticut	6	3,518	2,690	1,544	1,271	1,102	169	1,440	5,228
Delaware	2	744	535	304	219	214	5	224	4,126
District of Columbia	2	1,269	958	457	375	351	24	399	6,806
Florida	26	8,535	6,616	3,383	2,798	2,377	421	3,222	2,229
Georgia	8	4,264	3,673	2,014	1,657	1,440	217	1,875	1,986
Hawaii	5	1,010	802	430	341	258	83	426	3,798
Idaho	1	619	522	296	244	194	50	293	1,882
Illinois[f]	25	12,739	9,918	5,017	3,965	3,493	472	4,439	5,031
Indiana	9	2,227	1,786	841	682	562	120	804	1,719
Iowa	2	1,451	1,186	715	599	535	64	663	2,450
Kansas	4	1,001	830	469	383	337	46	429	1,792
Kentucky	4	1,431	1,168	534	435	364	71	505	1,687
Louisiana	5	1,517	1,135	600	502	434	68	571	1,621
Maine	1	513	441	229	191	167	24	216	2,216
Maryland	7	6,659	5,137	2,581	1,996	1,828	168	2,170	5,580
Massachu- setts[f]	9	10,178	8,424	4,011	3,263	2,985	278	3,548	7,366

Appendix Table H.2 Table Sample (*continued*)

Patient's Reporting Area of Residence	No. of ART Clinics[c]	No. of ART Procedures Performed	No. of ART Embryo-Transfer Procedures[d]	No. of ART Pregnancies	No. of ART Live-Birth Deliveries	No. of ART Singleton Live-Birth Deliveries	No. of ART Multiple Live-Birth Deliveries	No. of ART Live-Born Infants	ART Procedures per 1 Million Women Aged 15–44 years[e]
Michigan	11	3,939	3,184	1,730	1,426	1,130	296	1,728	2,102
Minnesota	5	3,066	2,694	1,499	1,239	1,061	178	1,418	2,874
Mississippi	2	579	485	262	220	196	24	245	979
Missouri	9	2,131	1,768	914	774	620	154	932	1,819
Montana	1	306	264	156	133	116	17	150	1,610
Nebraska	2	831	657	360	297	243	54	352	2,245
Nevada	5	1,181	996	571	447	388	59	509	2,005
New Hampshire	0	998	851	419	362	312	50	413	4,135
New Jersey[f]	19	10,562	8,317	4,799	3,940	3,599	341	4,285	6,158
New Mexico	2	367	342	185	159	132	27	187	928
New York	40	23,270	17,933	8,644	6,957	6,166	791	7,758	5,816
North Carolina	10	4,306	3,371	1,988	1,601	1,369	232	1,838	2,135
North Dakota	1	262	236	138	121	91	30	151	1,791
Ohio	11	4,687	3,727	2,002	1,637	1,443	194	1,837	2,127
Oklahoma	3	944	762	364	303	247	56	359	1,228
Oregon	3	1,273	1,144	752	641	525	116	761	1,571
Pennsylvania	15	7,082	5,586	2,883	2,317	2,084	233	2,554	2,971
Puerto Rico	3	222	194	96	67	49	18	85	338
Rhode Island[f]	1	950	806	328	273	250	23	296	4,544
South Carolina	4	1,713	1,315	695	566	483	83	645	1,774

Appendix Table H.2 Table Sample (*continued*)

Patient's Reporting Area of Residence	No. of ART Clinics[c]	No. of ART Procedures Performed	No. of ART Embryo-Transfer Procedures[d]	No. of ART Pregnancies	No. of ART Live-Birth Deliveries	No. of ART Singleton Live-Birth Deliveries	No. of ART Multiple Live-Birth Deliveries	No. of ART Live-Born Infants	ART Procedures per 1 Million Women Aged 15–44 years[e]
South Dakota	1	282	242	134	111	92	19	130	1,775
Tennessee	10	1,789	1,434	797	662	572	90	756	1,363
Texas	41	14,594	11,849	6,581	5,374	4,577	797	6,185	2,480
Utah	3	2,184	1,923	1,116	925	764	161	1,087	3,235
Vermont	2	368	301	143	109	94	15	123	3,232
Virginia	10	6,149	4,924	2,649	2,137	1,916	221	2,360	3,658
Washington	12	3,909	3,053	1,830	1,517	1,362	155	1,672	2,669
West Virginia	3	341	270	123	96	77	19	115	1,058
Wisconsin	6	2,027	1,683	903	801	664	137	941	1,870
Wyoming	0	169	148	90	74	56	18	93	1,569
Non-U.S. resident	–	7,075	5,910	3,522	2,972	2,425	547	3,529	—[g]
Total	**448**	**196,454**	**157,499**	**84,340**	**68,908**	**59,891**	**9,017**	**78,052**	**3,040**

ART, assisted reproductive technology.

[a]Total number of cycles reported to the CDC was 284,403. This report excludes 87,931 cycles in which egg or embryo banking was performed and 18 research cycles.

[b]In cases of missing residency data (0.3%), the patient's residence was assigned as the location where the ART procedure was performed.

[c]The ART procedures and outcomes by patient's reporting area of residence do not necessarily reflect the procedures and outcomes of the ART clinics within the reporting area because some patients seek treatment at a clinic in a location other than their area of residence.

[d]Embryo-transfer procedures include all procedures performed in which an attempt was made to transfer at least one embryo.

[e]On the basis of U.S. Census Bureau estimates (*Source: US Census Bureau. (2017). Annual estimates of the resident population for selected age groups by sex for the United States, states, counties, and Puerto Rico Commonwealth and municipios: April 1, 2010 to July 1, 2017.* U.S. Census Bureau, Population Division. https://data.census.gov/cedsci/table?q=United%20States&g=0100000US&tid=ACSST1Y2018.S0101&vintage=2018external icon).

[f]State with comprehensive insurance mandate requiring insurers to cover the costs associated with diagnosis and treatment of infertility inclusive of ART services for at least four oocyte retrievals.

[g]Non-U.S. residents were excluded from rate because the appropriate denominators were not available. (*Source:* From Sunderam, S., Kissin, D. M., Zhang Y., Jewett, A., Boulet, S. L., Warner, L., Kroelinger, C. D., & Barfield, W. D. (2020). Assisted reproductive technology surveillance—United States, 2017. *MMWR Surveillance Summaries,* 69(SS-9), 1–20.

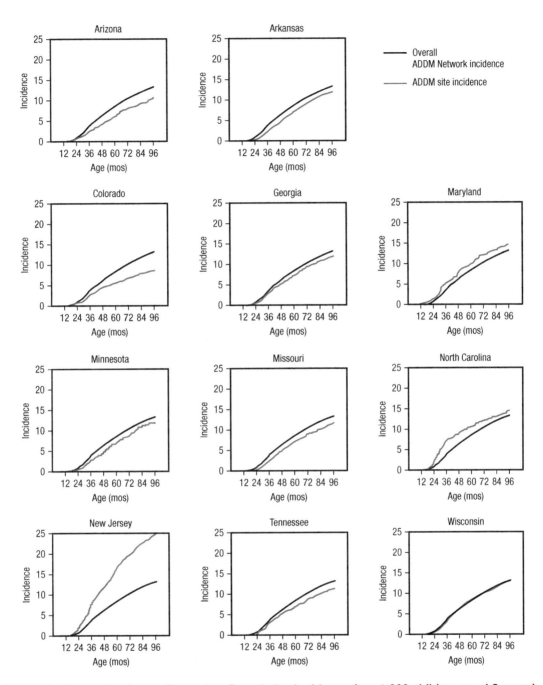

Appendix Figure H.1 Graph Example. Cumulative incidence (per 1,000 children aged 8 years) of autism spectrum disorder diagnoses; these data only include the portion of ADDM Network ASD cases with a documented diagnostic statement of ASD in the record. Children counted as ADDM Network cases without a documented ASD diagnosis (i.e., does not consider special education classifications or ICD codes) are not included], by age and site—Autism and Developmental Disabilities Monitoring Network, 11 sites, United States, 2016. ADDM, Autism and Developmental Disabilities Monitoring Network; ASD, autism spectrum disorder; ICD, International Classification of Diseases.

Source: Maenner, M. J., Shaw, K. A., Baio J, et al. (2020). Prevalence of autism spectrum disorder among children aged 8 years—Autism and developmental disabilities monitoring network, 11 sites, United States, 2016. *MMWR Surveillance Summaries, 69*(SS-4), 1–12. https://doi .org/10.15585/mmwr.ss6904a1

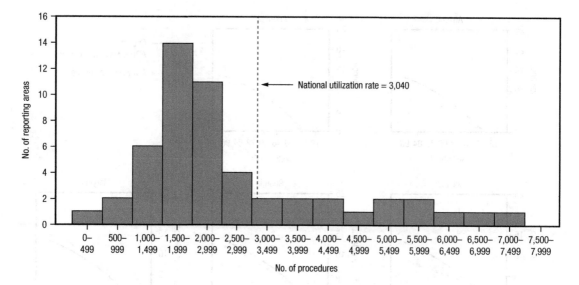

Appendix Figure H.2 Histogram Example. Number of reporting states and territories (total number of reporting states and territories: 52), by number of assisted reproductive technology procedures performed (total number of procedures: 196,454) among women of reproductive age (15–44 years; per 1 million women aged 15–44 years) in which at least one embryo was transferred — United States and Puerto Rico, 2017 [national utilization rate = (Total number of procedures performed/Female population aged 15–44 years) × 1,000,000].

Source: Sunderam, S., Kissin, D. M., Zhang, Y., Jewett, A., Boulet, S. L., Warner, L., Kroelinger, C. D., & Barfield, W. D. (2020). Assisted reproductive technology surveillance — United States, 2017. *MMWR Surveillance Summaries, 69*(SS-9), 1–20. https://doi.org/10.15585/mmwr.ss6909a1

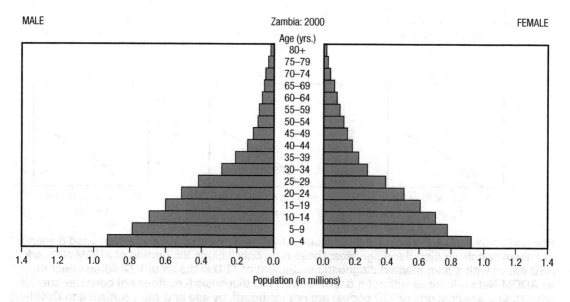

Appendix Figure H.3 Population Pyramid Example. Population distribution of Zambia by age and sex, 2000.

Source: U.S. Census Bureau [Internet]. (2004, September 10). IDB Population Pyramids. http://www.census.gov/ipc/www/idb/external icon

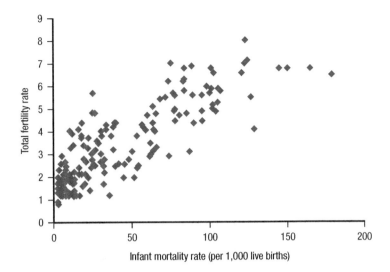

Appendix Figure H.4 Scatter Diagram Example. Correlation of infant mortality rate and total fertility rate among 194 nations, 1997.

Source: Population Reference Bureau [Internet]. (2004, December 13). *Datafinder*. http://www. prb.org/datafind/datafinder7.htmexternal icon

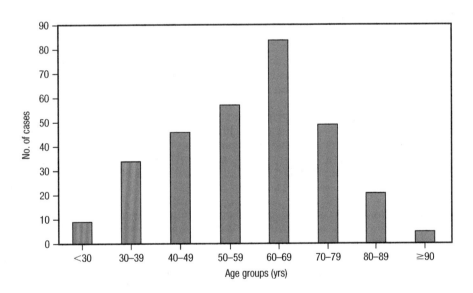

Appendix Figure H.5 Bar Chart Example.

Source: Romero, L., Pao, L. Z., Clark, H., et al. (2020). Health center testing for SARS-CoV-2 during the COVID-19 pandemic—United States, June 5–October 2, 2020. *MMWR Morbidity and Mortality Weekly Report, 69*, 1895–1901. https://doi.org/10.15585/mmwr.mm6950a3external icon

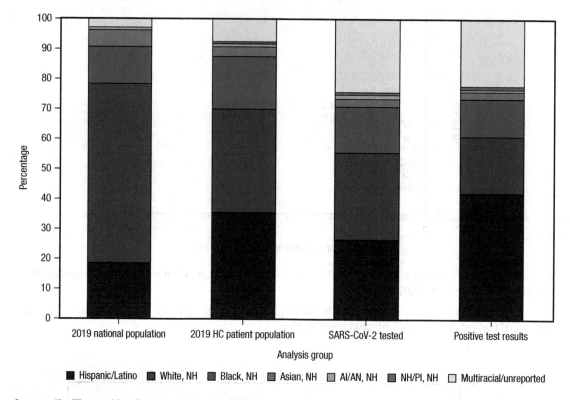

Appendix Figure H.6 Stacked Bar Chart Example. Racial/ethnic distribution of 2019 national (data from the 2019 American Community Survey https://data.census.gov/cedsci/table?d=ACS%201-Year%20Estimates%20Data%20Profiles&tid=ACSDP1Y2019. DP05&hide-Preview=falseexternal icon). Data include non-Hispanic NH/PI (0.2%), not visible in figure and do not include other races (0.3%). Persons with multiracial or unreported race/ethnicity have an unreported or non-Hispanic ethnicity and Health Resources and Services Administration (HRSA)–funded health center [HRSA–funded health centers include both Federally Qualified Health Centers (FQHCs) and Health Center Program Look-Alikes (i.e., meets all Health Care Center Program requirements but does not receive federal funding). During the COVID-19 pandemic, HRSA provided one-time COVID-19 funding to FQHCs and Health Center Look-Alikes to purchase, administer, and expand capacity for testing to monitor and suppress COVID-19 testing and response-related activities] patient populations (HRSA 2019 Uniform Data System. https://data.hrsa.gov/tools/data-reporting/program-data/nationalexternal icon) and persons who received testing and had positive SARS-CoV-2 test results (HRSA COVID-19 Survey, June 5–October 2, 2020. Data for the number tested or the number tested positive are aggregated by health centers before submission and cannot be deduplicated, which might inflate or misrepresent the number of patients tested or who had positive test results)—Health Center COVID-19 Survey, United States, June 5–October 2, 2020. AI/AN, American Indian/Alaska Native; COVID-19, coronavirus disease 2019; HC, health center; NH/PI, Native Hawaiian/Other Pacific Islander; NH, non-Hispanic.

Source: Romero, L., Pao, L. Z., Clark, H., et al. (2020). Health center testing for SARS-CoV-2 during the COVID-19 pandemic—United States, June 5–October 2, 2020. *MMWR Morbidity and Mortality Weekly Report, 69*, 1895–1901. https://doi.org/10.15585/mmwr.mm6950a3external icon

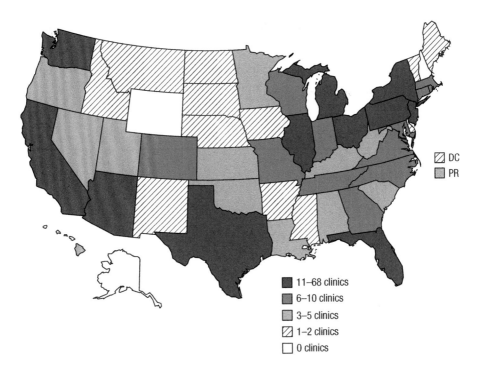

Appendix Figure H.7 Map Example. Location and number (in 2017, of the 498 clinics in the United States, 448 (90%) submitted data) of assisted reproductive technology clinics, by quartile—United States and Puerto Rico, 2017. DC, District of Columbia; PR, Puerto Rico.

Source: Sunderam, S., Kissin, D. M., Zhang, Y., Jewett, A., Boulet, S. L., Warner, L., Kroelinger, C. D., & Barfield, W. D. (2020). Assisted reproductive technology surveillance—United States, 2017. *MMWR Surveillance Summaries, 69*(SS-9), 1–20. https://doi.org/10.15585/mmwr.ss6909a1

END-OF-APPENDIX RESOURCES

BIBLIOGRAPHY

Centers for Disease Control and Prevention. (2012). *Principles of epidemiology in public health practice* (3rd ed.). https://www.cdc.gov/csels/dsepd/ss1978/SS1978.pdf

Fontaine, R. (2018). Describing epidemiologic data. In *The CDC field epidemiology manual.* https://www.cdc.gov/eis/field-epi-manual/chapters/Describing-Epi-Data.html

NATIONAL NOTIFIABLE INFECTIOUS DISEASES

Demetrius J. Porche

NATIONAL NOTIFIABLE INFECTIOUS DISEASES (CENTERS FOR DISEASE CONTROL AND PREVENTION, 2020)

- Anthrax
- Arboviral diseases, neuroinvasive and non-neuroinvasive
  - California serogroup virus diseases
  - Chikungunya virus disease
  - Eastern equine encephalitis virus disease
  - Powassan virus disease
  - St. Louis encephalitis virus disease
  - West Nile virus disease
  - Western equine encephalitis virus disease
- Babesiosis
- Botulism
  - Botulism, foodborne
  - Botulism, infant
  - Botulism, wound
  - Botulism, other
- Brucellosis
- Campylobacteriosis
- Cancer
- *Candida auris*, clinical
- Carbapenemase Producing Carbapenem-Resistant Enterobacteriaceae (CP-CRE)
  - CP-CRE, *Enterobacter* spp.
  - CP-CRE, *Escherichia coli*
  - CP-CRE, *Klebsiella* spp.
- Carbon monoxide poisoning
- Chancroid
- *Chlamydia trachomatis* infection
- Cholera
- Coccidioidomycosis
- Congenital syphilis
  - Syphilitic stillbirth
- Coronavirus disease 2019 (COVID-19)
- Cryptosporidiosis
- Cyclosporiasis
- Dengue virus infections
  - Dengue
  - Dengue-like illness
  - Severe dengue

- Diphtheria
- Ehrlichiosis and anaplasmosis
  - *Anaplasma phagocytophilum* infection
  - *Ehrlichia chaffeensis* infection
  - *Ehrlichia ewingii* infection
  - Undetermined human ehrlichiosis/anaplasmosis
- Foodborne disease outbreak
- Giardiasis
- Gonorrhea
- *Haemophilus influenzae*, invasive disease
- Hansen's disease
- Hantavirus infection, non-Hantavirus pulmonary syndrome
- Hantavirus pulmonary syndrome
- Hemolytic uremic syndrome, post-diarrheal
- Hepatitis A, acute
- Hepatitis B, acute
- Hepatitis B, chronic
- Hepatitis B, perinatal virus infection
- Hepatitis C, acute
- Hepatitis C, chronic
- Hepatitis C, perinatal infection
- HIV infection (AIDS has been reclassified as HIV Stage III)
- Influenza-associated pediatric mortality
- Invasive pneumococcal disease
- Lead, elevated blood levels
  - Lead, elevated blood levels, children (<16 Years)
  - Lead, elevated blood levels, adult (≥16 Years)
- Legionellosis
- Leptospirosis
- Listeriosis
- Lyme disease
- Malaria
- Measles
- Meningococcal disease
- Mumps
- Novel influenza A virus infections
- Pertussis
- Pesticide-related illness and injury, acute
- Plague
- Poliomyelitis, paralytic
- Poliovirus infection, nonparalytic
- Psittacosis
- Q fever
  - Q fever, acute
  - Q fever, chronic
- Rabies, animal
- Rabies, human
- Rubella
- Rubella, congenital syndrome
- Salmonella *paratyphi* infection (Salmonella enterica serotypes Paratyphi A, B [tartrate negative], and C [*S. paratyphi*])
- Salmonella typhi infection (S. enterica serotype typhi)
- Salmonellosis
- Severe acute respiratory syndrome-associated coronavirus disease

- Shiga toxin-producing Escherichia coli
- Shigellosis
- Silicosis
- Smallpox
- Spotted fever rickettsiosis
- Streptococcal toxic shock syndrome
- Syphilis
  - Syphilis, primary
  - Syphilis, secondary
  - Syphilis, early non-primary non-secondary
  - Syphilis, unknown duration or late
- Tetanus
- Toxic shock syndrome (other than streptococcal)
- Trichinellosis
- Tuberculosis
- Tularemia
- Vancomycin-intermediate *Staphylococcus aureus* and Vancomycin-resistant *S. aureus*
- Varicella
- Varicella deaths
- Vibriosis
- Viral hemorrhagic fever
  - Crimean-Congo hemorrhagic fever virus
  - Ebola virus
  - Lassa virus
  - Lujo virus
  - Marburg virus
  - New World arenavirus – Guanarito virus
  - New World arenavirus – Junin virus
  - New World arenavirus – Machupo virus
  - New World arenavirus – Sabia virus
- Waterborne Disease Outbreak
- Yellow Fever
- Zika virus disease and Zika virus infection
  - Zika virus disease, congenital
  - Zika virus disease, noncongenital
  - Zika virus infection, congenital
  - Zika virus infection, noncongenital

END-OF-APPENDIX RESOURCE

REFERENCE

Centers for Disease Control and Prevention. (2020). National notifiable diseases. https://wwwn.cdc
.gov/nndss/conditions/notifiable/2020/

COMMUNICABLE DISEASES

Oghenemaro C. Ugbeme

ADENOVIRAL KERATOCONJUNCTIVITIS

Clinical Features

Unilateral or bilateral inflammation of the conjunctivae and edema of the lids and periorbital tissue. Sudden onset with pain, photophobia, and blurred vision, and occasional low-grade fever, headache, malaise, and tender, inflamed preauricular lymph nodes. The cornea may exhibit several small, round subepithelial infiltrates about 7 days after onset that may eventually become erosions. Acute conjunctivitis may evolve to subepithelial opacities interfering with vision that may cause permanent scarring in severe cases.

Causative Agent

Adenovirus types 8, 19 and 37. The most severe disease manifestations have been found in types 5, 8 and 19.

Diagnosis

Virus identification in cultures inoculated with eye swabs or conjunctival scrapings. FA staining of scrapings and ELISA may also help with identification of the antigen.

Occurrence

Worldwide

Reservoir

Humans

Incubation Period

5 to 12 days

Transmission

Direct contact with eye secretions of an infected person. Indirect transmission occurs via contaminated surfaces, instruments, or solutions.

Risk Groups

Anyone with eye trauma and even minor eye manipulation can increase risk for infection.

Prevention

Adequate personal hygiene and avoid sharing towels, eye droppers, eye makeup, and other toilet articles. Education on minimizing hand-to-eye contact. Providers should perform effective handwashing prior to ophthalmologic procedures with proper sterilization of examination instruments after use. Any medicines or droppers that have come in contact with eyes should be discarded after use. Goggles should be used in high-risk areas.

Patient Management

Precautions should be implemented for drainage and secretions such as using separate towels and linens, and disinfection of items that have come in contact with secretions especially in the acute stages. Infected and uninfected persons should maintain separation or distance from each other.

None during acute stage, however topical corticosteroids may be used if any residual opacities occur and interfere with the patient's ability to perform daily and work tasks.

Amebiasis

Clinical Features

Fever, chills, mild abdominal comfort, bloody/mucoid diarrhea alternating with constipation

Causative Agent

Entamoeba histolytica, Entamoeba hartmanni, Escherichia coli

Diagnosis

Microscopic identification of trophozoites or cysts

Occurrence

Occurs in all age groups but less common in infants and young children. Females and males are also equally infected. Infection rates are higher in areas with crowding, poor sanitation, mental institutions and among male homosexuals.

Reservoir

Humans (chronically ill or asymptomatic carrier)

Incubation Period

2 to 4 weeks, but can be variable

Transmission

Person-to-person, fecal contaminated food or water, sexual via oral-anal contact

Risk Groups

Those living in areas of poor sanitation or where unsafe water or human fecal matter is used as fertilizer in agriculture, and consuming unsafe drinking water. Immigrants and travelers to endemic areas and persons engaging in oral-anal sexual activity.

Prevention

Sanitation education, effective hand washing practices, safe and proper disposal of human fecal matter, protection and treatment of public water supplies, and high-risk group education regarding sexual practices.

Patient Management

Isolation for hospitalized patients

Contacts and Environmental Management

Suspected contacts should have microscopic examination of fecal specimens and subsequently treated if results are positive. The use of condoms should be employed with sexual contact. Infected persons should refrain from using recreational water venues until treatment is completed.

Special Considerations

Disruption of normal sanitary methods and food management may lead to an outbreak.

Anthrax

Clinical Features

Clinical features occur in three forms depending on the route of infection: cutaneous, inhalation, or gastrointestinal. Cutaneous manifestations include initial itching of the affected site, lesion that is first papular and eventually becomes black eschar surrounded by edema. Inhalational symptoms are nonspecific and include fever, malaise, cough, or chest pain and may progress to respiratory distress, stridor, severe dyspnea, hypoxemia, diaphoresis, shock, and cyanosis. Gastrointestinal symptoms are rare, difficult to recognize, but include abdominal distress with pain, nausea and vomiting, fever, signs of septicemia and death.

Causative Agent

Bacillus anthracis

Diagnosis

Lab confirmation via recognition of the causative agent in blood, lesion exudates or smears, discharge by direct polychrome methylene blue stained smears, and bacterial DNA detection. Rapid detection methods include polymerase chain reaction (PCR) and anthrax lethal toxin detection in serum by mass spectrometry.

Occurrence

Infrequent, but primarily an occupational hazard of veterinarians, agriculture and wildlife workers, or workers who butcher animals or process meat, hides, hair, or wool. It is endemic in regions where anthrax is commonly encountered in animals such as Africa, Asia, South and Central America, and Southern and Eastern Europe.

Reservoir

Animals through ingestion of contaminated feed, water or dead carcasses of animals. Biting and nonbiting flies.

Incubation Period

Cutaneous anthrax is 5 to 7 days, inhalation anthrax is 1 to 43 days, and gastrointestinal anthrax is 1 to 6 days.

Transmission

Via contact with infected animals, their carcasses, or tissues or other parts of the animals such as the hair, wool, or hides. Ingestion of infected meat can also be a route of transmission. It can also be transmitted in the industrial process of tanning hides and processing wool or bone in poorly ventilated areas.

Risk Groups

Workers involved in industrial processing of hides, hair or wool, veterinarians, agricultural and wildlife workers, environmental investigators, lab workers, and remediation workers.

Prevention

Immunization of high-risk individuals and animals, implementation of effective prevention and control practices in animals and animal products, education of employees handling contaminated animal products, and proper ventilation of hazardous industries.

Patient Management

Patient isolation with proper disinfection of all items that come in contact with infected secretions. Initial intravenous (IV) therapy with two or more effective antimicrobial agents is also indicated. Postexposure prophylaxis (PEP) should follow inhalation exposure for persons at risk as soon as possible.

Contacts and Environmental Management

Assess adequacy of preventive measures in manufacturing plants and industries.

Special Considerations

Imported animals should be accompanied by international veterinary certificates to assure they are free from anthrax.

Aspergillosis

Clinical Features

Clinically compatible illness with serological evidence of antibody to *Bartonella henselae* by immunofluorescence assay (IFA) or enzyme immunoassay (EIA). Immunodetection and PCR are efficient in detecting *Bartonella* in biopsies or aspirates of lymph nodes.

Causative Agent

Aspergillus flavus, *Aspergillus fumigatus*, *Aspergillus nidulans*, *Aspergillus niger*, *Aspergillus clavatus*, and *Aspergillus versicolor*

Diagnosis

Diagnosis is based on radiographic, clinical, and laboratory findings.

Occurrence

Worldwide with occasional outbreaks in healthcare settings.

Reservoir

Decaying vegetation such as in piles of leaves or compost piles. It can sometimes be present in food, water, and air, both outdoors and indoors.

Incubation Period

2 days to 3 months

Transmission

By inhalation of airborne conidia

Risk Groups

Use of immunosuppressive or cytotoxic therapy poses high risk. Individuals with prolonged neutropenia or corticosteroid treatment, chronic granulomatous disease, transplant patients, and patients with HIV/AIDS are highly susceptible.

Prevention

Air quality improvement measures such as high efficiency air filtration may decrease incidence in hospitalized patients. Antifungal prophylaxis may be considered for high-risk conditions such as construction sites in health care settings.

Bacterial Conjunctivitis

Clinical Features

Lacrimation, irritation, and hyperemia of the palpebral and bulbar conjunctivae of one or both eyes. Followed by edema of the eyelids and mucopurulent discharge. Ecchymoses of the bulbar conjunctiva and marginal infiltration of the cornea with mild photophobia may occur in some cases.

Causative Agent

Haemophilus influenzae biogroup *aegyptius* (Koch-Weeks bacillus) and *Streptococcus pneumoniae* are the most important. Others are *H. influenzae* type b, *Moraxella* and *Branhamella* species, *Neisseria meningitidis*, and *Corynebacterium diphtheria*. In newborns, *H. influenzae* biogroup *aegyptius*, gonococci, *S. pneumoniae*, *Streptococcus viridans* and *Pseudomonas aeruginosa* may be rare causes of the disease.

Diagnosis

Microscopic examination of a stained smear, or a culture to exclude other agent.

Occurrence

Widespread and common worldwide especially in warmer climates, and commonly occurs with acute viral respiratory disease during cold seasons.

Reservoir

Humans

Incubation Period

24 to 72 hours

Transmission

Contact with discharges from conjunctivae or upper respiratory tracts of infected people, contaminated fingers, clothing, shared eye makeup and makeup applicators, multiple dose eye medications, and inadequately sterilized instruments such as tonometers.

Risk Groups

Children younger than 5 years are mostly affected but decreases with age. Older adults and immuno-compromised persons are also at risk especially for staphylococcal infections.

Prevention

Personal hygiene, hygienic care, and treatment of affected eye.

Patient Management

Children should not attend school during the acute stage. Drainage and secretions precautions should be implemented with subsequent disinfection of items in contact with these secretions. Treatment involves use of an ointment or eyedrops at site of infection containing fusidic acid, chloramphenicol, ciprofloxacin, gentamycin, or combination antibiotics such as polymyxin B with neomycin or trimethoprim.

Balantidiasis

Clinical Features

Affects the colon producing diarrhea or dysentery, abdominal colic, tenesmus, nausea, and vomiting. Dysentery can sometimes occur with stools containing blood, mucus, and a little pus.

Causative Agent

Balantidium coli

Diagnosis

Identification of trophozoites or cysts of *B. coli* in fresh feces, or trophozoites in fecal material obtained by sigmoidoscopy

Occurrence

Worldwide, although environmental contamination with feces may result in higher incidence

Reservoir

Swine, rats, and laboratory pigs

Incubation Period

Unknown, but may be only a few days

Transmission

Ingestion of contaminated food or water containing cysts from feces of infected host

Risk Groups

Immunocompromised

Prevention

Personal hygiene education for the general public. Food handlers may require education and supervision on safe food practices. Sanitary disposal of fecal matter. Minimize contact with swine feces.

Patient Management

10-day treatment with tetracycline to eliminate infection

Contacts and Environmental Management

Household members and suspected contacts should have microscopic examination of fecal matter. Investigate contact with swine and consider treating infected pigs with tetracycline.

Blastomycosis

Clinical Features

Acute infection presents with sudden onset of fever, cough, and pulmonary infiltrates in chest X-ray, with spontaneous resolution in 1 to 3 weeks. May present with infection already spread mainly to the skin and less often to the bone, prostate, or epididymis. Skin lesions begin as erythematous papules that become crusted or ulcerated and spread slowly. These lesions are commonly located on the face and distal extremities. Other symptoms include a low-grade fever, weight loss, and weakness. Disseminated disease is more common in immunocompromised patients.

Causative Agent

Blastomyces dermatitidis

Diagnosis

Confirmed by culture, deoxyribonucleic acid (DNA) probe, or visualization by direct microscopic examination. An enzyme immunoassay (EIA) test detects the antigen in urine, serum or bronchoalveolar lavage.

Occurrence

Uncommon, but endemic in the southern and southeastern United States

Reservoir

Moist soil in wooded areas along waterways, and in undisturbed places such as under porches or sheds. Common in dogs, and reported cats, a horse, a captive African lion, and sea lion.

Incubation Period

Weeks to months. 45-day median for symptomatic infections.

Transmission

Inhalation of conidia spore-laden dust of mold or saprophytic growth forms

Risk Groups

Rare in children, however males are more frequently affected than females. Immunocompromised at greater risk.

Prevention

Not yet fully understood

Patient Management

Itraconazole is the drug of choice. Amphotericin B is indicated for patients with severe illness or brain lesions, followed by itraconazole after condition has been stabilized.

Contacts and Environmental Management

Investigation of contacts and infection source not beneficial unless clusters of disease occur

Botulism

Clinical Features

Bilateral cranial nerve palsies, ptosis, diplopia, blurred vision, dysphagia, dysarthria, and ophthalmoplegia. GI symptoms such as nausea, vomiting, and diarrhea can occur in foodborne botulism. Infant manifestations include constipation, poor suck, altered cry, weakness, and loss of head control.

Causative Agent

Botulinum toxin

Diagnosis

Clinically diagnosed and laboratory confirmed by detecting the toxin in serum, stool, or wound cultures.

Occurrence

Case reports from the Americas, Africa, Asia, Australia, Europe, and the Middle East.

Reservoir

Soil, lake and marine sediments, agricultural products, and intestinal tracts of animals.

Incubation Period

2 hours to 8 days. Up to 30 days in infants for intestinal colonization.

Transmission

Foodborne and intestinal infection occurs by ingestion of preformed toxin in contaminated food. Wound infection occurs when *Clostridium botulinum* germinate and produce toxin within the wound. Inhalational infection occurs via inhalation of aerosolized botulinum neurotoxin. Iatrogenic infection can occur when commercial preparations for botulinum toxin are injected for cosmetic purposes and ophthalmologic disorders.

Risk Groups

General susceptibility, and those who consume improperly home-preserved foods.

Prevention

Proper food preparation practices. Avoid feeding infants honey. Thoroughly clean wounds contaminated by soil. Avoid injection doses above the recommendations of the manufacturers.

Patient Management

Immediate access to an intensive care unit to promptly recognize and manage respiratory failure. Treatment is supportive care and botulinum antitoxin. Wounds should be cleaned and/or debrided.

Contacts and Environmental Management

Thorough history should be taken to determine method of infection. Persons with foodborne illness and their contacts should be monitored for signs and symptoms with prompt treatment.

Special Considerations

A single case of foodborne illness should raise suspicion of an outbreak.

Brucellosis

Clinical Features

Irregular and variable fever, headache, weakness, profuse sweating, arthralgia, myalgia, fatigue, anorexia, and weight loss.

Causative Agent

Brucella abortus, Brucella melitensis, Brucella suis, Brucella canis, Brucella ceti, and *Brucella pinnipedialis*

Diagnosis

Microbiological isolation of *Brucella* species from blood, bone marrow, or other tissues or discharges.

Occurrence

Worldwide

Reservoir

Cattle, swine, goats, and sheep, but can occur in camels, bison, elk, equids, caribou, and some deer.

Incubation Period

1 to 2 months with a range of 5 days to 5 months

Transmission

Contact via mucous membranes and breaks in skin with animal tissue; blood; urine; vaginal discharges; aborted fetus; and ingestion of uncooked meat, raw milk, and dairy products from infected animals.

Risk Groups

Those working with infected animals or their tissues such as farmers, veterinarians, and slaughterhouse workers.

Prevention

Eliminate infection among domestic animals. Educate regarding the dangers of eating undercooked meat or unpasteurized dairy products. Educate high-risk populations about the dangers of exposure to infected animals. Hunters should be encouraged to use protective gear and practice good personal hygiene. Disinfect contaminated areas.

Patient Management

Drainage and secretion precautions if there are draining lesions. Treat with a combination of doxycycline and rifampicin or streptomycin for at least 6 weeks.

Contacts and Environmental Management

Trace infections to a common source, test and remove suspected animals, and disinfect affected areas.

Campylobacter Enteritis

Clinical Features

Diarrhea, abdominal pain, fever, malaise, nausea, and vomiting. Fever and malaise may precede diarrhea by a day or more. The severe abdominal pain is sometimes confused for appendicitis or inflammatory bowel disease. Blood and white blood cells are commonly observed in the stools.

Causative Agent

Campylobacter jejuni and *Campylobacter coli*

Diagnosis

Isolation of organisms from clinical specimens.

Occurrence

Worldwide. Highest incidence in males and children <5 years in industrialized countries, and children <2 years in developing countries.

Reservoir

Animals especially poultry and cattle, also puppies, kittens, swine, sheep, rodents and birds.

Incubation Period

2 to 5 days with a range of 1 to 10 days.

Transmission

Ingestion of organisms in undercooked meat, unpasteurized dairy products, or contaminated food or water, or direct contact with infected animals.

Risk Groups

Immunocompromised persons, and persons with decreased stomach acidity.

Prevention

Pasteurize milk, boil water, and thoroughly cook all food of animal origin. Recognize, prevent, and control infections among domestic animals and pets.

Patient Management

Enteric precautions in hospitalized patients. Rehydration and electrolyte replacement therapy in cases with dehydration.

Contacts and Environmental Management

Identify contaminated food or water sources to which others may have been exposed.

Cat Scratch Disease

Clinical Features

Malaise, granulomatous lymphadenitis, and variable fever patterns. Usually preceded by a cat scratch, lick, or bite that produces a red papular rash with regional lymph node involvement

Causative Agent

B. henselae

Diagnosis

Clinically compatible illness coupled with serological evidence of antibody to *B. henselae* by IFA or enzyme immunoassay (EIA). Immunodetection and PCR are efficient in detecting *Bartonella* in biopsies or aspirates in lymph nodes.

Occurrence

Worldwide, but uncommon. More in children and young adults. Majority of cases are seen during the late summer, fall and winter months.

Reservoir

Cats

Incubation Period

3 to 14 days from inoculation to primary lesion and 5 to 50 days from inoculation to lymphadenopathy

Transmission

Usually via cat scratch, bite, lick, or other exposure to a healthy, young cat or kitten. Cat fleas transmit the *B. henselae* among cats, but role clarity has yet to be established in direct transmission to humans. No person-to-person transfer.

Risk Groups

Children and young adults

Prevention

Thorough cleaning of cat scratches and bites may be helpful. Flea control is of high importance to prevent cat infection.

Patient Management

Treatment is not indicated in healthy patients. Azithromycin may lead to faster resolution of swelling in patients with extensive lymphadenitis. Doxycycline and rifampin are recommended for CSD-associated retinitis treatment. Treatment course with oral erythromycin or doxycycline longer than 3 to 4 months are indicated for immunocompromised patients with HIV infection.

Chancroid

Clinical Features

Clinically characterized by a single or multiple, painful, necrotic ulcers that bleed on contact. Found more often in uncircumcised men on the foreskin or the coronal sulcus that may cause phimosis. Accompanied by the lesions are painful and regional swollen lymph nodes. Painless lesions may occur on the vaginal wall or cervix in women, even though extragenital lesions have been reported in both sexes.

Causative Agent

Haemophilus ducreyi

Diagnosis

Culture and PCR are preferred for a definitive diagnosis

Occurrence

Mostly occurs in tropical and subtropical regions that include Africa and Southeast Asia. Outbreaks and endemic transmission occur in high-risk groups in industrialized countries.

Reservoir

Humans

Incubation Period

3 to 5 days, up to 14 days.

Transmission

The disease is highly transmissible until the lesions are completely healed. Direct sexual contact with open lesions and pus is the main mode of transmission. Nonsexual transmission may however still occur from contact with open lesions.

Risk Groups

Uncircumcised men, sex workers, and clients of sex workers. In industrialized countries, cases are associated with sex work, travel, or exposure to individuals from endemic areas.

Prevention

Consistent use of condoms or other protective methods to decrease risk of infection

Patient Management

Avoid sexual interactions until all lesions are completely healed. Treatment is a single dose of azithromycin or ceftriaxone in cases where non-compliance presents an issue. Otherwise, multiday treatment course using erythromycin and ciprofloxacin can be used. HIV-infected and uncircumcised cases may require a longer treatment period or therapy repetition.

Contacts and Environmental Management

All sexual contacts exposed within a 10-day period preceding symptom onset should be examined and treated.

Chlamydial Conjunctivitis

Clinical Features

Acute conjunctivitis with purulent discharge is usually seen in the newborn 5 to 12 days after birth spontaneously subsiding within a few weeks. Acute follicular conjunctivitis in children and adults occurs with preauricular lymphadenopathy on the affected side, hyperemia, infiltration, and slight mucopurulent discharge with superficial corneal involvement. Adults may experience a chronic phase with scanty discharge with symptoms persisting for more than a year if left untreated.

Causative Agent

C. trachomatis of serovars D through K. Feline strains of Chlamydia psittaci have also been an agent in human infections.

Diagnosis

Laboratory methods such as isolation in cell culture, antigen detection using IF staining of direct smears, EIA methods and DNA probe.

Occurrence

Sporadic cases are reported worldwide among sexually active adults. Neonatal conjunctivitis is common and occurs in about 35% of newborns exposed to maternal infection. Very few adults with genital chlamydial infection eventually develop chlamydial eye disease.

Reservoir

Humans for C. trachomatis, and cats for C. psittaci.

Incubation Period

5 to 12 days in newborns with a range of 3 days to 6 weeks. 6 to 19 days in adults.

Transmission

Transmitted during sexual intercourse with an infected person in adults. Eyes of the adult is usually infected by transmission of genital secretions to the eye by the fingers. Newborn conjunctivitis is acquired by direct contact with infectious secretions while moving through the birth canal. In utero infection can occur. The disease is highly transmissible while genital or ocular infection persist.

Risk Groups

Diabetics and infants of infected mothers

Prevention

Correct and consistent use of condoms to prevent sexual transmission. All persons, including pregnant women, infected with urethritis and cervicitis of chlamydial origin should be promptly treated. Infection should be quickly identified by culture or antigen detection in high-risk pregnant women to prevent subsequent transmission to the newborn. Routine prophylaxis for gonococcal ophthalmia neonatorum is effective against chlamydial infection and should be practiced.

Patient Management

Drainage and secretion precautions should be implemented for the first 96 hours after starting treatment. Nursery transmission should be prevented by following proper aseptic and handwashing techniques. Ocular and genital infections should be treated with erythromycin, tetracycline, azithromycin or ofloxacin. A 2-week erythromycin treatment regimen is recommended for treatment of neonatal ocular infections to eliminate risk of chlamydial pneumonia as well.

Contacts and Environmental Management

All sexual contacts of adult cases and parents of infected newborns should be examined and treated. Infected adults should be examined for evidence of ongoing co-infection with gonorrhea and/or syphilis.

Chlamydial Infections

Clinical Features

Although most presentations are asymptomatic, symptomatic presentations are sometimes difficult to distinguish from gonorrhea. Males present with urethritis evidenced as scanty mucopurulent discharge, dysuria, and urethral itching, while females present with cervicitis evidenced as mucopurulent endocervical discharge and cervical friability. Rectal infection can occur via anal intercourse or spread from the vagina. Some other manifestations include epididymitis in males, dysuria, pyuria, perihepatitis, bartholinitis and conjunctivitis. Spread of untreated infection from the cervix to the uterus, fallopian tubes, and ovaries can cause a symptomatic or acute pelvic inflammatory disease (PID)

Causative Agent

Mainly *Chlamydia trachomatis*, however other agents have been indicated including *Mycoplasma genitalium*, *Trichomonas vaginalis*, herpes simplex virus, adenovirus, *Ureaplasma urealyticum*, and enteric bacteria.

Diagnosis

Nucleic acid amplification tests

Occurrence

Worldwide

Reservoir

Humans

Incubation Period

7 to 14 days or longer.

Transmission

Through sexual contact with the penis, vagina, mouth, or anus of an infected partner. Exposure to the mother's infected cervix often results in neonatal infection.

Risk Groups

Sexually active individuals such as young adults, and those with multiple recent sex partners. Reinfection is common among women and is associated with an increased risk of PID.

Prevention

Health and sex education especially regarding condom use. Yearly, routine periodic screenings for all sexually active women 25 years and younger, older women with risk factors, and men who have receptive anal sex. It is also recommended at the first prenatal care visit for pregnant women.

Patient Management

Affected patients should abstain from sexual activity until they and their sexual partners have completed the antibiotic treatment (7-day abstinence period for a single dose, or post-completion of a 7-day treatment regimen). Doxycycline for 7 days or a single dose of azithromycin may be used. Alternative options are erythromycin, levofloxacin, and ofloxacin. All patients should be rescreened 3 months after treatment due to possibility of reinfection.

Contacts and Environmental Management

Exposed partners should be evaluated and treated within 60 days before symptom onset or diagnosis. Mothers of infants with chlamydial infection and their sex partners should also be evaluated and treated.

Cholera

Clinical Features

Sudden onset, profuse painless watery stools. Massive loss of fluid with nausea and vomiting. If left untreated, can progress to rapid dehydration, acidosis, circulatory collapse, hypoglycemia in children and renal failure.

Causative Agent

Vibrio cholerae

Diagnosis

Isolation of the agent from stool specimen

Occurrence

Areas with unsafe food and water supplies, poor hygiene and sanitation, and crowded living conditions.

Reservoir

Humans and the environment

Incubation Period

Few hours to 5 days, usually 2 to 3 days

Transmission

Ingestion of an infective dose in feces contaminated food or water

Risk Groups

Lowest socioeconomic groups, and persons with blood group O

Prevention

Prevention of fecal-oral transmission by providing safe drinking water, proper sanitation, and waste disposal, with proper handwashing hygiene. Completion of the oral vaccination series.

Patient Management

Enteric precautions with the hospitalized patient. Treatment is mainly adequate rehydration with oral rehydration solution (ORS) to replace fluid losses.

Contacts and Environmental Management

Patient surveillance of persons sharing food and drinks with a cholera patient for 5 days from exposure. Investigate infection possibilities from polluted drinking water and contaminated food.

Special Considerations

Educate the population at risk concerning the need to seek appropriate treatment of dehydration without delay. Provide safe water supplies. Ensure proper food-handling and preparation methods.

Chromomycosis

Clinical Features

Mycosis of the skin and subcutaneous tissues of the lower extremities. Initially appearing as a papule or nodule, it slowly progresses to neighboring tissues over a period of years eventually becoming large, nodular, verrucous, or cauliflower-like masses.

Causative Agent

Fonsecaea (Phialophora) pedrosi, Phialophora verrucosa, Cladosporium carrionii, Rhinocladiella aquaspersa, Botryomyces caespitatus, Exophiala spinifera, and *Exophial jeanselmei.*

Diagnosis

Microscopic examination of scrapings or biopsies from lesions

Occurrence

Worldwide, but mostly in tropical and subtropical regions such as Latin America, the Caribbean, Asia and Africa

Reservoir

Wood, soil, and decaying vegetation

Incubation Period

Unknown, likely months to years

Transmission

Inoculation via superficial, minor penetrating trauma/injuries. Not transmitted from person to person.

Risk Groups

Barefoot rural workers in tropical regions. Common among men aged 30 to 50 years.

Prevention

Wear shoes and protective clothing for protection against small puncture wounds.

Patient Management

Discharges from lesions and soiled articles should be effectively disinfected. Itraconazole is the treatment of choice.

Coccidioidomycosis

Clinical Features

May be asymptomatic or present with acute influenza-like symptoms such as fever, chills, cough, rash, and pleuritic pain. Some cases develop erythema nodosum. The primary infection may completely resolve, leave fibrosis with a pulmonary nodule with or without calcified areas or progress to a disseminated form of the disease. The disseminated form is characterized by lesions on any part of the body, especially in subcutaneous tissue, skin, bone, and meninges.

Causative Agent

Coccidioides immitis and *Coccidioides posadasii*

Diagnosis

Observation of the characteristic coccidioidal spherules on microscope examination or through culture of sputum, pus, urine, cerebrospinal fluid, or skin or organ lesion biopsies

Occurrence

Common in the arid and semiarid endemic areas of the Western Hemisphere

Reservoir

Soil

Incubation Period

1 to 4 weeks in primary infection. Dissemination may develop years after the primary infection.

Transmission

Inhalation of the arthroconidia from the soil and in laboratory accidents with the cultures

Risk Groups

Potential exposure can occur due to occupational environment. Pregnant women in the third trimester, persons of African or Filipino race/ethnicity, and immunocompromised persons are at greatest risk for the disseminated version of the infection.

Prevention

No practical prevention measures have been identified in endemic areas.

Patient Management

Proper disinfection of soiled articles. Though the primary infection spontaneously resolves after a few days or weeks without treatment, intravenous (IV) amphotericin B is used for severe pulmonary infections and fluconazole for any resulting meningeal infection.

Contacts and Environmental Management

Cases occurring in nonendemic areas should investigate and obtain residence, work exposure and travel history.

Special Considerations

Infection might be possible if large groups of susceptible people move or live in dusty areas where the fungus is prevalent.

Common Cold

Clinical Features

Coryza, sneezing, lacrimation, irritation of the nasopharynx, chills, and malaise lasting 2 to 7 days. Fever can occur in children under 3 years. Laryngitis, tracheitis or bronchitis may occur with serious complications like otitis media and sinusitis.

Causative Agent

Rhinoviruses in adults; parainfluenza viruses, respiratory syncytial virus (RSV), adenoviruses, certain enteroviruses, and other coronaviruses in adults.

Diagnosis

Cell or organ studies of nasal secretions may show a known virus. Epidemiological community data can inform the differential diagnosis. PCR can also be used to detect the virus.

Occurrence

Worldwide. Incidence rates rise in fall, winter, and spring. Incidence is higher in children under 5 years with a gradual decline with increasing age.

Reservoir

Humans

Incubation Period

Between 12 hours and 5 days, usually 48 hours.

Transmission

Direct contact or mucous membrane exposure to respiratory droplets. Indirect transmission occurs through hands and articles soiled with fresh nasal and throat discharges of infected persons.

Risk Groups

Universal susceptibility

Prevention

Practice good personal hygiene such as covering mouth when coughing and sneezing, and frequent handwashing. Avoid crowds and provide adequate ventilation. Avoid smoking and passive smoke exposure. Use masks.

Patient Management

Contact precautions should be implemented with droplet precautions added as necessary for the specific causative pathogen. Adequate disinfection methods should be performed for eating and drinking utensils with sanitary disposal of oral and nasal discharges.

Contacts and Environmental Management

Personal hygiene and infection control practices.

Cryptococcosis

Clinical Features

Primary pulmonary infection in healthy persons presents with fever and dry cough. In immunocompromised, signs and symptoms often develop after blood spreads the infection to the meninges with subacute or chronic meningitis; symptoms include headache, visual disturbance, and confusion. Other sites of disseminated infection are the kidneys, prostate, bone, and skin.

Causative Agent

Cryptococcus neoformans, *Cryptococcus grubii* and *Cryptococcus gattii*.

Diagnosis

Histology or cell culture, or evidence of the characteristic capsular halo or budding forms on microscopic examination of cerebrospinal fluid (CSF).

Occurrence

Worldwide and follows the AIDS epidemic epidemiology. Frequently affects adults more than children, and more males than females. *C. gattii* is more frequent in tropical and subtropical regions, and the Southern Pacific coast of the United States.

Reservoir

C. neoformans can be isolated from old pigeon nests, pigeon droppings, and soil from many parts of the world. Foliage and barks of many trees have shown colonies of *C. gattii*. Infection may also occur in cats, dogs, horses, camelids, and other animals.

Incubation Period

Unknown for *C. neoformans* and 2 to 13 days for *C. gattii*. Brain infection can be preceded by pulmonary disease for many years.

Transmission

Inhalation of fungal spores

Risk Groups

High susceptibility during corticosteroid or other immunosuppressive therapy, and by immune deficiency disorders such as HIV

Prevention

Fluconazole antifungal as a prophylaxis has been shown to decrease the incidence of infection.

Patient Management

Simultaneous disinfection of discharges and contaminated dressings. Treatment involves amphotericin B combined with 5-flucytosine as therapy of choice for disseminated infection. Treatment for meningitis involves long-term consolidation therapy following induction. Treatment for elevated intracranial pressure in patients with meningeal involvement involves the use of manometry and periodic therapeutic lumbar punctures.

Cryptosporidiosis

Clinical Features

Affects epithelial cells of the gastrointestinal (GI), biliary, and respiratory tracts. The major symptom is diarrhea that may sometimes be profuse and watery, with cramping and abdominal pain. The diarrhea is preceded by anorexia and vomiting in children. Symptoms are intermittent but eventually resolve in less than 30 days in otherwise healthy individuals. Infections in immunocompromised persons usually resolve when factors contributing to immunosuppression are improved upon or controlled.

Causative Agent

Cryptosporidium hominis and *Cryptosporidium parvum*

Diagnosis

Identification of oocysts in fecal smears or of life cycle stages of the parasites in intestinal biopsy secretions

Occurrence

Worldwide

Reservoir

Humans and various animals such as birds, fish, reptiles and mammals

Incubation Period

1 to 12 days is the probable range with a 7-day average.

Transmission

Fecal-oral from person-to-person and animal-to-person, waterborne and foodborne transmission.

Risk Groups

Children younger than 2 years, animal handlers, men who have sex with men, and those in close contact with infected individuals such as family members and day care workers

Prevention

Educate regarding personal hygiene especially for handwashing and food handling, and before eating and after toilet use. Feces should be disposed in a sanitary manner while exercising care with handling. Those in close contact with animals with diarrhea should be sure to wash their hands carefully. Water and water supplies should be boiled for 1 minute, and use of filters capable of removing small particles should be considered.

Patient Management

Enteric precautions should be implemented for hospitalized patients. Stress proper handwashing technique. Infected children should be excused from daycare facilities until the diarrhea resolves. Fluid and electrolyte replacement with ORSs should be implemented. Patients on immunosuppressants should consider safely reducing or stopping these medications especially in cases of severe symptoms. Nitazoxanide may be used as treatment in patients 1 year and older.

Contacts and Environmental Management

Feces of household members and suspected contacts should be microscopically evaluated.

Cytomegalovirus Disease (CMV)

Clinical Features

Usually occurs as an undiagnosed febrile illness without any specific characteristics. The worst form of the disease develops in infants infected in utero showing signs of severe generalized infection of the central nervous system and liver. Lethargy convulsions, jaundice, petechiae, purpura, hepatosplenomegaly, chorioretinitis, intracerebral calcifications, intrauterine growth restriction, and pulmonary infiltrates may occur. When the infection occurs later in life in a healthy person, it may look similar to mononucleosis and hepatitis. In immunocompromised patients, the disseminated infection causes pneumonitis; retinitis; GI tract disorders (gastritis, enteritis, colitis); and hepatitis. CMV is notably a common cause of post-transplant infection for organ and bone marrow transplants.

Causative Agent

Human (beta) herpesvirus 5 (human CMV)

Diagnosis

Viral isolation or PCR from urine or saliva samples from the newborn in the first 2 to 3 weeks of life. Multiple diagnostic modalities should be used in the adult due to high frequency of asymptomatic and recurrent infections. Use of viral isolation, CMV antigen detection and PCR detection can be used to demonstrate the virus in organs, blood, respiratory secretions, and urine.

Occurrence

Worldwide; more common among women than men, and associated with socioeconomic status or ethnic group in some countries

Reservoir

Humans

Incubation Period

Illness following transplant usually begins within 3 to 8 weeks. Perinatal or early postnatal infection is usually within 3 to 12 weeks after birth.

Transmission

Direct mucosal contact with infectious tissues; secretions; and excretions; including saliva, breast milk, cervical secretions, and semen. Fetal infection may occur in utero from maternal infection mostly due to maternal reactivation or reinfection. Perinatal infection occurs via exposure to cervical secretions at delivery, while postnatal infections occur via breast milk. Many children in daycare centers excrete CMV, which may represent a community reservoir.

Risk Groups

Fetuses, infants born prematurely or with low birth weight, patients with immunosuppressive conditions and transplant patients.

Prevention

Wash hands after diaper changes and toilet care of newborns and infants. Healthcare personnel should follow standard precautions. Daycare and preschool workers should observe strict hygiene methods. Transmission via transfusion of blood products can be avoided by freezing red blood cells in glycerol before administration. Avoid transplanting organs from CMV-seropositive donors to seronegative recipients.

Patient Management

Follow standard precautions in healthcare settings. Drugs for prophylaxis and treatment of CMV disease are ganciclovir IV or oral valganciclovir. Cidofovir IV, foscarnet IV and fomisiviren are used for the treatment of CMV retinitis in immunocompromised persons. Ganciclovir, valganciclovir, cidofovir and foscarnet when combined with anti-CMV immune globulin are used for pneumonitis and GI disease in immunocompromised persons.

Dengue

Clinical Features

Acute febrile illness with three phases: febrile, critical, and convalescent. Patients have sudden onset of fever for 2 to 7 days. Other manifestations are intense headache; arthralgia; myalgia; bone pain; retro-orbital pain; anorexia; vomiting; macular or maculopapular rash; and minor hemorrhagic manifestations including petechiae, ecchymosis, purpura, epistaxis, bleeding gums, hematuria, or a positive tourniquet test. Warning signs of progression to severe dengue occur in the late febrile phase and include persistent vomiting, severe abdominal pain, mucosal bleeding, difficulty breathing, signs of hypovolemic shock, and rapid decline in platelet count with an increase in hematocrit. Hemorrhagic manifestations such as hematemesis, hematochezia, and melena may occur as well, especially in cases of prolonged shock. As plasma leakage subsides, the convalescent phase begins. Extravasated fluids reabsorb, hemodynamic status restabilizes, and diuresis ensues. Patients may develop a generalized erythematous rash with circular areas of nonerythematous skin that may desquamate and be pruritic.

Causative Agent

Dengue viruses

Diagnosis

Single serum specimen obtained during the febrile phase of the illness to detect DENV and immunoglobulin class M (IgM) anti-DENV. Reverse transcriptase PCR (RT-PCR) can detect DENV ribonucleic acid (RNA). DENV can also be detected by immunoassay for the nonstructural protein 1 (NS1) antigen that is present in the viremic period.

Occurrence

Endemic in most countries in the tropics and subtropics, with epidemic experience occurring at 2 to 5 years intervals. More than one serotype circulates in certain island locations, and usually 2 or more serotypes circulate simultaneously.

Reservoir

DENV is maintained in a human/*Aedes aegypti* mosquito cycle in endemic regions with or without human symptoms. A sylvatic monkey/mosquito cycle exists and may spill over to human populations of southeastern Asia and western Africa.

Incubation Period

3 to 14 days

Transmission

Bite of infective mosquitoes

Risk Groups

People of all ages living in dengue endemic areas. Incidence is highest in children, though there are increasing numbers of adults recently in both rural and urban areas. Infants infected at 6 to 12 months of age born to previously dengue infected mothers are at an increased risk for severe dengue.

Prevention

Prevent mosquito bites by eliminating mosquito vector larval habitats such as water-holding containers close to inside human habitation. Manage and treat mosquito production sites with larvicides as appropriate. Use repellents, screening, and productive clothing to prevent against bites. Chemoprophylaxis or antiviral agent for prevention or treatment. Cases should be identified in a timely manner with implementation of good patient management practices to prevent morbidity and mortality. Educate the public about warning signs.

Patient Management

Standard/bloodborne infection precautions. Use mosquito bed net that are preferably insecticide-impregnated. Patients should be kept well-hydrated and avoid aspirin use or other nonsteroidal anti-inflammatory drugs to control fever. Monitor patients for early signs of shock, occult bleeding, and resolution of plasma leak to avoid prolonged shock, end-organ damage, and fluid overload. In cases of refractory shock, IV colloids and/or blood or blood products may be required.

Contacts and Environmental Management

Determine the patient's place of residence 2 weeks prior to onset of illness and search for unreported or undiagnosed cases in the same household or area.

Special Considerations

Use indoor insecticide sprays to decrease mosquito populations

Diphtheria

Clinical Features

Primarily involves the mucous membranes of the upper respiratory tract, skin, or other mucous membranes of the conjunctivae, vagina, or ear. There is an asymmetrical greyish white membrane with surrounding inflammation. In moderate to severe cases of respiratory diphtheria, the throat may be moderately to severely sore with enlarged and tender cervical lymph nodes that give rise to a "bull neck" appearance with marked swelling of the neck. Pharyngeal membranes may extend into the trachea causing airway obstruction. Other symptoms are myocarditis, heart block, and progressive congestive heart failure beginning a week after onset of symptoms. Neurologic complications may occur about 2 weeks after onset of illness and can mimic Guillain-Barre syndrome. Respiratory diphtheria presents with streptococcal pharyngitis, Vincent angina, infectious mononucleosis, oral syphilis, oral candidiasis, and adenoviruses.

Causative Agent

Toxin-producing strains of *C. diphtheriae.*

Diagnosis

Observation of an asymmetrical, adherent grayish membrane associated with tonsillitis, pharyngitis, or a serosanguinous nasal drainage. Diagnosis is confirmed by bacteriological examination of lesions.

Occurrence

Occurs in colder months in temperate zones. In tropical regions, the inapparent, cutaneous and wound diphtheria version is more common.

Reservoir

Humans

Incubation Period

2 to 5 days

Transmission

Contact with a patient or carrier, or contact with articles soiled with discharges from lesions of infected people including raw milk that has served as a vehicle

Risk Groups

Nonimmunized or underimmunized children younger than 15 years and other underimmunized populations.

Prevention

Educate about importance of immunization. Control is effective with widespread diphtheria immunization, and vaccination schedule should be followed according to age-appropriate guidelines. The recommended vaccine schedule is three primary doses given intramuscularly at 6, 10 and 14 weeks of age and a diphtheria, tetanus, pertussis booster at 1 to 6 years of age. Those at higher risk of patient exposure such as healthcare workers should ensure full immunization with a booster dose of tetanus and diphtheria (Td) every 10 years. Immunization recommendations are the same for healthy and immunocompromised persons alike.

Patient Management

Droplet precautions for pharyngeal diphtheria and contact isolation for cutaneous diphtheria, until 2 cultures from both throat and nose taken at least 24 hours apart and at least 24 hours after cessation of antibiotic therapy, fail to grow C. diphtheria. In absence or unavailability of culture, droplet precautions may end after 14 days of antibiotic therapy. Disinfection of all articles in contact with and soiled with discharges of the patient. Diphtheria antitoxin given IM is the treatment for respiratory diphtheria, administered after sensitivity testing has been performed. Procaine penicillin G (IM) or parenteral erythromycin is recommended until patient can swallow comfortably. Oral erythromycin or penicillin V may be used for a 14-day period. Prophylactic treatment may employ the use of a single dose of benzathine penicillin G (IM) or a 10-day course of erythromycin.

Contacts and Environmental Management

All close contacts should have swabs taken from nose and throat for culture of causative agent with prophylactic treatment with erythromycin or benzathine implemented. Adult contacts whose occupation involves handling food especially milk or work closely with nonimmunized children should be excluded from work until treated and tests confirm them not to be carriers. Previously immunized persons should receive a booster dose of diphtheria toxoid if more than 5 years has elapsed since their last dose. Nonimmunized persons should have a primary series initiated.

Dwarf Tapeworm

Clinical Features

Asymptomatic, or may cause enteritis with or without diarrhea, abdominal pain, pallor, weight loss, and weakness.

Causative Agent

Hymenolepsis nana

Diagnosis

Identification of eggs in feces

Occurrence

Cosmopolitan

Reservoir

Humans and rodents

Incubation Period

Variable. Mature worms develop in 2 weeks.

Transmission

Autoinfection via feces or person-to-person transmission. Ingestion of food and water contaminated with eggs. Directly from fecal contaminated fingers. Ingestion of insects such as mealworms, larval fleas, and beetles.

Risk Groups

Immunodeficient groups and malnourished children

Prevention

Personal hygiene and handwashing education. Safe disposal of feces. Provide and maintain clean toilet facilities. Protect food and water from human and rodent fecal contamination. Treat infected patients. Eliminate rodents from home environment.

Patient Management

Safe disposal of feces. Treat with praziquantel, niclosamide, or nitazoxanide.

Contacts and Environmental Management

Fecal examination of family or institution members.

Special Considerations

Outbreaks in schools and institutions should be controlled by treating infected persons, and special attention to personal and group hygiene.

Ebola-Marburg Viral Diseases

Clinical Features
Sudden onset of fever, malaise, myalgia, and headache followed by pharyngitis, vomiting, diarrhea, and a maculopapular rash. Severe forms may present with hepatic damage, renal failure, CNS involvement, and terminal shock with multiorgan dysfunction.

Causative Agent
Ebola and Marburg viruses

Diagnosis
Direct detection of virus in blood or tissue samples by virus isolation, PCR, or ELISA

Occurrence
Africa, UK, and Russia

Reservoir
Forest-dwelling fruit bats for Ebola virus; cave-dwelling fruit bats for Marburg virus; swine

Incubation Period
5 to 15 days

Transmission
Via manipulation of infected dead wild mammals in the rainforest. Close contact with bats or spending time in bat-inhabited area like caves or mines. Person-to-person transmission through direct contact with blood, urine, vomitus, feces, secretions, organs, or semen.

Risk Groups
All ages and those in close proximity to infected patients, secretions or specimens

Prevention
Use of protective methods with sexual intercourse for 3 months or until semen is free of virus.

Patient Management
Strict patient isolation procedures along with their body fluids and excreta should be maintained. Personal protective equipment should be used whenever interacting with the patient. Proper disinfection with heating or chemical methods should be used for objects coming in contact with the patient after use.

Contacts and Environmental Management
Identify all contacts within 3 weeks after the onset of illness. Establish close surveillance of contacts via body temperature checks at least twice daily for 3 weeks after exposure.

Enterobiasis

Clinical Features
Most common feature is perianal itching leading to disturbed sleep patterns, irritability, and secondary infection of scratched skin. Others include vulvovaginitis, salpingitis, and pelvic and liver granuloma. Appendicitis and enuresis have been reported as well.

Causative Agent
Enterobius vermicularis

Diagnosis
Presence of worms or their eggs in the perianal region seen 2 to 3 hours after the person goes to sleep. Eggs can be observed by applying a transparent adhesive tape to the perianal region and examining the tape microscopically for eggs. Examination needs to be repeated three or more times before accepting a negative result. Female worms may be found in feces and in the perianal region during vaginal or rectal examinations.

Occurrence

Worldwide across all socioeconomic classes. Prevalent in warmer climate and in school-age children.

Reservoir

Humans

Incubation Period

1 to 2 months

Transmission

Direct transfer of infective eggs by hand from anus to mouth of the same or another person, or indirectly through clothing, bedding, food, or other contaminated articles. Dust borne infection can occur in heavily contaminated areas. A person can self-reinfect or be reinfected by eggs from another person.

Risk Groups

High prevalence in domiciliary institutions. Children younger than 18 months and their caretakers, and people who are institutionalized.

Prevention

Educate on personal hygiene, especially handwashing with soap and water after defecation and changing diapers, and before eating or preparing food. Discourage nail biting and scratching the anal area. Daily morning bathing with showers should be encouraged over tub baths. Change to clean undergarments and nightwear, and bedsheets frequently. Reduce overcrowding in living areas. Provide adequate toilet facilities and maintain cleanliness.

Patient Management

Change linen and underwear of infected person daily for several days after treatment. Boil bed clothing or use washing machine and dryer on hot setting. Children's toys should be cleaned regularly. Albendazole, mebendazole, or pyrantel pamoate can be given as single dose treatments to be repeated 2 to 4 weeks after to ensure treatment of any reinfection. Family members can be concurrently treated whether symptomatic or not without prior testing.

Contacts and Environmental Management

Remove sources of infection by treating cases. Examine all members of an affected family or institution. Clean and vacuum house daily for several days after treatment of cases.

Special Considerations

Multiple cases in schools and institutions can best be controlled through systematic treatment of all infected individuals and household contacts.

Enteroviral Vesicular Stomatitis With Exanthem (Hand, Foot, and Mouth Disease), Enteroviral Vesicular Pharyngitis (Herpangina)

Clinical Features

Hand, foot, and mouth is a brief, mild, febrile illness with papulovesicular rashes over the palms and soles, with or without painful mouth ulcers. Rash may involve the buttocks, knees, or elbows in infants and younger children. Herpangina manifests similarly, but with mouth ulcers affecting the posterior oral cavity. Common to both are odynophagia and dehydration.

Causative Agent

Enteroviruses

Diagnosis

Viral RNA detection via RT-PCR

Occurrence

Worldwide

Reservoir

Humans

Incubation Period

3 to 5 days

Transmission

Direct contact with nasal and oral secretions, vesicular fluid and stools of infected individuals, and contaminated toys and surfaces

Risk Groups

Groups of children

Prevention

Implement crown control measures to prevent person-to-person contact. Isolate infected children. Promote handwashing with soap and water.

Patient Management

Enteric precautions should be implemented. Treat with analgesia, antipyretics, IV rehydration, supportive management. Communicate risks to parents, guardians, and child caregivers and educate them about warning signs (refusal to eat, persistent vomiting, drowsiness, startling or myoclonic jerks).

Contacts and Environmental Management

Follow-up with contacts for manifestations of hand, foot, and mouth disease. Clean contaminated surfaces and soiled articles with soap and water, then with a dilute solution of chlorine-containing bleach for 5 minutes.

Special Considerations

Mandatory reporting of cases in some countries. Isolate diagnosed cases and all children with fever pending diagnosis, paying attention to handling of respiratory secretions and feces.

Epidemic Louse-Borne Typhus Fever

Clinical Features

Sudden onset of headache, chills, malaise, fever, and general pains. Macular eruption everywhere except face, palms, or soles. Cough and tachypnea with confusion, drowsiness, coma, seizures, and hearing loss.

Causative Agent

Rickettsia prowazekii

Diagnosis

Thrombocytopenia and elevated liver enzymes are common. IFA is the most accurate method of diagnosis.

Occurrence

Worldwide in unhygienic conditions with lice infestation

Reservoir

Humans

Incubation Period

1 to 2 weeks

Transmission

Rubbing feces or crushed lice into the bite or into superficial abrasions.

Risk Groups

General susceptibility

Prevention

Apply effective insecticide powder to clothes and skin of persons living in conditions favoring louse infestation. Improve living conditions with provisions for bathing and washing clothes. Treat persons at risk prophylactically by applying residual insecticide to clothing, and directly to skin.

Patient Management

Treat with doxycycline or chloramphenicol.

Contacts and Environmental Management

Immediate contacts should be kept under surveillance for 2 weeks. Insecticide powder should be applied to clothing and beddings of contacts. Trace the infection to the immediate source.

Special Considerations

Mandatory reporting required. In widespread infections apply residual insecticide to everyone in the community. As a bioweapon, it is infectious by aerosol with a high case-fatality rate.

Erythema Infectiosum

Clinical Features

Low-grade or no fever, and sporadically or in epidemics. A distinctive characteristic is an erythema of the cheeks associated with a lace-like rash on the trunk and extremities fading and recurring when exposed to sunlight or heat. The rash affected area on the skin and palm/sole may itch. Polyarthropathy without a rash may occur in adults. It is symmetrically distributed and involves the joints of the hands, ankles, knees, and wrists.

Causative Agent

Human parvovirus B19

Diagnosis

Detection of parvovirus B19 specific IgM antibodies or by a rise in immunoglobulin class G (IgG) antibody titers. Viral DNA detection by nucleic acid amplification by PCR.

Occurrence

Worldwide. Common in children and occurs in winter and spring in temperate zones.

Reservoir

Humans

Incubation Period

4 to 20 days to development of rash

Transmission

Primarily through respiratory secretions. From mother to fetus and transfusion of blood and blood products

Risk Groups

Universal susceptibility in persons with blood group P antigen

Prevention

Efforts should focus on preventing complications in susceptible groups. Susceptible women who are pregnant or plan to and are in close contact to people with the infection should be advised about the potential for acquiring the infection and the potential complications to the fetus. Healthcare workers should be reminded of the importance of good infection control measures.

Patient Management

Children should be excluded from school or daycare activities while fever or rash is present. IV immunoglobulin (IG) can be used to treat chronic anemia in persistent infections and may be needed for additional IVIG therapy.

Contacts and Environmental Management

Exposed pregnant women should be offered B19 IgG and IgM antibody testing to determine susceptibility and counseling regarding fetal risks.

Genitourinary Gonococcal Infection (Gonorrhea, Gonococcal Urethritis, Gonococcal Vulvovaginitis, Gonococcal Cervicitis, Gonococcal Bartholinitis, Clap, Strain, Gleet, Dose, GC)

Clinical Features

Males present with purulent discharge from the urethra with dysuria. Females present with mucopurulent cervicitis, and bleeding after intercourse. Pharyngeal, anorectal infections with pruritis, tenesmus and discharge may also occur.

Causative Agent

Neisseria gonorrhoeae

Diagnosis

Gram stain of discharge, cell culture, or tests that detect gonococcal nucleic acid.

Occurrence

Worldwide in men, women, and sexually active young adults and adolescents.

Reservoir

Humans

Incubation Period

1 to 14 days

Transmission

Contact with exudates of infected persons resulting from sexual activity

Risk Groups

Persons who engage in unprotected sex

Prevention

Treatment is IM ceftriaxone with oral azithromycin or oral doxycycline. Due to increased risk of concurrent HIV infection, patients should be counseled and tested.

Patient Management

Refrain from sexual intercourse until antimicrobial therapy is complete, with the same rule for previous infected sexual contacts. Contact precautions implemented for newborn infants and children until 24 hours of antimicrobial therapy has been administered.

Contacts and Environmental Management

Interview patients and notify sexual partners, with offer of subsequent treatment in the case of infection. Infants of infected mothers must be treated prophylactically.

Giardiasis

Clinical Features

Can be asymptomatic, present with acute diarrhea self-limited in 2 to 4 weeks, lead to intestinal symptoms such as chronic diarrhea, steatorrhea, abdominal cramps, bloating, frequent loose and pale greasy stools, fatigue, malabsorption, and weight loss.

Causative Agent

Giardia lamblia

Diagnosis

Identification of cysts or trophozoites in feces or duodenal fluid. At least three negative results are needed to rule out diagnosis of giardiasis.

Occurrence

Worldwide with children affected more frequently than adults. Prevalence is higher in areas of poor sanitation and in institutions where children are not toilet-trained. Endemic infections in temperate regions occur in July through October among children younger than 5 years and adults aged 25 to 39 years.

Reservoir

Humans, wild and domestic animals such as cats, dogs, cattle, and beavers

Incubation Period

3 to 25 days or longer. Average is 7 to 10 days.

Transmission

Drinking water from unfiltered surface water sources or shallow wells, swimming in freshwater bodies, and consuming fecal contaminated food. Person-to-person transmission occurs from ingestion of cysts in fecal contaminated drinking and recreational water more than food.

Risk Groups

Persons with HIV infection

Prevention

Educate families, personnel, and inmates of institutions on personal hygiene, safe sex practices, and the need for washing hands frequently. Fecal matter should be disposed of in a sanitary manner. Public water supplies should be protected against human and animal feces. Boil emergency drinking water supplies.

Patient Management

Enteric precautions should be implemented. Fecal matter and soiled articles should be adequately disinfected. Metronidazole or tinidazole are treatment drugs of choice, but nitazoxanide, furazolidone, paromomycin and quinacrine can be used as alternatives.

Gonococcal Ophthalmia Neonatorum

Clinical Features

Unilateral or bilateral redness and swelling of conjunctivae with purulent discharge occurring within 1 to 5 days of birth.

Causative Agent

N. gonorrhoeae

Diagnosis

Microscopic evaluation, nucleic acid amplification, or culture

Occurrence

Worldwide

Reservoir

Infection of maternal cervix

Incubation Period

1 to 5 days

Transmission

Contact with infected birth canal at birth

Risk Groups

Newborns with infected mothers

Prevention

Ocular prophylaxis at birth with erythromycin or tetracycline ointments. Prevention of maternal infection, or diagnosis and treatment with infection. Ceftriaxone IV or IM for infants of untreated mothers.

Patient Management

Prompt diagnosis and treatment. Contact isolation for the first 24 hours after administration of treatment therapy. Treatment is a single dose of IV or IM ceftriaxone.

Contacts and Environmental Management

Examination and treatment of mothers and their sexual partners.

Granuloma Inguinale

Clinical Features

Commonly affects the skin and mucous membranes of the external genitalia, inguinal, and anal regions. Indurated papules or nodules eventually lead to slowly spreading, nontender, hypertrophic granulomatous, ulcerative, or sclerotic lesions that are nonfriable, beefy red granulomas with rolled edges that form a fibrous tissue.

Causative Agent

Klebsiella granulomatis

Diagnosis

Demonstration of intracytoplasmic gram-negative, rod-shaped organism in stained smears of granulation tissue or biopsy samples.

Occurrence

Endemic in tropical and subtropical areas such as Australia, southern India, and Papua New Guinea.

Reservoir

Humans

Incubation Period

1 and 16 weeks

Transmission

Direct contact with lesions during vaginal and anal sexual activity

Risk Groups

Frequently seen in more males than females, and lower socioeconomic groups.

Prevention

Barrier methods during sexual activity, especially during vaginal and/or anal contact.

Patient Management

Avoid close contact until lesions are fully healed. Exercise care in disposing discharges from lesions and soiled articles. The recommended adult treatment is a 3-week course of doxycycline at minimum, unless pregnant or breastfeeding.

Contacts and Environmental Management

Examination of sexual contacts

Group A Streptococcal (GAS) Infections

Clinical Features

Pharyngitis, tonsillitis, impetigo or pyoderma, scarlet fever, puerperal fever, septicemia, erysipelas, cellulitis, mastoiditis, otitis media, pneumonia, peritonsillitis, wound infections, toxic-shock like syndrome.

Causative Agent

Streptococcus pyogenes

Diagnosis

Isolation of organism from affected tissues. Identification of GAS antigen in pharyngeal secretions.

Occurrence

Temperate zones and semitropical areas

Reservoir

Humans

Incubation Period

1 to 3 days for pharyngitis, 7 to 10 days for impetigo.

Transmission

Respiratory droplets or direct contact with patients or carriers

Risk Groups

Patients with skin breakdown, those with chronic underlying medical conditions, and the elderly

Prevention

Hand hygiene, and antibiotic prescription completion. Pasteurize milk and prevent infected people from handling milk or dairy products. Infection control practices should be implemented with GAS outbreaks.

Patient Management

Antibiotics should be completed for 10 days to prevent development of rheumatic heart disease. Treatment involves use of oral or IM penicillin G, oral amoxicillin, cephalosporin, clindamycin, clarithromycin, or azithromycin. Monthly injections of long-acting penicillin G should be given for at least 5 years to prevent reinfection.

Contacts and Environmental Management

Search for and treat carriers.

Special Considerations

Prophylaxis administration may be given to close contact groups such as the military to terminate spread.

Group B Streptococcal (GBS) Sepsis of the Newborn

Clinical Features

Sepsis, pneumonia, meningitis, osteomyelitis, and septic arthritis

Causative Agent

Streptococcus agalactiae

Diagnosis

Culture and isolation of GBS from blood, CSF, or other sterile body fluid.

Occurrence

Worldwide

Reservoir

Humans

Incubation Period

1 to 6 days after birth

Transmission

Transmitted during the intrapartum period or after rupture of membranes (ROM) more than 18 hours before delivery.

Risk Groups

Babies born prematurely when there is premature rupture of membranes (ROM) ≥ 18 hours before delivery, or when their mothers have fever during labor.

Prevention

Identify candidates for intrapartum chemoprophylaxis according to risk factors (delivery under 37 weeks, intrapartum temperature ≥ 100.4F, and ROM for 18 hours or more). Screen all pregnant women for GBS at 35 to 37 weeks gestation with the offer of antibiotics during labor.

Patient Management

Isolate patients in maternity wards and nurseries. Therapeutic use of antibiotics for infants with clinically suspected sepsis.

Contacts and Environmental Management

Administer IV penicillin or ampicillin to women with GBS infection at the onset of and throughout labor. Alternative agents are clindamycin and cefazolin.

Hemophilus Meningitis

Clinical Features

Meningitis, epiglottitis, bacteremia, lower respiratory tract infection, sudden onset with fever, vomiting, lethargy, and meningeal irritation, bulging fontanelle in infants or stiff neck and back in older children. Progressive stupor or coma is common.

Causative Agent

H. influenzae

Diagnosis

Isolation of organism from blood or CSF

Occurrence

Worldwide. Most prevalent among children aged 2 months to 3 years.

Reservoir

Humans

Incubation Period

Probably 2 to 4 days

Transmission

Droplet infection, throat and nasal discharges during infectious period.

Risk Groups

Universal susceptibility is assumed.

Prevention

Routine childhood immunization.

Patient Management

Respiratory isolation for 24 hours after start of chemotreatment. Ampicillin has been the drug of choice, but due to bacterial resistance ceftriaxone, cefotaxime, or chloramphenicol are now recommended.

Contacts and Environmental Management

Prophylaxis treatment using rifampicin should be given to all household contacts with children less than 1 year or with a child 1 to 3 years who is inadequately immunized. Contacts younger than 6 years should be observed for signs of infection such as fever. Parents should be educated about the risk of secondary cases in siblings younger than 4 years and the need for quick evaluation and treatment if fever or stiff neck develops.

Hemorrhagic Conjunctivitis Adenoviral

Clinical Features

Adenoviral features include lymphoid follicles, conjunctivitis lasting 7 to 15 days and small subconjunctival hemorrhages. Sometimes occurs with upper respiratory disease, fever, and minor corneal epithelial inflammation. Enteroviral features include sudden onset with redness, swelling, and pain bilaterally. Petechiae may occur on the bulbar conjunctiva that enlarges to form confluent subconjunctival hemorrhages. Some neurological complications may begin a few days to a month after conjunctivitis, often leave residual weakness.

Causative Agent

Adenoviruses and picornaviruses (most prevalent is enterovirus 70 and a variant of coxsackievirus A24).

Diagnosis

Laboratory confirmation via viral isolation from conjunctival swabs in cell culture, rising antibody titers, detection of viral antigens through IF, or identification of viral nucleic acid by DNA probe.

Occurrence

Widespread and common worldwide in warmer climate regions

Reservoir

Humans

Incubation Period

For adenovirus infection, 4 to 12 days with an 8-day average. Enteroviral infection is 12 hours to 3 days.

Transmission

Direct or indirect contact with discharge from infected eyes. Person-to-person transmission is most noticeable in families, transmission may also occur in poorly chlorinated swimming pools and via respiratory droplets. Epidemics are commonly associated with overcrowding and poor hygiene especially in school-age children.

Risk Groups

Populations associated with overcrowding such as those living in institutions

Prevention

Prevention methods are incredibly important as there is no treatment for this disease. Personal hygiene should be highly emphasized. Strict asepsis in eye clinics should be utilized in addition to proper handwashing before examining and in between patients, and during procedures. Adequate chlorination of swimming pools as well as school closures in outbreaks should be implemented.

Patient Management

Drainage and secretions precautions with disinfection of items that have come in contact with secretions. Restrict contact with cases while disease is still active.

Contacts and Environmental Management

Locate other cases to determine a common source of infection, if possible.

Special Considerations

Standards of hygiene should be improved and overcrowding should be limited as much as possible.

Herpesviral Infections (Herpes Simplex, Genital Herpes, Alphaherpesviral Disease, Herpesvirus Hominis, Human Herpesvirus 1 and 2)

Clinical Features

Herpes viruses establish latency and persist for life after a primary infection. Latent infection may be reactivated with or without symptoms. If symptoms, present they may be localized or systemic. Oral herpes presents with fever and malaise lasting 1 week or more, with gingivostomatitis and vesicular lesions in the oropharynx. Reactivation is preceded by tingling prior to appearance of vesicles, commonly causes fever blisters and cold sores on the face or lips, and is precipitated by trauma, fever or other disease process.

Causative Agent
HSV-1 and HSV-2

Diagnosis
Viral isolation and HSV DNA detection by PCR

Occurrence
Worldwide

Reservoir
Humans

Incubation Period
2 to 12 days

Transmission
Contact with HSV-1 or HSV-2 in saliva or genital secretions with transmission to various sites via genital-genital, oral-genital, oral-anal, or anal-genital contact.

Risk Groups
Persons engaging in frequent unprotected sex and neonates born to women with genital HSV infection.

Prevention
Health care workers should wear gloves when in direct contact with the mucous membranes of an infected individual. Appropriate and consistent condom use in sexual practices. Partners of infected persons should be notified, evaluated, and treated accordingly.

Patient Management
Contact isolation for neonatal and disseminated of primary severe and recurrent lesions, and for drainage and secretion precautions. Patients with genital herpes should avoid sexual contact with uninfected partners when lesions are present. Treatment options for acute manifestations are trifluridine, acyclovir, ganciclovir, idoxuridine, or vidarabine.

Contacts and Environmental Management
Serologic testing should be performed for the infected person's partner.

Histoplasmosis Capsulati

Clinical Features
Four clinical forms of the disease are recognized: acute respiratory, disseminated histoplasmosis, chronic disseminated disease, and chronic pulmonary form. The acute respiratory symptoms include mild respiratory illness to temporary incapacity with general malaise, fever, chills, headache, myalgia, chest pains, and nonproductive cough. Occasional erythema multiforme and nodosum may be observed. Late findings can include multiple, small, scattered calcifications in the lung, hilar lymph nodes, spleen, and liver. Acute disseminated histoplasmosis symptoms include debilitating fever, GI symptoms, bone marrow suppression, hepatosplenomegaly, lymphadenopathy, and a rapid course. The chronic disseminated disease includes symptoms such as low-grade intermittent fever, weight loss, weakness, hepatosplenomegaly, endocarditis, meningitis, mucosal ulcers of the mouth, larynx, stomach or bowel, and Addison's disease. The chronic pulmonary form includes resembling chronic pulmonary tuberculosis with cavitation.

Causative Agent
Histplasma capsulatum

Diagnosis

Confirmed by culture, DNA probe, or visualizing the fungus in stained smears of ulcer exudates, bone marrow, sputum, or blood.

Occurrence

Commonly in geographic foci over the Americas, Africa, eastern Asia, and Australia. Prevalence increases from childhood to age 15 years, with more prominence of the chronic pulmonary form in males. Outbreaks in endemic areas have occurred in individuals exposed to bird, chicken, bat droppings, or contaminated soil.

Reservoir

Soil with high organic content, bird and bat droppings in chicken houses, bat caves and pigeon roosts.

Incubation Period

3 to 17 days

Transmission

Fungus growth in soil produces microconidia with subsequent infection occurring as a result of inhaling airborne microconidia

Risk Groups

Opportunistic infection in those with compromised immunity even though susceptibility is general

Prevention

Minimize dust exposure in contained environments possibly by spraying with water or oil, and using protective masks.

Patient Management

Disinfection of soiled articles. Mild infection may resolve on its own, however treatment options are amphotericin B, itraconazole, and corticosteroids.

Contacts and Environmental Management

Investigate household and occupational contacts for evidence of infection from a common environmental source.

Special Considerations

A possible hazard exists if large groups move through, live in, or disturb soil in mold prevalent areas.

HIV Infection and AIDS

Clinical Features

AIDS is the late clinical stage of infection with HIV. Several weeks after infection with HIV the individual develops an acute mononucleosis illness lasting for a week or 2 and may be free of symptoms for years before other manifestations develop. Development of opportunistic infections.

Causative Agent

HIV-1 and HIV-2

Diagnosis

Detection of HIV-1/2 antibodies or HIV-1 p24 antigen. A three-test strategy is recommended where three sequential reactive results from three different assays are required to confirm HIV positivity.

Occurrence

Worldwide

Reservoir

Humans

Incubation Period

Variable

Transmission

Person-to-person contact via unprotected penile-vaginal or penile-anal intercourse, the use of HIV-contaminated injecting and skin piercing equipment like shared needles and syringes, transmission from mother to child during pregnancy, delivery, or breastfeeding.

Risk Groups

Persons engaging in frequent unprotected sex, injecting drug use, and healthcare workers through injury with needles and other sharp objects.

Prevention

PEP with a combination of antiretroviral drugs are available and sometimes recommended after HIV exposure. Only administer medically necessary injections, and exercise care with its disposal after use. Preventive prophylaxis therapy.

Patient Management

Universal precautions for hospitalized patients. Use germicides effective against HIV and M. tuberculosis to disinfect equipment contaminated with blood or body fluids contaminated with blood. Treatment is early diagnosis, medical evaluation, and constant evaluation of CD4+ cell count. Manage associated opportunistic infections according to national guidelines.

Contacts and Environmental Management

Notify contacts and source of infection. Sexual and needle-sharing partners should not donate blood, plasma, organs, tissues, cells, or breast milk.

Hookworm

Clinical Features

Anemia and a variety of symptoms proportional to degree of iron deficiency. Heavy infections present with iron deficiency anemia and hypochromic, microcytic anemia.

Causative Agent

Ancylostoma duodenale, Ancylostoma ceylanicum, Ancylostoma braziliense, Ancylostoma caninum, and *Necator americanus*

Diagnosis

Identification of hookworm eggs and larvae in a stool sample with microscopic techniques

Occurrence

Endemic in tropical and subtropical regions where facilities for sanitary disposal of human feces are not available and soil, moisture, and temperature favor development of infective larvae.

Reservoir

Humans for *A. duodenale* and *N. americanus*. Cats and dogs for *A. ceylanicum, A. braziliense,* and *A. caninum.*

Incubation Period

A few weeks to many months.

Transmission

Eggs in feces are deposited on the ground and hatch under favorable conditions. Larvae develop, become infectious and cause human disease once it penetrates the skin, especially of the foot, producing a characteristic dermatitis (ground itch). Transmission can occur through breastmilk and contaminated soil.

Risk Groups

People living in areas with warm and moist climates, where sanitation and hygiene are poor, and who walk around barefoot, or are in some way in direct contact with contaminated soil.

Prevention

Create sanitary disposal methods of feces in the community. Examine and treat persons coming from endemic to nonendemic areas. A preventive chemotherapy strategy using mebendazole or albendazole as treatment has been recommended by the WHO.

Patient Management

Safe disposal of feces to prevent soil contamination. Treatment options include albendazole, mebendazole, or pyrantel pamoate. Follow-up stool examination should be done after a 2-week treatment course, with treatment repetition as needed. Iron supplementation, or transfusion in severe anemia, should be implemented with deworming.

Contacts and Environmental Management

Contacts and source of infection should be investigated.

Infectious Mononucleosis

Clinical Features

Fever, sore throat, lymphadenopathy, and splenomegaly

Causative Agent

EBV

Diagnosis

Lymphocytosis >50% and abnormal liver function tests

Occurrence

Worldwide, but primarily in industrialized countries

Reservoir

Humans

Incubation Period

4 to 6 weeks

Transmission

Person-to-person through saliva via the oropharyngeal route

Risk Groups

Reactivation of EBV in immunodeficient persons

Prevention

Handwashing, and avoid drinking beverages from a common container to minimize contact with saliva.

Patient Management

Nonsteroidal anti-inflammatory drugs (NSAIDs) or low dose steroids given in increasing amounts over a week.

Kawasaki Syndrome

Clinical Features

High fever, unresponsive to antibiotic treatment, increased irritability and mood change, unilateral cervical lymphadenopathy, bilateral nonexudative conjunctivitis, "strawberry tongue," dry fissured or erythematous lips, limb changes such as presence of edema, erythema, generalized desquamation, and polymorphous erythematous exanthem.

Causative Agent

Unknown, but suspected to be caused by *Staphylococcus aureus* or group A streptococci.

Diagnosis

No laboratory test, but an elevated erythrocyte sedimentation rate (ESR), C-reactive protein (CRP), and elevated platelet counts above normal are common laboratory features. Six clinical signs are part of the diagnostic criteria: fever lasting 5 days or more; bilateral conjunctival redness; changes in the lips and oral cavity (reddening of lips, strawberry tongue, diffuse injection of the oral and pharyngeal mucosa); polymorphous exanthem; changes in the peripheral extremities (reddening of palms and soles, indurative edema in the initial stage, and membranous desquamation from fingertips); and acute nonpurulent cervical lymphadenopathy.

Occurrence

Worldwide

Reservoir

Unknown

Incubation Period

Unknown

Transmission

Unknown, but limited to the pediatric age group

Risk Groups

Children younger than 5 years, males, and Asian ancestry

Prevention

Unknown

Patient Management

Treatment is high-dose IVIG within the first 10 days of onset and should even be considered even if fever duration is greater than 10 days. High-dose aspirin is recommended during the acute phase followed by a low dose for up to 2 months.

Legionellosis

Clinical Features

There are two distinct clinical manifestations, Legionnaires' disease, and Pontiac fever; both present with anorexia, malaise, myalgia, headache, and fever. Legionnaires' disease presents with pneumonia and nonproductive cough. Pontiac fever presents with fever and cough.

Causative Agent

Legionellae gram-negative bacilli.

Diagnosis

Legionnaires' is diagnosed by isolating the causative organism from a lower respiratory specimen, with a urine specimen sometimes used. Pontiac fever is diagnosed by identifying the symptoms consistent with the disease.

Occurrence

North and South America, Asia, Africa, Australia, and Europe

Reservoir

Water supply systems such as potable showers, whirlpool spas, and decorative fountains

Incubation Period

Legionnaires' disease is 2 to 10 days, while Pontiac fever is 5 to 72 hours.

Transmission

Air and waterborne transmission

Risk Groups

Increasing age, smoking, diabetes mellitus, chronic lung disease, renal disease, malignancy, and compromised immunity, and affects more females than males. Outbreaks are observed more among travelers and hospitalized patients.

Prevention

Avoid conditions that enhance legionella growth. Proper disinfection methods should be used for whirlpool spas and drinking water supplies. Biocides should be used to limit organism growth and formation of protective biofilm. Tap water should not be used in respiratory therapy devices.

Patient Management

Legionnaires' can be treated using a respiratory fluoroquinolone or a macrolide. Pontiac fever is self-limiting and does not require antimicrobial therapy.

Contacts and Environmental Management

Additional case finding to find more cases

Special Considerations

Identify common exposures and review maintenance logs for water systems during an outbreak to detect potential sources of infection.

Leprosy

Clinical Features

There are two forms of the disease, tuberculous and lepromatous. Tuberculoid leprosy is characterized by large, flat plaques with irregular borders and asymmetric distribution. Lepromatous leprosy is characterized by numerous symmetric lesions, with small, smooth hyperpigmented papules and plaques with or without loss of sensation. Nerve involvement may occur as sensory, motor and/or autonomic neuropathies. The manifestations can include two acute adverse events—reversal reactions and erythema nodosum leprosum (ENL). ENL is characterized by appearance of tender, erythematous subcutaneous nodules on normal skin accompanied by fever, malaise, anorexia, arthralgia, and edema.

Causative Agent

Mycobacterium leprae

Diagnosis

Complete skin examination

Occurrence

Relatively declining incidence, but still prevalent in the Republic of the Marshall Islands, the Federated States of Micronesia and Kiribati

Reservoir

Humans and armadillos.

Incubation Period

A few weeks to 30 years, average of 3 to 10 years.

Transmission

Close contact, and possibly from nasal mucosa and respiratory secretions.

Risk Groups

Persons living in endemic areas, genetic factors, and patients with advanced HIV disease

Prevention

Early detection and prompt initiation of multidrug therapy (MDT). Evaluation and treatment of infected household contacts.

Patient Management

Isolation is unnecessary and should be avoided to prevent stigmatization. Hospitalization should be limited to those in need of corrective procedures for deformities and ulcer treatment. Combined chemotherapy regimens are effective treatment options, and can be used with drugs such as rifampicin, dapsone and clofazimine. Corticosteroids and thalidomide may also be used as treatment options.

Contacts and Environmental Management

Examination and follow-up of close contacts

Lyme Disease

Clinical Features

Distinctive skin lesion called erythema migrans of at least 5 cm in diameter, systemic flu-like symptoms with stiff neck, migratory arthralgias and lymphadenopathy, and neurologic, rheumatologic and cardiac involvement in different combinations over months to years. Neurologic abnormalities can include aseptic meningitis, facial palsy, chorea, cerebellar ataxia, motor or sensory radiculoneuritis, or encephalitis. More severe symptoms can include encephalopathy, polyneuropathy or leukoencephalitis. Cardiac abnormalities can include atrioventricular block and acute pyopericarditis or cardiomegaly. Rheumatologic abnormalities can include swelling and pain in larger joints.

Causative Agent

Borrelia burgdorferi, Borrelia afzelii, Borrelia bavariensis, Borrelia garintii, Borrelia spielmanii, Borrelia bissetti, Borrelia lusitaniae, and *Borrelia valaisiana.*

Diagnosis

Diagnosis can be made in patients presenting with erythema migrans rash with or without the knowledge of a tick bite in endemic regions. Other patients presenting with Bells's palsy or arthritis may also be diagnosed. Diagnosis should be supported by serologic testing such as EIA or IFA.

Occurrence

USA, Canada, Europe, Russia, China, and Japan. More frequently in the late spring or summer peaking in June or July.

Reservoir

Small rodents like squirrels and birds

Incubation Period

3 to 32 days after exposure

Transmission

Tickborne and blood transfusions

Risk Groups

All persons are susceptible.

Prevention

No blood donation from those suspected with Lyme disease. Avoid tick-infested areas when possible, otherwise minimize exposure by wearing clothing that covers arms, legs, and use tick repellants. Shower soon after being outdoors and check for ticks on body and remove ticks promptly.

Patient Management

Carefully remove ticks from patients. Treat with amoxicillin, doxycycline, cefuroxime axetil, or erythromycin. Lyme arthritis can be treated with previously mentioned agents, but the neurological abnormalities should be treated with IV ceftriaxone or IV penicillin for 3 to 4 weeks.

Contacts and Environmental Management

Determine source of infection when disease occurs outside endemic areas.

Lymphogranuloma Venereum

Clinical Features

Consists of three stages. The first stage is characterized by a small, painless papule or ulcer at the site of inoculation. The second stage involves extension to the regional lymph nodes draining the primary lesion with or without pus formation. In men, inguinal and/or femoral buboes may adhere to the skin and cause sinus formation. In women, pelvic nodes are more frequently affected with extension to the rectum and rectovaginal septum. Left untreated, it can become a chronic inflammation with fibrosis and lymphatic obstruction leading to colorectal strictures, fistulas, lymphedema, and genital elephantiasis. Rectal exposure can cause proctocolitis, rectal discharge, anal pain, constipation fever and/or tenesmus.

Causative Agent

C. trachomatis of genotypes L-1, L-2, or L-3.

Diagnosis

Direct detection of chlamydial organisms is swabs from legions or bubo aspirates by direct immuno-fluorescence or nucleic acid detection.

Occurrence

Worldwide especially in tropical and subtropical regions. Endemic in parts of Africa, India, Southeast Asia, Latin America, and the Caribbean. Occurs more frequently in men than women.

Reservoir

Humans

Incubation Period

3 to 30 days

Transmission

Anal, vaginal, or oral sex

Risk Groups

Persons in tropical or subtropical climates, and sexually active persons

Prevention

Safe sex precautions

Patient Management

Refrain from sexual contact until active infection has been completely treated. Careful disposal of discharges from lesions and soiled articles. Treatment can involve use of doxycycline or erythromycin orally for 21 days.

Contacts and Environmental Management

Search for, test, and treat recent sexual contacts in the last 60 days of confirmed or suspected cases.

Malaria

Clinical Features

Fever, chills, headache, muscular aching, weakness, vomiting, cough, diarrhea, and abdominal pain. Severe manifestations include impaired consciousness, prostration, convulsions, deep breathing and respiratory distress, circulatory collapse and shock, acute kidney failure, and evidence of other vital organ dysfunction.

Causative Agent

Plasmodium falciparum, Plasmodium vivax, Plasmodium ovale, and *Plasmodium malariae.*

Diagnosis

Microscopy, rapid diagnostic tests (RDTs), PCR-based assays, and serological tests.

Occurrence

Tropical Africa, southwestern Pacific, forested areas of South America, southeastern Asia, and in parts of the Indian subcontinent.

Reservoir

Humans, African apes, and South American monkeys.

Incubation Period

9 to 14 days for *P. falciparum*, 12 to 18 days for *P. vivax* and *P. ovale*, and 18 to 40 days for *P. malariae*.

Transmission

Bite of an infective female *Anopheles* sp. Mosquito.

Risk Groups

Universal susceptibility except individuals with the inherited sickle cell trait (heterozygotes).

Prevention

Avoid being bitten by mosquitoes; take antimalarial drugs as chemoprophylaxis to prevent infection becoming clinical disease; and immediately seek diagnosis and treatment if a fever develops 1 week or more after entering an endemic area and up to 3 months after departure. For community measures in endemic areas, protect individuals against mosquito bites and decrease the intensity of transmission with the use of insecticides and larval control methods.

Patient Management

Prompt treatment of all forms of malaria is recommended to prevent irreversible complications. Treatment involves the use of IV or IM artesunate, or alternatives such as IM artemether, IV or IM quinine dihydrochloride, or parenteral quinidine with careful electrocardiographic monitoring and vital signs assessment. Artemisinin-based combination therapies (ACTs) is now used as the first line of treatment for uncomplicated falciparum malaria.

Contacts and Environmental Management

Determine history of previous infection or possible exposure. Investigate and treat all persons sharing a needle, for instance.

Special Considerations

Full coverage vector control measures should be implemented.

Measles

Clinical Features

Prodromal fever, conjunctivitis, coryza, cough, and small spots with bluish-white centers on an erythematous base on the buccal mucosa (Koplik spots). A red rash appears on the face around the third to seventh day that becomes generalized, lasts 4 to 7 days and ends in brawny desquamation. Leukopenia and decreased serum vitamin A are common.

Causative Agent

Measles virus

Diagnosis

WHO defines a clinical case as anyone with a fever, maculopapular rash, cough, coryza or conjunctivitis, with confirmation by lab testing in every case.

Occurrence

Cases have decreased with the availability of vaccines.

Reservoir

Humans

Incubation Period

14 days, average of 7 to 21 days

Transmission

Airborne by droplet spread, and direct contact with throat or nasal secretions of infected persons

Risk Groups

Anyone unimmunized

Prevention

Public education to complete the two vaccine doses to confer immunity for infants, children, adolescents and young adults

Patient Management

Keep children out of school for 4 days after appearance of rash. Quarantine of institutions, wards or dorms may be helpful. Complications should be managed; vitamin A supplementation replaces body reserves, prevents blindness, and decreases measles fatality.

Contacts and Environmental Management

Postexposure may be administered to those without contraindications. Investigate contacts and infection source.

Meningococcal Meningitis

Clinical Features

Sudden onset of fever, intense headache, nausea, vomiting, stiff neck, photophobia, petechial rash with pink macules or occasional vesicles. Invasive disease is characterized by one or more clinical syndromes including meningitis, bacteremia, and sepsis. The most severe form is meningococcemia and presents with petechial rash, hypotension, disseminated intravascular coagulation, and multiorgan failure.

Causative Agent

N. meningitidis

Diagnosis

Recovery and culture of meningococci from a sterile site like the CSF or blood.

Occurrence

Europe and North America, with higher incidence in winter and spring

Reservoir

Humans

Incubation Period

2 to 10 days

Transmission

Direct contact and respiratory droplets from the nose and throat.

Risk Groups

Travelers to epidemic areas, Hajj pilgrims, military groups, immunocompromised persons, crowding, low socioeconomic status, exposure to tobacco smoke, and concurrent infection of the upper respiratory tract.

Prevention

Vaccination

Patient Management

Respiratory isolation for 24 hours after start of chemotreatment. Concurrent disinfection of discharges from the nose and throat and associated soiled articles. Treatment should be implemented as soon as presumptive diagnosis is made, and involves the use of parenteral ceftriaxone or penicillin; ampicillin and chloramphenicol may also be used.

Contacts and Environmental Management

Household, daycare, and other contacts should be watched closely for early signs of illness especially fever and provided with prophylaxis treatment.

Special Considerations

Forced crowding may create outbreaks. Decrease overcrowding and increase ventilation of living areas.

Middle Eastern Respiratory Syndrome

Clinical Features

Severe respiratory disease, mild influenza-like illness to severe respiratory illness. Immunocompromised patients may present with gastric involvement. Coinfections with other respiratory viruses have been reported.

Causative Agent

MERS-CoV

Diagnosis

Nucleic acid detection for upper and lower respiratory tract samples. Persons must have positive tests in at least two different PCR targets on the viral genome.

Occurrence

Worldwide with direct/indirect link to the Middle East

Reservoir

Bats

Incubation Period

Suspected to be between 2 to 14 days.

Transmission

Person-to-person transmission via respiratory droplets, direct contact, and fomites.

Risk Groups

Comorbidities such as diabetes, immunosuppression, and heart disease. Contact with an infected person. Healthcare workers involved in aerosolizing procedures such as intubation or nebulization.

Prevention

Wear a face mask with eye protection, and wash hands frequently before and after patient contact. Droplet precautions should be implemented. Healthcare workers involved in aerosolizing procedures should use protective equipment such as gloves and long-sleeved gowns. Early case identification.

Patient Management

Use of antibiotics is recommended at admission until the treatable causes of ARDS has been excluded. Strict droplet and airborne precautions should be implemented. Disposable equipment should be used wherever possible. Visitors should be kept to a minimum with personal protective equipment used under supervision.

Contacts and Environmental Management

Close contacts should be identified and placed under active surveillance for 10 to 14 days with self-monitoring for respiratory symptoms.

Special Considerations

Infection control in healthcare settings prevents further transmission of MERS-CoV to healthcare workers and patients.

Molluscum Contagiosum

Clinical Features

Smooth, firm, and dome-shaped papules; flesh-colored, white or translucent lesions. Lesions in adults are on the lower abdominal wall, pubis, genitals, or inner thighs. In children, it mostly occurs on the trunk, face, and proximal extremities. Lesions are occasionally itchy with a linear orientation.

Causative Agent

Molluscum contagiosum virus (MSV)

Diagnosis

Lesions viewed by Dermatoscopy show orifices and vessels in crown or radial patters are suggestive of molluscum contagiosum.

Occurrence

Worldwide

Reservoir

Humans

Incubation Period

19 to 50 days

Transmission

Direct skin-to-skin and sexual contact with contaminated objects or environments.

Risk Groups

All age groups, but more often in children

Prevention

Avoid contact with affected patients, and sharing bathtubs, bath towels, or sponges.

Patient Management

Infected persons with visible lesions should be excluded from close contact with other unless lesions can be fully covered. Treatment falls into three types of therapies: ablative (cryotherapy, curettage, salicylic acid, trichloroacetic acid); immunomodulatory (imiquimod, cimetidine); and virucidal (topical cidofovir).

Contacts and Environmental Management

Examine sexual partners as applicable. Disinfect surfaces and objects regularly handled by children with lesions.

Special Considerations

Suspend direct contact activities and disinfect surfaces as epidemic control measures.

Monkeypox

Clinical Features

Resembles ordinary or modified smallpox. Lymphadenopathy is a prominent feature.

Causative Agent

Species of the genus *Orthopoxvirus*

Diagnosis

Identification of the characteristic lesion, history of direct or indirect contact with animals of West and Central African origin.

Occurrence

Reported in Democratic Republic of Congo (DRC). Affects all age groups, majorly children <16 years.

Reservoir

Humans, primates, squirrels

Incubation Period

7 to 17 days

Transmission

Contact with affected animal, and person-to-person contact.

Risk Groups

Hunters in tropical rainforests of West and Central Africa and their families, lab workers, and others directly or indirectly exposed to rodent populations of West and Central Africa.

Prevention

Vaccination. Limit contact with infected patients and animals.

Patient Management

Manage patients symptomatically. Place patients under strict infection control measure and sterilize any tools used in patient management. Physical contact should be avoided until lesions have completely healed.

Contacts and Environmental Management

Self-monitoring and examination by a medical worker if signs and symptoms emerge.

Mumps

Clinical Features

Fever; swelling and tenderness of one or more salivary glands; unilateral or bilateral parotitis; prodromal symptoms (myalgia, anorexia, malaise, headache, and low-grade fever); sensorineural hearing loss; pancreatitis; and aseptic meningitis.

Causative Agent

Mumps virus

Diagnosis

Positive serological test for mumps-specific IgM antibodies, viral detection by RT-PCR, or isolation of mumps virus from a buccal swab or CSF.

Occurrence

Unvaccinated populations

Reservoir

Humans

Incubation Period

16 to 18 days

Transmission

Droplet spread and direct contact with saliva of infected person

Risk Groups

Immunity is long-lasting and develops after infection.

Prevention

Encourage vaccination for susceptible individuals.

Patient Management

Respiratory isolation for 5 days after onset of parotitis. Concurrent disinfection of articles soiled with nose and throat secretions.

Contacts and Environmental Management

Immunize susceptible contacts to decrease likelihood of infection from future exposures. Exclude susceptible persons from school or work from the 12th to the 25th day after exposure if other susceptible persons are present.

Mycoplasma Pneumonia

Clinical Features

Gradual onset with headache, malaise, cough, sore throat, pleuritic chest pain, scant sputum that increases in amount over time, patchy infiltration of lungs, and leukocytosis. Pharyngitis may occur and progress to tracheobronchitis or pneumonia.

Causative Agent

Mycoplasma pneumoniae

Diagnosis

Molecular diagnostics such as PCR assays using respiratory tract specimens

Occurrence

Worldwide

Reservoir

Humans

Incubation Period

6 to 32 days

Transmission

Droplet inhalation and direct contact with an infected person

Risk Groups

School-age children and young adults

Prevention

Avoid overcrowding in living areas.

Patient Management

Hand hygiene and cough etiquette. Treatment options are azolides, erythromycin, or tetracycline.

Contacts and Environmental Management

Investigation of contacts and source of infection to allow treatment of clinical infection among family members.

Special Considerations

Antimicrobial agents may be used prophylactically, but there is a lack of evidence to fully support use.

Norovirus Infection

Clinical Features

Nausea, vomiting, diarrhea, abdominal pain, myalgia, headache, malaise, low-grade fever, or a combination of these symptoms.

Causative Agent

Noroviruses

Diagnosis

RT-PCR assays for detection on stool samples and vomitus.

Occurrence

Worldwide and common

Reservoir

Humans

Incubation Period

About 10 to 50 hours

Transmission

Fecal-oral route, direct person-to-person contact, and indirect transmission via contaminated food, water, or environmental surfaces. Vomitus-oral transmission occurs via aerosolized particles.

Risk Groups

Older adults >65 years, young children <5 years, and immunocompromised persons.

Prevention

Use of hygienic measures applicable to diseases transmitted via the fecal-oral route. Hand hygiene using soap and water, environmental disinfection, and exclusion of ill individuals to prevent spread. Use of alcohol-based hand sanitizers in addition to handwashing measures.

Patient Management

Contact precautions. Treatment is mainly supportive with fluid and electrolyte replacement for dehydration.

Contacts and Environmental Management

Identify means of infection spread in outbreaks. Isolate ill individuals to reduce further exposure.

Other Acute Febrile Respiratory Illnesses

Clinical Features

Fever, cough, increased respiratory rate, chills, headache, general aches, malaise, anorexia, and gastrointestinal. Some other localizing symptoms occur in the respiratory tract such as rhinitis, pharyngitis, tonsillitis, laryngitis, laryngotracheitis, bronchitis, bronchiolitis, pneumonitis, or pneumonia.

Causative Agent

RSV, parainfluenza viruses, human metapneumovirus, adenoviruses, rhinoviruses, certain coronaviruses and enteroviruses.

Diagnosis

Isolation of the causative agent from respiratory secretions by fluorescent antibody (FA), enzyme-linked immunosorbent assay (ELISA), and radioimmunoassay tests.

Occurrence

Worldwide. Greatest incidence in fall and winter in temperate regions, while during wet and colder seasons in tropical regions.

Reservoir

Humans

Incubation Period

1 to 10 days depending on the pathogen.

Transmission

Oral contact or droplet spread, from hands, eating utensils, napkins/handkerchiefs, or other articles soiled with fresh respiratory discharges of an infected person.

Risk Groups

Universal susceptibility with higher frequency and severity of occurrence in infants, children, older adults, and immunocompromised persons.

Prevention

Practice good personal hygiene such as covering mouth when coughing and sneezing, and frequent handwashing. Avoid crowds and provide adequate ventilation. Avoid smoking and passive smoke exposure. Use masks.

Patient Management

Contact precautions should be implemented with droplet precautions added as necessary for the specific causative pathogen. Adequate disinfection methods should be performed for eating and drinking utensils with sanitary disposal of oral and nasal discharges.

Contacts and Environmental Management

Personal hygiene and infection control practices.

Pediculosis and Phthiriasis

Clinical Features

Severe itching and excoriation of the scalp or body. Secondary infection may lead to lymphadenitis.

Causative Agent

Pediculosis capitis (head louse), *Pediculosis corporis* (body louse), and *Phthirus pubis* (crab louse), adult lice, nymphs, and eggs.

Diagnosis

Visualizing a live nymph or adult louse in hair or scalp using a fine-toothed louse comb. Body lice is diagnosed by finding eggs and crawling lice in the seams of clothing, and pubic lice is diagnosed by finding nits or crab lice on hair in the pubic region.

Occurrence

Worldwide. Head lice is more common among children in schools. Body lice is prevalent among populations with poor personal hygiene, especially in cold regions where heavy clothing is worn and bathing is infrequent, or people cannot change clothes.

Reservoir

Humans

Incubation Period

Three-stage life cycle: eggs, nymphs, and adults. Eggs 7 to 10 days. Nymphs 9 to 12 days for head and body lice, and 13 to 17 days for crab lice. Adults 1 month.

Transmission

Direct contact with infected persons and their personal belongings for head and body lice. Pubic lice is through sexual contact.

Risk Groups

Children, especially during play or group activities, and persons in close contact with each other in crowded areas and poor hygiene.

Prevention

Public education about the diagnosis, treatment, and prevention of lice. Avoid all types of contact with infected persons and their belongings. Perform direct inspection of body and clothing for evidence of lice when indicated.

Patient Management

For head lice, use topical permethrin cream rinse (1%), piperonyl butoxide/pyrethrins, Spinosad suspension (0.9%), ivermectin lotion (0.5%), or benzoyl alcohol lotion (5%). For pubic lice, use piperonyl butoxide/pyrethrins topical or lindane shampoo. For body lice, clothing and bedding should be washed with hot water or dusted with pediculicides like 1% malathion and 0.5% permethrin.

Contacts and Environmental Management

Examine household and close personal contacts and treat those infected at the same time.

Special Considerations

Mass treatment with epidemics. Impregnate clothes and personal belongings with repellants or permethrin.

Pertussis

Clinical Features

Paroxysmal cough and inspiratory whoop. Initial catarrhal stage consists of upper respiratory infection with irritating cough. Paroxysms develop and increase in intensity before gradually improving and include repeated violent coughing each followed by a high-pitched inspiratory whoop. Paroxysms end with expulsion of clear, tenacious mucus followed by vomiting.

Causative Agent

Bordetella pertussis

Diagnosis

Clinical suspicion in the presence of signs and symptoms. Confirmation requires presence of the organism in nasopharyngeal specimens obtained during the catarrhal and early paroxysmal stages.

Occurrence

Endemic and common in children worldwide

Reservoir

Humans

Incubation Period

9 to 10 days

Transmission

Direct contact with discharges from respiratory mucous membranes of infected persons by airborne route.

Risk Groups

Susceptibility is universal for nonimmunized persons. Highest incidence is in infants.

Prevention

Immunity is conferred by administering three doses of the vaccine given in combination with diphtheria and tetanus toxoids.

Patient Management

Respiratory isolation for known cases. Suspected cases should be excluded from the presence of young children and infants until the person has received 5 days of antibiotics. Treatment options are erythromycin, clarithromycin, and azithromycin.

Contacts and Environmental Management

Under-immunized patients <7 years may be excluded from schools, day care centers, and public gatherings for 21 days after last exposure or until infected persons have received 5 days of antibiotic treatment. Immunization status of contacts should be verified and updated.

Special Considerations

Review the need for a booster dose or ensure completion of primary immunization of infants and young children before they travel to other countries if possible.

Plague

Clinical Features

Three possible presentations: bubonic, septicemic, and pneumonic. All phases begin with fever, chills, malaise, myalgia, nausea, prostration, sore throat, and headache. With bubonic plague, lymphadenitis develops along with buboes that may be tender, inflamed and suppurate. The septicemic form involves bloodstream dissemination to various parts of the body, endotoxic shock and disseminated intravascular coagulation. The pneumonic form results from a secondary lung infection.

Causative Agent

Yersinia pestis

Diagnosis

Visualization of bipolar staining in microscopic examination of specimen aspirated from a bubo, sputum, or CSF. Examination by FA, ELISA, PCR, or dipstick formats.

Occurrence

Areas with persistent wild rodent infection

Reservoir

Wild rodents and other mammals such as rabbit, wild carnivores, and domestic cats.

Incubation Period

1 to 7 days

Transmission

Human handling of infected animals and domestic pets carrying the agent, and careless manipulation of laboratory specimens.

Risk Groups

General susceptibility but increased in persons living in areas with poor rodent sanitation practices, hunters, trekkers, veterinary staff, and farmers.

Prevention

Public education in enzootic areas on modes of human and domestic animal exposure, rat-proofing buildings, fumigation methods and practices, and prevent rodent access to food and shelter. Public should also be educated on appropriate storage and disposal of food, garbage, and refuse. Rodent population should be surveyed periodically to determine possibility of epizootics. Wear gloves when handling wildlife.

Patient Management

Avoid living in rodent-infested dwellings and treat clothing and personal belongings with appropriate insecticide. Human cadavers and animal carcasses should be handled with great care. Treatment options are streptomycin, gentamicin, tetracycline, and chloramphenicol.

Contacts and Environmental Management

Those in contact with infected persons should be provided with chemoprophylaxis and observed for 7 days. Search for dead rodents and fleas and submit them for lab analysis.

Pneumococcal Meningitis

Clinical Features

Sudden onset with high fever, lethargy or coma, and signs of meningeal irritation.

Causative Agent

S. pneumoniae

Diagnosis

Isolation of organism from blood or CSF

Occurrence

Worldwide. Most prevalent among children aged 2 months to 3 years.

Reservoir

Humans

Incubation Period

Probably 1 to 4 days

Transmission

Droplet spread and contact with respiratory secretions. Direct contact usually results in nasopharyngeal carriage of the organism rather than the disease.

Risk Groups

Young infants, the elderly, asplenic and hypogammaglobulinemic patients. Predisposing factors include cochlear implantation and basilar fracture.

Prevention

Vaccination

Patient Management

Concurrent disinfection of nasal and throat secretions. Treatment involves the use of penicillin, ceftriaxone, or cefotaxime

Contacts and Environmental Management

Protection of contacts is not necessary unless in an outbreak.

Pneumococcal Pneumonia

Clinical Features

Sudden onset, high fever, rigors, pleuritic chest pain, dyspnea, tachypnea, and productive cough with "rusty" sputum.

Causative Agent

S. pneumoniae

Diagnosis

Isolation of pneumococci from blood or pleural fluid. Lab findings include leukocytosis and elevated CRP. Chest X-ray shows lobar or segmental consolidation that may be bronchopneumonic.

Occurrence

Community acquired cause for all ages, but mostly endemic to the elderly and those with underlying medical conditions.

Reservoir

Humans

Incubation Period

Not well determined, may be 1 to 3 days

Transmission

Droplet spread

Risk Groups

Infants, elderly, persons with underlying illnesses. Malnourished.

Prevention

Avoid overcrowding. Prevent malnutrition and encourage physical activity. Provide vaccinations where available and necessary.

Patient Management

Respiratory isolation for hospitalized patients, hand hygiene and cough etiquette, and presumptive initiation of antibiotic treatment with penicillin G or ampicillin.

Contacts and Environmental Management

None

Special Considerations

Immunizations as necessary. Crowding of populations in temporary housing increases risk of infection especially for the very young and elderly.

Pneumocystis Pneumonia

Clinical Features

Dyspnea on exertion, dry, nonproductive cough, and fever. Chest X-ray shows bilateral diffuse interstitial infiltrates.

Causative Agent

Pneumocystis jiroveci

Diagnosis

Presence of the organism in sputum, bronchoalveolar lavage, or transbronchial or open lung biopsy.

Occurrence

Worldwide

Reservoir

Humans

Incubation Period

Unknown

Transmission

Unknown in humans

Risk Groups

Increased susceptibility with prematurely born persons, chronic debilitating illness, and disease or treatments impairing immune defenses

Prevention

Prophylaxis treatment with trimethoprim-sulfamethoxazole, atovaquone, dapsone with immunocompromised patients

Patient Management

Trimethoprim-sulfamethoxazole is the treatment of choice.

Contacts and Environmental Management

Indicated use of prophylaxis with immunocompromised patients.

Pneumonia Due to C. trachomatis

Clinical Features

Insidious onset with cough, lack of fever, patchy infiltrates on chest X-ray with hyperinflation, eosinophilia, and elevated IgM and IgG.

Causative Agent

C. trachomatis

Diagnosis

Direct FA tests, enzyme immunoassays, DNA probes, and nucleic amplification systems.

Occurrence

Coincides with worldwide distribution of genital chlamydial infection.

Reservoir

Humans

Incubation Period

In infants from 1 to 18 weeks of age

Transmission

From infected cervix to the infant during birth

Risk Groups

Infants of mothers with chlamydial infection

Prevention

Same as chlamydial conjunctivitis

Patient Management

Universal precautions in hospitals and nurseries. Treatment is use of oral erythromycin with sulfisoxazole as an alternative.

Contacts and Environmental Management

Examine and treat parents with infection.

Poliomyelitis

Clinical Features

Acute onset of flaccid paralysis (affecting the legs more than the arms), infection beginning in GI tract spreading to regional lymph nodes, fever, malaise, headache, nausea, and vomiting, severe muscle pain, and stiffness of neck and back.

Causative Agent

Poliovirus types 1, 2, and 3

Diagnosis

Isolation of poliovirus from stool samples, CSF, or oropharyngeal secretions.

Occurrence

Historically occurred worldwide. It is primarily a disease of infants and young children. Importation from endemic areas remains a threat.

Reservoir

Humans, especially those with inapparent infections like children

Incubation Period

7 to 14 days, but possibly 3 to 35 days.

Transmission

Person-to-person via fecal-oral route, may also be spread in food and other materials contaminated with feces.

Risk Groups

Non-immunized groups, minority populations, migrants, unregistered children, nomads, refugees, urban poor, and those in geographic proximity to endemic areas.

Prevention

Four doses of the oral polio vaccine (OPV) at 6, 10, and 14 weeks of age in addition to the dose at birth is recommended. Primary immunization for previously nonimmunized adults traveling to endemic/high-risk areas.

Patient Management

Enteric precautions in the hospital setting. Communities should provide modern and adequate sewage disposal systems. No treatment has been discovered; however, experts should pay attention to complications of paralysis such as decreasing respiratory ability to promptly provide respiratory assistance.

Contacts and Environmental Management

Immunization of family and other close contacts. A single case occurrence should prompt investigation for additional cases in an area to facilitate response.

Special Considerations

A single case of poliomyelitis is a public health emergency requiring immunization within the geographical area of occurrence.

Rabies

Clinical Features

Onset is preceded by a sense of apprehension, headache, fever, malaise, and sensory changes at the site of animal bite. Often seen with excitability and aero- and/or hydrophobia with spasms of swallowing muscles, delirium, and occasional convulsions. May present with paralysis of limbs and respiratory muscles with preserved consciousness.

Causative Agent

Lyssaviruses

Diagnosis

Postmortem confirmation via FA staining of brain tissue or viral isolation in cell cultures. Antemortem diagnosis is also made by FA staining of viral antigens in frozen skin secretions taken from the back of the neck at the hairline, and detection of viral antibodies in serum and CSF.

Occurrence

Worldwide

Reservoir

All mammals such as dogs, coyotes, foxes, raccoons, and other carnivores. Dogs are the primary reservoir in developing countries.

Incubation Period

3 to 8 weeks

Transmission

Mostly dogs to humans in developing countries. Usually due to spillover infection to domestic animals from wild carnivores in developed countries.

Risk Groups

Veterinarians and their technicians, animal control staff, wildlife researchers, cavers, staff of quarantine kennels, rehabilitators, and lab and field personnel working with rabies virus.

Prevention

Vaccinate all owned dogs, cats, and other pets. Placing pets on leashes in public areas. Active surveillance should be implemented for animal rabies. Detain and observe animals (stray or ownerless) that have bitten a person for 10 days. Vaccinate individuals at high risk of exposure. Prevent rabies after animal bites with first aid procedures, passive immunization, and vaccination.

Patient Management

Avoid salivary secretions or tears of a rabid patient during the illness. Intensive supportive medical care should be implemented as treatment for the infected patient.

Contacts and Environmental Management

Perform risk assessment and provide PEP to contacts who are bitten by the patient, or who have an open wound or mucous membrane to the patient's saliva or tears.

Special Considerations

Perform mass immunization of wildlife with baits containing the vaccine.

Rotavirus Infection

Clinical Features

Vomiting, fever, watery diarrhea, and severe dehydration

Causative Agent

Rotavirus belonging to the *Reoviridae* family.

Diagnosis

ELISA

Occurrence

Infants in industrialized and developing countries

Reservoir

Humans

Incubation Period

24 to 72 hours

Transmission

Fecal-oral with possible contact or respiratory spread

Risk Groups

Greatest susceptibility between 6 to 24 months of age

Prevention

Vaccination for all children worldwide. Inactivated by chlorine, but not other disinfectants. Prevent exposure of infants and young children to individuals with acute gastroenteritis across all settings and maintain sanitary practices.

Patient Management

Frequent handwashing. Sanitary disposal of diapers. Oral rehydration therapy, or IV fluids in cases with vascular collapse or uncontrolled vomiting have been proven as effective treatment options.

Contacts and Environmental Management

Source should be identified in high-risk populations and those with the risk of prolonged rotavirus shedding.

Rubella

Clinical Features

Children present with few or no symptoms. Adults present with low-grade fever, headache, malaise, mild coryza, conjunctivitis, diffuse maculopapular rash, and postauricular, occipital, and posterior cervical lymphadenopathy that precedes the rash.

Causative Agent

Rubella virus

Diagnosis

Lab confirmation of positive rubella-specific IgM ELISA test on blood specimen obtained within 28 days after rash onset.

Occurrence

Worldwide in the absence of immunization

Reservoir

Humans

Incubation Period

14 to 17 days with a range of 14 to 21 days

Transmission

Direct contact with nasopharyngeal secretions of infected people, or droplet spread. Infants may spread the virus in urine as well.

Risk Groups

Permanent immunity after infection

Prevention

Public education on transmission modes as well as immunization importance. Single vaccine dose to confer immunity. IM IG given within 72 hours of exposure may decrease clinical disease, viral shedding and viremia rate in exposed susceptible persons.

Patient Management

Droplet isolation for hospitalized patients. Children and adults should be excluded from activities with others for 7 days after rash onset.

Contacts and Environmental Management

Identify pregnant contacts, especially those in first trimester to be serologically tested for susceptibility or early infection, with relevant advice given.

Special Considerations

WHO-recommended case definition of a suspected case is anyone with fever, maculopapular rash, and adenopathy. Promptly report all confirmed and suspected cases.

Salmonellosis

Clinical Features

Sudden onset of diarrhea, abdominal pain, fever, nausea, and vomiting. Infection may begin as acute enterolitis and develop into septicemia or focal infection. If the agent localizes to a specific site, it may cause abscess, septic arthritis, osteomyelitis, cholecystitis, endocarditis, meningitis pericarditis, pneumonia, cystitis, or pyelonephritis.

Causative Agent

Nontyphoidal *Salmonella* bacteria

Diagnosis

Isolation from feces or blood during acute stages of the illness

Occurrence

Worldwide

Reservoir

Domestic and wild animals, poultry, reptiles, amphibians, swine, cattle rodents, pets and humans

Incubation Period

6 to 72 hours, usually 12 to 36 hours.

Transmission

Direct or indirect contact with infected animals or their environments. Can occur via ingestion of contaminated water, or food of animal origin such as milk and eggs. Person-to-person fecal-oral transmission can occur especially in the presence of diarrhea.

Risk Groups

Universal susceptibility

Prevention

Food safety and personal hygiene education. Food industries should implement adequate and proper food-handling measures. Public health agencies should regularly inspect and supervise abattoirs, butcher shops and food-processing plants for sanitation policies and procedures.

Patient Management

Stress proper handwashing methods. Enteric precautions should be implemented for hospitalized patients. Rehydration and electrolyte replacement are indicated as treatment options. Ciprofloxacin may also be used for treatment. Provide patient education on prevention of foodborne illness in patient waiting rooms.

Contacts and Environmental Management

Culture stools of contacts involved in food handling, direct patient care, or care of young children and the elderly

Special Considerations

Mandatory case reporting required in all countries.

Scabies

Clinical Features

Evidence of papules, vesicles, or tiny linear burrows containing mites and their eggs. Intense itching especially at night. Prominent lesions around finger webs, anterior surfaces of wrists and elbows, anterior axillary folds, and belt line and thighs. Affects the nipples, abdomen, and the lower portion of the buttocks of women, the external genitalia in men, and the head, neck, palms and soles in infants.

Causative Agent

Sarcoptes scabiei var hominis

Diagnosis

Clinical examination of papules. Microscopic identification of the mite, eggs, or mite feces.

Occurrence

Widespread and endemic in many countries

Reservoir

Humans

Incubation Period

2 to 6 weeks in persons without previous exposure. 1 to 4 days after exposure in persons with previous infection.

Transmission

Direct contact with infected skin, and sexual contact. Contact with beddings and undergarments of infected persons.

Risk Groups

Household members and sexual partners of persons with scabies and conditions where close body and skin contact is common.

Prevention

Early diagnosis and treatment of infected persons and their contacts

Patient Management

Isolation from school or work until the day after treatment. Hot cycles of the washer and dryer will kill mites and eggs. Treatment of choice is 5% topical permethrin, 10% crotamiton and 1% lindane.

Contacts and Environmental Management

All affected members or contacts should be treated simultaneously to avoid reinfestation.

Special Considerations

Can be a potential nuisance in situations of overcrowding.

Seasonal Influenza

Clinical Features

Fever, dry cough, headache, myalgia, prostration, coryza and sore throat

Causative Agent

Influenza A, B, and C

Diagnosis

RT-PCR assay specimens from throat, nasal, and nasopharyngeal secretions, or tracheal aspirates

Occurrence

Yearly in adolescents and school-age children of industrialized countries.

Reservoir

Aquatic birds

Incubation Period

2 days

Transmission

All transmission routes

Risk Groups

All age groups with greatest risk in children <2 years, adults >64 years, individuals with chronic medical conditions, immunocompromised persons, pregnant women and those with neuromuscular/neurologic conditions

Prevention

Masks. Antiviral agents (e.g., oseltamivir and zanamivir) to supplement vaccines in outbreaks.

Patient Management

Patient isolation or cohorting with adequate spacing. Early treatment with medications indicated within 48 hours of symptom onset.

Contacts and Environmental Management

Antiviral prophylaxis for contacts

Severe Acute Respiratory Syndrome (SARS)

Clinical Features

Fever above 100.4F; lower respiratory tract illness symptoms (cough, dyspnea, shortness of breath); chest X-rays showing lung infiltrates consistent with pneumonia or adult respiratory distress syndrome (ARDS). Cases can become severe and progress to respiratory distress.

Causative Agent

SARS-coronavirus (CoV)

Diagnosis

Diagnosis of exclusion and based on a history of animal host exposure, SARS-CoV-related lab work and/or travel to southern China or another area with increased likelihood of animal-to-human transmission in the presence of pneumonia. Clinical illness needs to be present along with definitive lab test for SARS-CoV infection. Respiratory and stool samples may be collected for nucleic acid detection by RT-PCR or viral isolation during the first and second weeks of illness.

Occurrence

Worldwide

Reservoir

Himalayan masked palm civet as animal-to-human transmission. Cave-dwelling Chinese horseshoe bats.

Incubation Period

2 to 10 days

Transmission

Person-to-person by direct contact and respiratory droplets

Risk Groups

Contact with persons infected with SARS-CoV

Prevention

Wear a face mask with eye protection, and wash hands frequently before and after patient contact. Wide-spectrum disinfectants should be widely available at appropriate locations and concentrations.

Patient Management

Use of antibiotics is recommended at admission until the treatable causes of ARDS has been excluded. Strict droplet and airborne precautions should be implemented. Disposable equipment should be used wherever possible. Visitors should be kept to a minimum with personal protective equipment used under supervision.

Contacts and Environmental Management

Trace contacts and inform them about the signs, symptoms and means of transmission of SARS. Place contacts under surveillance for 10 days and educate about monitoring for fever by performing daily temperature checks.

Special Considerations

Reemergence of SARS will necessitate regular updates and travel recommendations by WHO. Strict adherence to biosafety procedures should be stressed in labs.

Shiga Toxin-Producing *E. coli* (STEC)

Clinical Features

Diarrhea ranging from mild and non-bloody to virtually all blood, severe abdominal cramps, and hemolytic uremic syndrome (HUS).

Causative Agent

STEC producing cytotoxins called Shiga toxins 1 and 2

Diagnosis

Specimen culture

Occurrence

North America, Europe, Japan, Australia, and the southern area of South America

Reservoir

Cattle, sheep, goats, deer, humans

Incubation Period

2 to 10 days

Transmission

Ingestion of food contaminated with ruminant feces and direct contact with infected animals and their environment

Risk Groups

All age groups. Frequently diagnosed in children 1 to 4 years. Older adults are at the greatest risk of death from infection.

Prevention

Pasteurize milk, other dairy products, juices, and ciders. Thoroughly wash fruits and vegetables to be eaten raw or peel the skin before consuming. Cook beef adequately and use a meat thermometer to measure temperature. Purify public water supplies, and boil before use if necessary.

Patient Management

Enteric precautions should be taken during illness. Prompt rehydration is recommended to decrease the severity of colitis and monitor development of HUS.

Contacts and Environmental Management

Infected persons should not handle food, or provide child or patient care until two successive negative fecal samples or rectal swabs are obtained.

Shigellosis

Clinical Features

Acute involvement of the small intestine and colon, loose stools accompanied by fever, nausea, toxemia, vomiting, cramps, and tenesmus.

Causative Agent

Shigella strains from Groups A, B, C, and D.

Diagnosis

Isolation of shigella from feces or rectal swabs.

Occurrence

Endemic in tropical and temperate climates.

Reservoir

Humans

Incubation Period

1 to 3 days but may range from 12 to 96 hours up to 1 week.

Transmission

Direct or indirect fecal-oral transmission from symptomatic patient or asymptomatic carrier. May also be spread through contaminated food and water, and sexual contact especially in men who have sex with men.

Risk Groups

Children <10 years old, the elderly, debilitated, malnourished patients, and those infected with HIV. Crowded areas and areas where contact with fecal material is possible such as in prisons and child-care centers.

Prevention

Promote careful handwashing with soap and water. Use of barriers during oral-, digital-, and genital-anal contact, accompanied by washing hands and genitals with soap before and after sexual contact.

Patient Management

Early recognition and report of outbreaks in childcare centers and institutions are especially important. Fluid and electrolyte replacement with signs of dehydration. Ceftriaxone and azithromycin are used as possible treatment agents. Enteric precautions implemented during acute illness.

Contacts and Environmental Management

Ill contacts should be excluded from handling food and from caring for others until diarrhea ceases and one or more negative stool cultures are obtained 24 hours apart and at least 48 hours after discontinuation of antibiotics. Investigate water and food supplies using general sanitation measures.

Smallpox

Clinical Features

Rash appearing first on the face and extremities, then the trunk with sudden onset fever, malaise, headache, prostration, severe backache, and occasional abdominal pain and vomiting. 2 to 4 days later fever resolves, with the rash progressing through various stages of macules, papules, vesicles and pustules, then crusted scabs falling off after 3 to 4 weeks.

Causative Agent

Variola virus

Diagnosis

Viral isolation on chorioallantoic membranes or tissue culture from scrapings of lesions, vesicular or pustular fluid, from crusts and sometimes blood.

Occurrence

Formerly worldwide, but no known human cases since 1979.

Reservoir

Humans

Incubation Period

7 to 19 days; commonly 10 to 14 days to onset of illness and 2 to 4 days more to rash onset.

Transmission

Droplet spread or skin inoculation.

Risk Groups

Universal susceptibility to unvaccinated. Smallpox research patients.

Prevention

Based on vaccination within a 4-day period after exposure.

Patient Management

Vaccination, identification and isolation of cases, and supportive treatment.

Contacts and Environmental Management

Vaccination of contacts and those living in immediate vicinity, surveillance of contacts, and isolation of contacts who developed fever.

Special Considerations

A single case could represent an outbreak.

Staphylococcal Disease in Hospital Nurseries

Clinical Features

Skin lesions develop secondary to colonization of the nose, umbilicus, circumcision site, rectum, or conjunctivae, and are initially vesicular turning seropurulent surrounded by an erythematous base.

Causative Agent
Same as for Staphylococcal Disease in the Community

Diagnosis
Same as for Staphylococcal Disease in the Community

Occurrence
Worldwide

Reservoir
Humans

Incubation Period
4 to 10 days

Transmission
Hands of hospital personnel.

Risk Groups
General newborn susceptibility.

Prevention
Use of aseptic technique and use of alcohol-based hand rubs before contact with each infant in nurseries. Routine application of antibacterial substances such as chlorhexidine to the umbilical stump while in the hospital.

Patient Management
Contact isolation precautions. Cleanse skin and apply a topical antibiotic such as mupirocin ointment three times a day.

Contacts and Environmental Management
Same as for Staphylococcal Disease in the Community.

Special Considerations
Wash cribs, beds, and other furniture with an approved disinfectant.

Staphylococcal Disease in the Community

Clinical Features
"Scalded skin syndrome," fever, malaise, headache, and anorexia. Lesions may seed into the bloodstream causing lung abscess, osteomyelitis, arthritis, endocarditis or meningitis.

Causative Agent
Various strains of *S. aureus*

Diagnosis
Isolation of the organism on culture.

Occurrence
Worldwide with the highest incidence seen with poor hygiene and crowded areas, and among children.

Reservoir
Humans

Incubation Period
Variable and indefinite

Transmission

Autoinfection, contact with a person with purulent lesion or asymptomatic carrier.

Risk Groups

Newborn and chronically ill, in addition to the elderly, debilitated persons, drug abusers, those with diabetes mellitus, cystic fibrosis, chronic renal failure, agammaglobulinemia, disorders of neutrophil function, neoplastic disease and burns.

Prevention

Treat initial cases promptly.

Patient Management

Avoid contact with infants and debilitated persons. Identify any draining lesions. Treat lesions by cleaning skin followed by a topical antimicrobial agent. Use penicillinase-resistant penicillin, cephalosporin, or clindamycin for severe infections.

Contacts and Environmental Management

Determine nasal carrier status of the strain among family members or healthcare workers.

Staphylococcal Disease on the Medical and Surgical Wards

Clinical Features

Lesions resembling furuncles, stitch abscesses or surgical wounds, septic phlebitis, acute or chronic osteomyelitis, pneumonia, meningitis, endocarditis, or sepsis.

Causative Agent

S. aureus

Diagnosis

Isolation of *S. aureus* associated with compatible clinical illness.

Occurrence

Worldwide

Reservoir

Humans

Incubation Period

4 to 10 days

Transmission

Hands of hospital personnel

Risk Groups

Hospitalized surgical patients

Prevention

Use of narrow-spectrum antimicrobials for simple staphylococcus infections for short treatment durations. Enforce strict aseptic technique. Promote hand hygiene compliance with alcohol-based hand rubs throughout the hospital.

Patient Management

Patient isolation in a private room. Antimicrobials to be used as determined by antibiotic sensitivity tests.

Contacts and Environmental Management

Suspect epidemic spread in the presence of two or more cases, and initiate investigation. Review and enforce strict aseptic techniques.

Syphilis

Clinical Features

Primary stage is characterized by an indurated, painless ulcer called a chancre at the site of exposure developing 3 weeks after contact with an infectious person's lesions. Chancres commonly occur on the penis, vulva, mouth, or perianal skin. Subsequently a macular-to-papulosquamous skin lesion develops on the trunk, palms, and soles. Glistening white-to-red patches are seen in the mouth, and condylomata lata are seen in the genital area. The secondary stage manifests as fever, sore throat, malaise, and generalized lymphadenopathy. If untreated, tertiary syphilis develops but remains latent for the remainder of the patient's life. Untreated pregnant women may transfer the infection to her fetus causing prematurity, stillbirth, neonatal death, or a spectrum of congenital syphilis manifestations at birth.

Causative Agent

Treponema pallidum

Diagnosis

Positive rapid plasma reagin with positive *T. pallidum* particle agglutination test for patients without prior history of infection. A fourfold increase in nontreponemal test titer compared to previous titers is seen in cases of reinfection.

Occurrence

Worldwide

Reservoir

Humans

Incubation Period

10 days to 3 months, usually 3 weeks

Transmission

Direct contact with the primary or secondary lesion of an infected person via sexual contact during oral, vaginal, or anal sex. Transmission may occur without either partner being aware of the infection.

Risk Groups

General susceptibility

Prevention

Decrease number of sexual partners, establish mutual monogamous partnerships, and practice use of barrier methods to decrease risk of infection. Screen all patients with high index of suspicion and high-risk groups such as sex workers. Pregnant women should be screened at their first prenatal visit, in the third trimester, and at delivery. Cases should be interviewed to identify contacts with notification and treatment to follow.

Patient Management

Test for other STIs. Universal precautions with blood and lesion exudates. All parents should receive parenteral long-acting penicillin. Abstain from sexual contact until treatment is completed, lesions disappear, and sexual partner has also been treated.

Contacts and Environmental Management

Identification, notification, testing, and treatment of sexual contacts or partners should be implemented, with the patient's stage of disease taken into consideration.

Tetanus

Clinical Features

Generalized tetanus is characterized by painful muscular contractions induced by sensory stimuli (hyperextension of the body, opisthotonos, and "risus sardonicus") and abnormal rigidity.

Causative Agent
Clostridium tetani

Diagnosis
No proven method of consistent diagnosis.

Occurrence
Worldwide

Reservoir
Harmless in the environment, intestines of horses and other animals.

Incubation Period
3 to 21 days

Transmission
Introduced via a puncture wound contaminated with soil, street dust, or animal or human feces. Through lacerations and burns or injected contaminated drugs.

Risk Groups
Workers in contact with soil, sewage, and domestic animals; members of the military and policemen; adults with diabetes mellitus; and unvaccinated women of reproductive age and their newborns.

Prevention
Emphasize clean deliveries and increase tetanus toxoid immunization coverage in women of child-bearing age. Tetanus prophylaxis may be needed to manage patient with wounds based on assessment findings.

Patient Management
Prophylaxis treatment if indicated. Maintain an adequate airway and use sedation as indicated.

Tinea Barbae and Tinea Capitis (Ringworm of the Beard and Scalp)

Clinical Features
Small area of erythema spreading peripherally leaving scaly patches of temporary baldness. Infected hairs may become brittle and break off easily.

Causative Agent
Various species of *Microsporum* and *Trichophyton*

Diagnosis
Scalp examination under ultraviolet (UV) light for yellow-green fluorescence

Occurrence
Australia, the UK, eastern United States, Puerto Rico, Mexico, and western Africa.

Reservoir
Humans, dogs, cats, and cattle

Incubation Period
10 to 14 days

Transmission
Direct skin-to-skin contact, or indirect contact from backs of seats, barber clippers, toilet articles, clothing and hats contaminated with hair of infected persons or animals.

Prevention
Public education, especially parents, about the danger of acquiring infection from infected individuals and animals. Survey heads of children with UV light before school attendance.

Patient Management

Selenium sulfide or ketoconazole shampoos to help remove scale. Oral griseofulvin, terbinafine and itraconazole are also effective agents.

Contacts and Environmental Management

Study household members and pets for signs of infection with subsequent treatment provided.

Tinea Cruris and Tinea Corporis (Ringworm of the Groin, Perianal Region and the Body)

Clinical Features

Flat, spreading, ring-shaped or circular lesion with a raised edge. This edge may be reddish, vesicular, or pustular, and may be dry and scaly or moist and crusted.

Causative Agent

Most species of *Microsporium, Trichophyton*, and *Epidermophyton floccosum*

Diagnosis

Scrapings from the lesion margins, clearing in 10% potassium hydroxide, and examining microscopically or under UV microscopy.

Occurrence

Worldwide and frequent. More males affected than females.

Reservoir

Humans, farm animals, and soil.

Incubation Period

4 to 10 days

Transmission

Direct or indirect contact with skin and scalp lesions of infected people or animals, contaminated floors, shower stalls, benches, and similar articles.

Risk Groups

All humans, mostly in men

Prevention

Wash and dry clothes with hot water and fungicidal agent. Maintain cleanliness in dressing rooms and public showers.

Patient Management

Exclude infected persons from swimming pools. Effective and frequent laundering of clothing. Thorough bathing with soap and water and application of topical fungicide.

Contacts and Environmental Management

Examine all contacts and household pets, and treat infections as necessary.

Toxoplasmosis

Clinical Features

Lymphadenopathy only, or may resemble infectious mononucleosis with fever, lymphadenopathy, and lymphocytosis. A maculopapular rash, generalized skeletal muscle involvement, cerebritis, chorioretinitis, pneumonia, myocarditis can be seen in immunocompromised persons.

Causative Agent

Toxoplasma gondii

Diagnosis
Based on clinical signs and supportive serological results.

Occurrence
Worldwide in mammals and birds. Human infection is common.

Reservoir
Cats, soil contaminated with cat feces.

Incubation Period
10 to 23 days

Transmission
Transplacental infection. Children consuming infective oocysts in from sandboxes and playgrounds. Eating raw or undercooked infected meat or vegetables. Ingesting water contaminated with feline feces.

Risk Groups
Primarily those ingesting undercooked or contaminated meat.

Prevention
Educate pregnant persons about preventive measures such as using irradiated meats or cooking to 150F before eating. Wash hands thoroughly before eating and after handling raw meat, or soil contaminated with cat feces. Domestic cats should be discouraged from hunting. Avoid drinking untreated water.

Patient Management
Treat with pyrimethamine combined with sulfadiazine and folinic acid for 4 weeks for those with symptomatic disease

Contacts and Environmental Management
Determine antibody titers in mother and child in congenital cases. Determine common exposure to cat feces, soil, untreated water, raw meat, or unwashed vegetables.

Trachoma

Clinical Features
Conjunctivitis with presence of lymphoid follicles, conjunctival inflammation producing superficial vascularization of the cornea and scarring of the conjunctiva. Scarring causes lid deformities and in-turning of eyelashes that may result in visual impairment and blindness.

Causative Agent
C. trachomatis

Diagnosis
Clinical observation of the disease-specific signs. Confirmation can be made by PCR.

Occurrence
Worldwide, mostly in poor rural communities in developing countries

Reservoir
Humans

Incubation Period
5 to 12 days

Transmission
Direct contact with infectious ocular or nasopharyngeal discharges on fingers or indirect contact with fomites such as towels or clothes.

Risk Groups
General susceptibility

Prevention
Provide appropriate community-based mass treatment with oral or tropical azithromycin.

Patient Management
Surgery for those with trichiasis. Disinfection of contaminated fomites. Drainage and secretion precautions for hospital patients.

Contacts and Environmental Management
Investigation of contacts and source of infection.

Trichomoniasis

Clinical Features
Mild to moderate genital inflammation, pruritus, vaginitis, urethritis, or prostatitis. Pain during urination or sexual intercourse, malodorous genital discharge appearing white, clear, yellow, or green.

Causative Agent
T. vaginalis

Diagnosis
Nucleic acid amplification test for genital secretions or urine specimens. Motile parasite can be viewed on a "wet mount" within 20 minutes of genital secretion specimen collection.

Occurrence
Worldwide

Reservoir
Humans

Incubation Period
5 to 28 days after initial infection, but asymptomatic infections can persist for years.

Transmission
Sexual transmission via contact with genital secretions.

Risk Groups
Increasing age and immunocompromised persons

Prevention
Symptomatic women should be tested. High-risk asymptomatic patients may benefit from screening and treatment. Condom use can reduce risk of acquiring or transmitting the disease and other STIs.

Patient Management
Curable with a single oral dose of nitroimidazole antimicrobial agent.

Contacts and Environmental Management
Concurrent treatment of sexual partners.

Tuberculosis (TB)

Clinical Features
Latent TB causes no outward manifestations but is characterized by microscopic lesions in the lungs that heal and leave small pulmonary or tracheobronchial lymph node calcifications. Active TB may affect lymph nodes, pleura, genitourinary tract, bones and joints, meninges, GI tract and peritoneum, and pericardium. Common symptoms are cough (initially nonproductive, but eventually with purulent sputum), fatigue, fever, night sweats, and weight loss.

Causative Agent
Mycobacterium tuberculosis (MTB) complex

Diagnosis
Latent TB detected via tuberculin skin testing and/or blood tests (QuantiFERON-TB Gold In-Tube). Active TB is diagnosed based on the presence of acid-fast bacilli (AFB) in the microscopic examination of sputum specimen.

Occurrence
Worldwide

Reservoir
Primarily humans

Incubation Period
Latent TB is 2 to 10 weeks after infection. Active TB develops within 18 months after initial infection.

Transmission
Coughing, sneezing, or singing (all via droplet transmission).

Risk Groups
Active TB is highest in children <3 years, adolescents, young adults, the very old, and immunocompromised persons who are HIV positive.

Prevention
Primary prevention includes prompt diagnosis and treatment, public education regarding mode of spread, symptoms, methods of control, importance of early diagnosis, and continued adherence to treatment plan, and reduce the conditions that increase the risk of infection and disease progression such as poor living conditions, smoking and indoor air pollution. Secondary prevention includes treatment of latent TB infections, screening for active and extrapulmonary TB.

Patient Management
Patients with active pulmonary TB should be taught to cover both nose and mouth when coughing or sneezing and can be achieved through the use of face masks. Adult patients with active pulmonary TB should be placed in airborne-infection isolation rooms with negative pressure ventilation. Treatment involves supervised use of INH, RIF, pyrazinamide (PZA), and ethambutol (EMB) to ensure patient receives all prescribed drugs. Cultures should be obtained monthly to evaluate response to treatment.

Contacts and Environmental Management
Investigate potentially exposed contacts. Treatment for latent TB is indicated by positive TST or IGRA results. Close contacts at high-risk of developing active pulmonary or extrapulmonary TB should be started on presumptive treatment.

Tularemia

Clinical Features
Skin ulcer, regional lymphadenopathy, painful pharyngitis, transudative pleural effusion, purulent conjunctivitis, punctate palpebral ulcers, sudden high fever, chills, fatigue, general body aches, headache, and nausea.

Causative Agent
Francisella tularensis

Diagnosis
Serological demonstration of a fourfold rise in antibody titers between acute and convalescent sera

Occurrence
Regionally throughout the northern hemisphere

Reservoir

Wild animals, rabbits, voles, muskrats, beavers, and some domestic animals.

Incubation Period

3 to 5 years

Transmission

Insect-to-human infection, handling infected animal tissues, ingestion of contaminated food or water, and inhalation of contaminated aerosols.

Risk Groups

Hunters, trappers, sheep shearers, veterinarians, forest rangers, game wardens, hikers, campers.

Prevention

Avoid bites of ticks, fleas, and mosquitoes by using repellants. Cook meat of wild animals thoroughly. Avoid handling meat and vegetables together. Take appropriate precautions when handling cultures of *F. tularensis*.

Patient Management

Universal precautions during patient care. Treat with aminoglycosides, ciprofloxacin or tetracyclines. Persistent lymphadenopathy with pus formation may require drainage.

Contacts and Environmental Management

Investigate the source of infection in every case.

Typhoid Fever and Paratyphoid Fever

Clinical Features

Sustained fever, marked headache, and malaise. Other symptoms include anorexia, relative brady-cardia, splenomegaly, nonproductive cough, rose spots on trunk, constipation more than diarrhea in adults. Nonsweating fevers, parotitis, and slight deafness may also occur.

Causative Agent

Salmonella enterica

Diagnosis

Organism isolation from blood, urine, and feces early in disease onset.

Occurrence

Worldwide

Reservoir

Humans and domestic animals

Incubation Period

3 days to more than 60 days, usual range of 8 to 14 days. 1 to 10 days for paratyphoid fever.

Transmission

Ingestion of food and water contaminated by feces or urine of patients and carriers.

Risk Groups

Preschool children, children 5 to 19 years, international travelers to endemic areas, and individuals with gastric achlorhydria.

Prevention

Prevention is based on access to safe water and proper sanitization, and on following safe food-handling practices.

Patient Management

Enteric precautions during illness. Treat with fluoroquinolones, oral chloramphenicol, amoxicillin, trimethoprim-sulfoxazole, azithromycin, ceftriaxone, or brief high-dose corticosteroid medications.

Contacts and Environmental Management

Determine actual or probable source of infection to determine possible chain of transmission

Special Considerations

Search for case/carrier who was the source of infection and source through which infection was transmitted. Chlorinate suspected water supplies or boil before use. Immunization is advised for international travelers to endemic areas.

Varicella/Herpes Zoster (VZV)

Clinical Features

Fever, generalized, pruritic maculopapulovesicular rash with lesions at various developmental stages. Lesions are more abundant on the trunk and proximal extremities, but may appear on the scalp, axilla, mucous membranes of the mouth and upper respiratory tract, and the conjunctivae. Herpes zoster is a local manifestation of latent VZV and presents as a unilateral rash affecting thoracic, cervical, and ophthalmic dermatomes. Lesions here are identical to varicella but are deeper and more closely aggregated. Rash lasts about 7 to 10 days and heals within 2 to 4 weeks. Postherpetic neuralgia is a common complication of herpes zoster.

Causative Agent

Human (alpha) herpesvirus 3 (VZV)

Diagnosis

Viral strain identification may be needed.

Occurrence

Worldwide

Reservoir

Humans

Incubation Period

10 to 21 days

Transmission

Person-to-person by direct contact, airborne spread of vesicle fluid from skin lesions, infected aerosolized upper respiratory tract secretions, and indirectly through soiled articles by discharges from vesicles and mucous membranes of infected people.

Risk Groups

Infants, adolescents, adults, immunocompromised persons, and pregnant women.

Prevention

Varicella vaccination, and herpes zoster vaccines for healthy older adults ≥50 years of age.

Patient Management

Infectious persons should be isolated and excluded from school, work or other public places until lesions are crusted. Treatment choices include acyclovir, valacyclovir, or famciclovir. Postherpetic neuralgia may be treated with amitriptylin, gabapentin, pregabalin, or carbamazepine.

Contacts and Environmental Management

All contacts should be evaluated to determine the need for PEP. Those exposed and eligible for vaccination should receive the vaccine promptly to prevent further transmission. Quarantine may be required for 8 to 21 days after exposure.

Special Considerations

Deaths may be reportable to local health authorities. Infectious cases should be isolated and immunized promptly.

Viral Meningitis

Clinical Features

Sudden onset of fever, headache with meningeal involvement, and CSF findings are pleocytosis, increased protein, normal sugar, and absence of bacteria. Certain rashes such as a rubella-like, vesicular, and petechial rashes. Some residual signs may include weakness, muscle spasm, insomnia and personality changes may occur and persist for a year or longer.

Causative Agent

Enteroviruses (such as coxsackieviruses and echoviruses), arboviruses, adenovirus, lymphocytic choriomeningitis, measles, herpes simplex, and varicella viruses

Diagnosis

Based on epidemiological patterns, patient characteristics, and laboratory information. Viral agents may be detected while in early stages from nasopharyngeal and oropharyngeal swabs, stool, CSF, and blood/serum.

Occurrence

Worldwide. Increases in late summer and early fall, while late spring may be due to mumps.

Reservoir

Varies according to the causative agent.

Incubation Period

Varies according to the causative agent.

Transmission

Varies according to the causative agent.

Risk Groups

Varies according to the causative agent.

Prevention

Varies according to the causative agent.

Patient Management

Enteric precautions for 7 days after illness onset, unless nonenteroviral diagnosis is established. Treatment is supportive, however acyclovir may be used if the cause is herpes simplex virus.

Contacts and Environmental Management

Immunization is indicated and dependent on the causative agent. Risk of infection can be lowered with good personal hygiene, environmental and item disinfection, and avoiding close contact with an infected person.

Special Considerations

Reporting depends on the causative agent.

Warts (Verruca Vulgaris, Common Wart, Condylomata Acuminatum, Papilloma Venerum, Palmar Wart, Plantar Wart, Periungal Wart)

Clinical Features

Diverse skin and mucous membrane lesions characterized by growths or changes in the epithelium. Common locations are the genitals and skin, but can also occur in the throat, respiratory tract, mouth and conjunctivae.

Causative Agent

Genital warts are caused by nononcogenic HPV types 6 and 11, but can also cause warts on the uterine cervix, vulva, vagina, penis, anus, scrotum, and rectum.

Diagnosis

Based on visual examination findings, though histological exam or biopsy may be needed if lesion presents atypically.

Occurrence

Worldwide

Reservoir

Humans

Incubation Period

2 to 3 months, range is 1 to 20 months

Transmission

Direct skin-to-skin contact, and commonly via sexual intercourse

Risk Groups

Verruca vulgaris commonly affects children, while genital warts affect sexually active adults.

Prevention

Avoid direct contact with lesions on another individual. Using condom may decrease sexual transmission. Prophylactic vaccination with quadrivalent HPV (types 6, 11, 16 and 18) have proven effective against infection in males and females aged 9 to 26 years.

Patient Management

Provider administered treatment include curettage, trichloroacetic acid, cryotherapy with liquid nitrogen, and surgical debulking if necessary. Patient administered treatments include imiquimod 5% or 3.75% cream, sinecatechins 15% ointment, or different types of podophyllotoxin 0.5% and salicylic acid.

Contacts and Environmental Management

Sexual contacts should be examined for genital warts and other sexually transmitted diseases.

West Nile Virus (WNV)

Clinical Features

Symptomatic manifestations include febrile illness with headache, myalgia or arthralgia, GI tract symptoms, and a transient maculopapular rash. Meningitis, encephalitis, or acute flaccid paralysis progressing to respiratory paralysis requiring mechanical ventilation may occur. WNV encephalitis may present with seizures, mental status changes, focal neurologic deficits, or movement disorders.

Causative Agent

Family *Flaviviridae* and genus *Flavivirus*

Diagnosis

Identification of anti-WNV IgM antibodies in serum or CSF

Occurrence

Every continent except Antarctica

Reservoir

Mosquitoes, birds, humans, other mammals

Incubation Period

2 to 6 days, but ranges from 2 to 14 days

Transmission

Bite of infected mosquitoes, blood transfusion, and solid organ transplantation

Risk Groups

Favorable environmental conditions, season and human activities.

Prevention

Vector prevention methods. Horse WNV vaccines in certain countries. Screening of blood and organ donations.

Patient Management

Primary treatment is supportive. Standard precautions are sufficient.

Contacts and Environmental Management

Search for unreported or unrecognized cases when someone may have been exposed during the 2 weeks prior to disease onset should be considered.

Special Considerations

Use mosquito repellants and eliminate established and potential breeding grounds.

Yellow Fever

Clinical Features

Sudden onset of fever, chills, backache, headache, general muscle pain, prostration, nausea, and vomiting. Pulse may be slow and weak, disproportionate to the elevated temperature (Faget sign).

Causative Agent

Family *Flaviviridae* and genus *Flavivirus*

Diagnosis

Isolation of virus, demonstration of the viral antigen in tissues, or demonstration of viral RNA in blood or tissue by RT-PCR.

Occurrence

Influenced by the transmission cycle present in the area.

Reservoir

Humans and *Aedes* mosquitoes

Incubation Period

3 to 6 days

Transmission

Bite of infective *Aedes* mosquitoes

Risk Groups

Unvaccinated travelers to endemic regions, forest workers in endemic areas, and those living in A. aegypti-infested areas not vaccinated.

Prevention

Maintain human and nonhuman primate disease surveillance, vaccinate persons at risk, and implement mosquito surveillance and control.

Patient Management

Treatment is supportive.

Contacts and Environmental Management

Unvaccinated family members and contacts should be immunized promptly. Inquire about contacts and areas visited by the patient 3 to 6 days before onset to detect focus of yellow fever. Apply insecticide to patient's living quarters. Investigate mid febrile illnesses and unexplained deaths suggesting yellow fever.

Special Considerations

Animal quarantine may be required for 12 weeks.

END-OF-APPENDIX RESOURCE

BIBLIOGRAPHY

Heymann, D. (2014). *Control of communicable disease manual* (20th ed.). APHA Press.

INDEX